PROTECTING AMERICAN HEALTH CARE CONSUMERS

Eleanor DeArman Kinney

Protecting American

Health Care Consumers

Duke University Press   Durham & London

2002

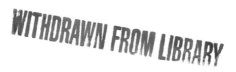

© 2002 Duke University Press

All rights reserved   Printed in the United States of America on acid-free paper ∞

Designed by C. H. Westmoreland   Typeset in Plantin Light and Frutiger display by

Keystone Typesetting, Inc.   Library of Congress Cataloging-in-Publication Data

appear on the last printed page of this book.

In loving memory of my father,

DR. THOMAS D. KINNEY,

who taught me how to live and write, and

with loving thanks to my mother,

DR. ELEANOR ROBERTS KINNEY,

for all her unfailing support throughout

my life

Contents

Acknowledgments

There have been many who have helped me with this book in many very different ways. First, I would like to thank my husband, Charles M. Clark, M.D., my mother, Eleanor R. Kinney, Ph.D., and my children, Jennie, Brian, and Margaret, for their support in innumerable ways for this project. I would also like to thank the staff at the Center for Law and Health at the Indiana University School of Law—Indianapolis for their invaluable help, including my research assistants Julie Reed, Andrij Susla, Jeffrey Kerner, Greg Gulick, Kristen Meyer, Helaine Hatter, Narendra Pleas, Erica Franklin, Teresa Hall, Robyn Daugherty, Jodi Herron, Kyle Ferrell, Faith Long, and Alejondra Conconi. I would especially like to thank Nobuko Kudo for her excellent work on the preparation of the index and the final proofreading of this book. I would also like to thank Claudia Porretti and Phyllis Bonds, the current and former administrators of the Center for Law and Health, as well as my colleague Dr. David Orentlicher, the co-director of the center. Without the assistance of these people, this book would never have been completed.

Many others provided me space and resources for my work on this book. In that regard, I would like to thank the administration of the Indiana University School of Law—Indianapolis for both financial and moral support for the completion of the book. I would also like to thank my colleagues at the Institute of Latin American Integration at the National University of Law Plata in La Plata, Argentina, for the wonderful atmosphere in which to work and complete much of the work on this book. I would also like to thank the Council on International Exchange of Scholars for my Fulbright Fellowship for teaching and research in Argentina, which supported my work in Argentina.

Finally, many colleagues and friends offered extensive comments and suggestions on drafts of chapters of this book that were extremely helpful in focusing and improving them. In particular, I would like to thank Professors Gary Spitko, Ron Krotozinski, Andy Klein, and Dan Cole of my faculty for their support and comments. I would also like to thank colleagues from other schools and institutions for their invaluable assistance as well, including Marc Rodwin of the Suffock University School of Law, Bill Sage of the Columbia University School of Law, Fran Miller of the

Boston University School of Law, Cynthia Farina of the Cornell University School of Law, Randy Bovbjerg of the Urban Institute, and Bonnie Lefkowitz, formerly of the U.S. Department of Health and Human Services. I am especially grateful to Tim Jost of the Ohio State University School of Law and Tom Sargentish of the Washington College of Law at American University for their careful reviews. I would also like to thank my editor, Valerie Mullholland, and my other colleagues at the Duke University Press, for their encouragement, support, and excellent editorial assistance.

1 : Introduction

Following tremendous changes in health-care financing and delivery in the United States in recent years, the protection of the interests of individuals who need and seek affordable, high quality health care services is a critical and controversial issue. Two factors have precipitated the fierce debate on this issue. First, many more Americans get health insurance coverage and health care through capitated managed care plans that, by definition, affirmatively and aggressively manage the cost and utilization of enrollees' health-care services. Second, the number and proportion of Americans who do not have health insurance coverage remains a major problem following a period of unprecedented economic growth.

Clearly, many Americans do not like managed care and fear that the quality of their health care suffers as a consequence of the movement toward managed care in the American health-care sector.[1] Numerous recent polls suggest that Americans are more concerned about their health care and its quality, price, and availability today than in previous times. For example, in a recent poll for the Kaiser Family Foundation, a majority of respondents believed that managed care plans would be more concerned with saving money than providing high quality care to plan enrollees.[2] Journalistic reports[3] and widely publicized court decisions[4] about coverage denials for gravely ill people in prepaid managed care plans have fueled concerns as well. In sum, the issue of patient protection in managed care plans resonates deeply with the American public. One upshot of this trend is pressure on employers to offer looser forms of managed care plans.[5] Another has been calls for the reform of managed care plans and the expansion of health insurance coverage to protect the interests of all consumers.

Despite the attention that consumer concerns about managed care plans and health care generally have received, there is little consensus on what should be done politically or otherwise to address these problems. Many states have enacted various types of consumer protection measures targeted at managed care plans. However, Congress, despite serious consideration of multiple proposals in the 105th and 106th Congresses, could not pass patient protection legislation. As this book goes to press, the 107th is considering similar legislation.

This inability to reach consensus, particularly at the federal level, may be due to several factors that often come into play with efforts to address systemic problems in the health-care sector. First, there is no agreement on the nature of the problem to be solved or on whether there is, in fact, a problem. Many would argue that managed care plans are operating in a desirable manner and that disappointed consumers have unreasonable expectations about the amount and quality of health care that plans should provide. Second, even assuming agreement on the nature of the problem, many would part company when it comes to designing solutions. Some would argue that solutions should be private and market oriented. Others might concede that government has a regulatory role. This latter group would probably divide on whether states and/or the federal government should take the lead, whether the federal government should act in concert with the states, or whether either should be involved at all in crafting such regulatory solutions. Finally, well-financed health sector constituencies have vigorously advocated their version of patient protection legislation, preventing the development of compromise positions necessary for legislation and other reform.

Unfortunately, the current debate over patient protection has failed to address the concerns of certain individuals with an interest in health care in need of protection—namely, people without health insurance coverage. The vigorous debate on how and whether government should provide health insurance coverage for the poor and uninsured in the early years of the Clinton administration waned with the failure of President Clinton's health care reform initiative. The mid-1900s saw two federal initiatives to expand coverage—first, tighter regulation of private insurer underwriting and marketing practices and, second, expanded federal-state coverage for poor children. These measures have not assured complete coverage for all Americans or enhanced procedural protections of health-care interests for the uninsured. Yet the number of uninsured in the population continues to grow. Like a thunderhead on the horizon, the growing number of uninsured portends a serious future threat to the security of health insurance coverage for all Americans.

The subject addressed in this book is procedural protection of the health-care interests of all Americans within the institutions that provide and pay for that health care. The current patient protection debate has focused in large part on procedural measures as primary strategies for protecting the interests of consumers in managed care plans. The focus of these procedural reforms has been on adjudicative procedures targeted at resolving patient concerns and publication of plan information including coverage policy, plan and provider performance in providing high quality care, and contractual incentives for providers to save costs. This book takes a much more global perspective and focuses on all types of health-care concerns of all types of consumers, including the uninsured. For the debate to date over patient protection and procedural reform has been incomplete. It has only addressed concerns of members of health plans and not the concerns of the uninsured or concerns, such as medical malpractice, that may involve a provider rather than a health plan.

Further, the debate has largely ignored the procedural protections for individuals in the processes for making policies that define the content, quality, and cost of health-care services as well as access to health-care services. A central thesis of this book asserts that reform of policymaking procedures is the key procedural reform for protecting the interests of American health-care consumers. For policies defining the content, quality, and cost of health-care services are often at the heart of Americans' concerns about their health care. Policies often govern the outcome of adjudicative procedures before courts, agencies, and private alternative dispute resolution tribunals.

THE THEORETICAL CONTEXT FOR PROCEDURAL PROTECTIONS

Procedural protections for individuals who need, seek, and use health-care services should be placed in a theoretical context that informs choices for the design and implementation of such protections both now and in the future. This theoretical context boils down to the question of what procedures treat health-care consumers justly and also produce just results.

What is justice is a philosophical question that has challenged moral and legal philosophers throughout history. Daily, this question challenges lesser figures—such as lawyers, judges, legislators, administrators, and citizens— as they grapple with making policies and decisions in limited contexts that inevitably affect the overall allocation of health-care resources.

This book does not take on the jurisprudential task of developing a theory of justice for the allocation of health-care services in a developed society. Other scholars have thoughtfully examined this question more systematically and completely.[6] Specifically, since the 1960s, when government became more involved in the financing and delivery of health-care services, scholars have addressed the question of whether and how to ration health-care services in a just manner in the face of escalating health sector costs that consume ever greater proportions of the nation's resources.[7] In the early 1980s, the President's Commission for the Study of Ethical Problems in Medicine and Biomedical and Behavior Research convened experts in philosophy, health policy, and law to explore the ethical dimensions of securing access to health-care services. The published work of this commission provides a wealth of scholarship on the underlying philosophical questions regarding justice and health care.[8] Subsequent excellent work has ably summarized and developed different theories of justice and health care.[9]

Most philosophical theories of justice proceed from the principle attributed to Aristotle that equals must be treated equally and unequals treated unequally and then specify material principles that determine just how equals and unequals, respectively, should be treated to achieve justice.[10]

Also, most theories of justice distinguish between distributive and procedural justice. This distinction is important for understanding justice and health care and the issue of consumer protection explored in this book. Distributive justice pertains to the distribution of benefits and burdens among members of a society. Procedural justice pertains to the characteristics of the process by which decisions about the allocation of benefits and burdens in a society are made.

Fairness is a central criterion for both procedural and distributive justice. John Rawls's seminal work, *A Theory of Justice,* which has dominated liberal political philosophy in the United States in the last decades of the twentieth century, posits justice as fairness and then explicates how the principle of fairness plays out to achieve justice.[11] The philosopher Norman Daniels aptly describes the concept of fairness in prevailing views of justice in liberal political philosophy as essentially equality of opportunity: "Liberal political philosophy has relied on what is essentially a *procedural* notion, equality of opportunity, to justify a system in which unequal outcomes are thought morally acceptable. It is morally acceptable that there be winners and losers, even in races where the prize is a share of important social goods, provided the race is *fair* to all participants."[12] This definition of *fairness* is particularly useful for the inquiry of this book, which is primarily concerned with procedural justice. It also captures the prevailing understanding of fairness in the social mores of American society today.

Of note, disparate visions of distributive justice lie at the root of the current health policy debate in the United States. Depending on the material principles invoked to govern the treatment of all individuals in a particular theory of justice, visions of distributive justice can be quite different. For example, a governing principle that promotes equality yields far different conclusions than does a governing principle promoting liberty.[13]

Distributive justice is not easily conceived when it comes to health care. Whether a society, or entities within a society, decides to provide health insurance coverage for those unable to pay for coverage or care is a complex political and moral judgment. Decisions whether and how to expand public health insurance coverage for needy populations are generally policy decisions that legislatures make in democratic societies. Legislatures can use a variety of approaches to expand coverage, including public programs that offer incentives encouraging private entities to provide the needed goods and services. Further, the individual and collective decisions of private purchasers of health care, such as individuals, employers, insurers, and managed care organizations, and government agencies, as stewards of public health insurance programs, have enormous implications for the allocation of health-care services to individuals in need and thus for distributive justice regarding health care.

Further, the issue of distributive justice and health care is strongly influenced by judgments of the medical profession about the content and quality of appropriate health-care services. Physicians determine the appropriate amount and content of health-care services for individuals in clinical contexts. Further, the medical profession, both collectively (as formally organized) and individually, shapes the decisionmaking of health plan sponsors about health plan benefits and coverage. All these decisions are predicated on collective professional judgments about appropriate clinical care. These judgments, in turn, are heavily influenced by the professional norms and the culture of medical practice as well as by economic incentives.

This book is chiefly concerned with procedural justice. Procedural justice promises only that important policies and decisions will be made in processes striving for procedural regularity and fairness. Specifically, how should institutional arrangements and procedures for making and publicizing relevant policies and adjudicating disputes over health care be designed to ensure fairness for consumers in protecting their legitimate interests in health care?

However, procedural justice is inherently limited. No amount of procedural justice will assure that the uninsured will get health-care services for which they are unable to pay. Fair procedures do not and cannot address either the underlying problems of structural inequities in current systems for financing and delivering health-care services or the content of substantive entitlements that generally determine who should get public or private health insurance coverage. Procedural justice affects the "fair" allocation of resources or other substantive outcomes only when such results are enhanced by fair procedures for making policies and decisions about these matters. Nevertheless, these limitations of procedural justice do not justify ignoring the issue of how to design and implement procedural protections for the legitimate and real interests of uninsured individuals in health care.

Further, the dominant role of the medical profession in determining the content and quality of medical care has crucial implications for procedural justice as well. As explained in this book, physicians and other health-care professionals develop the medical standards that are applied in health-care decisionmaking about coverage and quality and, in particular, adjudicating disputes over health-care services. Only genuine understanding of this role of the medical profession in defining the content and quality of medical care will elicit the true nature of procedural justice for health care.

THE SCOPE OF THE BOOK

The book addresses the entire range of procedural protections for consumers in the American health-care sector. It focuses chiefly on consumer concerns about access to and quality and cost of health-care services as they represent the majority of consumer concerns of interest to public policy. Also, owing to the importance of policies regarding the content, quality, and cost of health-care services, a full treatment of procedural protections must include a consideration of making and publicizing relevant policy. Thus, this book considers the procedures for making policies that define the content, quality, and cost of health-care services.

This book proceeds from the theory that complete and effective patient protection flows not just from better hearing and appeal procedures for individual cases. Rather, true protection, in today's rapidly changing health-care sector, is best accomplished through sound policies that define the content and quality of health-care services appropriately and set prices fairly.

The book also is ever mindful of the fact that over 16 percent of the American population is uninsured.[14] Consequently, the many policies, particularly those for health plans, do not apply to this substantial group of health-care consumers. Yet there are policies that do apply to these consumers, policies that govern the corporate obligations and practices of those public and private hospitals that are programmatically committed and/or mandated by statute or mission to serve the poor and uninsured. These policies are made in very diverse and private processes to which consumers have virtually no access. Procedural protections for uninsured consumers are more difficult to conceptualize but arguably more important in terms of achieving true justice for all American consumers of health care.

The first four chapters of the book provide important background needed for understanding the full dimensions of procedural protections described and proposed subsequently. Chapter 1 has presented some of the overarching theoretical issues facing the debate over procedural protections for individuals seeking health care in the United States. Chapter 2 provides a brief overview of the patient protection debate as it has evolved to the present day as well as of the major patient protection proposals and legislation. Chapter 3 presents relevant history that provides insight into the evolution of the health sector and the current state of health insurance coverage in the United States. This history, and the organization of health insurance coverage in the United States, is crucial in understanding the extant policymaking processes as well as the balkanized system for tapping and resolving the concerns of individuals about their health care. Chapter 4 discusses the relevant law and theory—regulatory law, corporate and associated tax law, administrative law, contract law, and tort law—that shape the design of current procedural protections for health-care consumers. Chapter 4 suggests that, while helpful, this current law and theory constrains imagining more genuine and innovative procedural protections for health-care consumers.

The substance of the book begins in chapter 5. This chapter identifies the universe of consumer concerns about health care and develops a typology of these concerns. The typology includes a description of how consumer concerns are manifested initially and resolved ultimately.

Chapters 6 and 7 address policymaking in the health-care sector. Chapter 6 describes the history of the quest for health-care quality that has driven the movement to develop medical standards of care to define the content, quality, and price of health-care services. Chapter 6 also includes a taxonomy of the different types of policies governing the quality and cost of health-care services as well as access to health-care services for individuals. Chapter 7 then describes the current procedures to make relevant policies that generate or govern consumer concerns in place today. This chapter emphasizes that most policies of concern to health-care consumers are made in private policymaking processes of private medical organizations and accrediting bodies that are beyond the scope of law governing development of policies by public administrative agencies. Rulemaking process and publication requirements have historically been important ingredients in ensuring the accuracy, accountability, and accommodation of interests in public policy. However, when policy is made by private organizations, do consumers and other interested parties have adequate opportunities to influence the content of this policy, as they do in public policymaking processes?

Chapter 8, based on the typology of consumer concerns presented in chapter 5, describes and analyzes the current processes for tapping and resolving consumer concerns and complaints about health care, including extralegal mechanisms given that not all consumer disputes find their way into legal processes for adjudication and resolution. This chapter also critiques current processes and emphasizes the need for reforms. This book argues that the current legal systems for identifying and resolving consumer concerns are balkanized and incomprehensible to most consumers and inaccessible to many, particularly those without health insurance. Indeed, throughout this discussion are addressed the special problems of the uninsured, who because they are not enrolled in health plans do not have the benefit of pressing concerns through most existing grievance-and-appeal procedures.

Chapter 9 addresses theoretical considerations that must be taken into account when crafting reforms of procedures both for making policy and for adjudicating disputes. Particular attention is accorded the problems of the uninsured, who do not have access to many of the grievance-and-appeal as well as administrative review procedures that are available to members of health plans. This chapter proposes principles for making better policies governing health care as well as principles to guide the design of procedures for the adjudication and resolution of individual consumer disputes. The chapter closes with a call for more empirical research on the nature of consumer concerns and their disposition.

Chapter 10 concludes the book with a vision of better procedural processes for American consumers of health care and includes concrete ideas for how reforms, based on the principles enunciated in chapter 9, might be designed. The chapter emphasizes the book's major theme—that true reform requires better integration of policymaking and adjudication in ways that facilitate the protection of individuals who need, seek, and receive health-care services. The book closes with the observation that procedural justice will always be limited in its ability to provide true protection of the interests of consumers in access to high quality and affordable health care if distributive justice is compromised because a substantial portion of the population is uninsured.

Finally, this book refers to both *patients* and *consumers* and intends to include all Americans who clearly have a strong and legitimate interest in health care. Neither term completely captures the situation of individual Americans with respect to protecting their interests in health care. Consumer rights, it has been said, "focus on purchasing decisions before a provider relationship is formed," while patient rights "focus on the relationship between patients and physicians (and other providers) and the type and quality of care provided."[15] Clearly, the term *patients* excludes those individuals who are not in the process of receiving health-care services but still have very real interests in health care to protect. And, while the term *consumer* captures all individuals who may need or use health-care services at any point in time and have an interest in health care warranting protection, it connotes a knowledgeable purchaser with choices. This is not the state of affairs for all Americans, even those with health insurance coverage. Thus, the terms *patient* and *consumer* are used as seems appropriate, but always with the understanding that this book, first and foremost, is addressing the interests of individuals in health care.

However, the term *consumers* clearly includes patients in a physician-patient relationship. While patients are receiving care, they are making judgments about that care, just as consumers make judgments about their purchases and choices. Indeed, recognizing that a patient is also a consumer acknowledges the power of patients to make choices about their care. There is no theoretical reason that the obligations of physicians in the treatment of consumers who are also patients are compromised by a patient's status as a consumer. Consequently, this book will use both terms in talking about all individuals with an interest in health-care services warranting protection. That interest is access to necessary and high quality health-care services at a reasonable cost.

2 : The Patient Protection Debate

The current debate over patient protection and managed care has involved many diverse constituencies and their interest groups, legal and health policy scholars, and state and federal policymakers. Much of the debate has been responsive to state and federal legislative proposals for the protection of patients in managed care plans. Since the mid-1990s, there has been much legislative and regulatory activity at both the state and the federal level regarding protections for patients in managed care plans in the light of reports of problems with managed care.

The current patient protection debate has its origins in the demise of the Clinton health reform initiative in 1994. The Clinton initiative sought to establish managed competition among integrated delivery networks under a regulatory framework that would expand coverage and control costs.[1] This regulatory framework also sought to ensure that competition proceeded on the basis of cost and quality rather than predatory practices that compromised care and hurt patients. The proposed legislation gave great attention to the procedural protections for health-care consumers.[2] Following the failure of the Clinton initiative in 1994 and the subsequent move of the American health-care sector toward prepaid managed care independent of protective regulation, the patient protection debate took on greater urgency.

Resulting legislative proposals and enacted legislation have contained similar patient protection strategies. From a substantive perspective, these strategies address four basic concerns regarding managed care plans: (1) the use of provider networks that limit patient choice and provider participation; (2) restrictions on benefits through utilization and strict coverage determinations; (3) utilization management measures that often involve unexpectedly strict coverage determinations; and (4) financial incentives to providers and patients to limit utilization.[3]

With respect to procedural reforms, proposed and enacted legislation has focused on four main issues: (1) reformed grievance-and-appeal procedures within health plans; (2) use of external review for disputes involving disputed medical issues; (3) better disclosure and publication of relevant information about health plan policies and performance; and (4) improvement of civil liability rules and remedies for federally regulated health plans. Procedural reforms, in general, have not addressed the processes for making policies that health plans and providers use to define the content, quality, and cost of health-care services for patients.

Further, enacted and proposed patient protection legislation has not addressed the particular problems of the uninsured in assuring protection of their interests in health care. For proposed procedural reforms have been confined primarily to enrollees in health plans. There has been little attention to the procedures in place in other institutions that enable the uninsured to voice concerns about their health care and obtain relief where their interests in health care have been inappropriately invaded.

PRIVATE REFORM PROPOSALS

With so much legislative action at both the state and the federal level, the interest groups representing concerned constituencies have been intensely involved in the patient protection debate. In addition to representing the interests of constituencies before legislative bodies and courts, these organizations have also developed imaginative and sound ideas for reforms. Private foundations have supported these efforts and have funded the convening of constituency group representatives and other experts to conceptualize the best procedural protections for managed care.[4]

The consumer advocacy community has been particularly vocal in the patent protection debate.[5] Among the most important groups dedicated to health reform advocacy participating in the debate are the National Health Law Program, the Public Citizen Health Research Group, the Center for Medicare Advocacy, and the Center for Health Care Rights. Also important are groups representing specific types of consumers with strong interests in health, such as Families USA, the American Association of Retired Persons, the National Senior Citizens Law Center, and the Children's Defense Fund, as well as organizations dedicated generally to consumer advocacy, such as the Consumers Union. Many of these organizations have joined forces in an umbrella organization, the Coalition for Consumer Protection and Quality in Health Care Reform, to enhance their advocacy and lobbying efforts in connection with the Clinton health reform initiative and the subsequent patient protection debate.

Consumer organizations have been extraordinarily prolific in their analysis of patient protection legal and policy issues.[6] Most work of advocates has focused on improved grievance-and-appeal procedures for health plans, external medical review, and improved civil remedies. This work has not addressed procedural issues in relevant policymaking processes except to call attention to the need for improved disclosure and publication of plan policies regarding health-care services and quality performance information.

The health insurance and managed care industries have also been vocal participants in the debate over procedural protections. In addition, several health plan executives have suggested reform approaches.[7] The prevailing concern of the managed care industry has been exposure to tort liability and the lifting of protections from tort liability for employer-sponsored health plans (discussed in chaps. 3 and 8) that now prevail. Health insurers and other managed care organizations (MCOs) have also been concerned about the additional cost of procedural protections for plan beneficiaries such as external review of medically related disputes.

The provider community has also actively participated in the debate with multiple proposals and input. The American Hospital Association put forward several procedural reform proposals.[8] The American Medical Association collaborated with the American Bar Association and the American Arbitration Association in the development of a prominent proposal entitled *Health Care Due Process Protocol*.[9] The task force that prepared this report proposed use of arbitration and other alternative dispute resolution methodologies in resolving consumer disputes with managed care plans.

GOVERNMENT INITIATIVES

In terms of legislative accomplishments, the real leadership in health-care consumer protection legislation has come from states. The 105th and 106th Congresses actively considered but did not pass patient protection legislation. As this book goes to press, the 107th Congress is considering patient protection legislation.

State Patient Protection Legislation

States have been very active in legislating consumer protections for state-regulated health plans of MCOs, including health maintenance organizations (HMOS).[10] As noted above, these various reform proposals have focused on problems with limited provider networks, benefit restrictions, management of service utilization, and inappropriate financial incentives for providers to limit services.[11]

In terms of procedural protections, many states have proposed and adopted two major strategies that are particularly important. First is external medical review for complaints from enrollees in managed care plans. A majority of states have mandated some type of external medical review of consumer grievances for state-regulated health plans.[12] Second, Texas and other states have tried to clarify and expand tort liability for managed care plans. Specifically, these statutes establish an independent statutory basis for tort liability for HMOs with respect to medical decisions for enrollees regardless of the sponsorship of the enrollee's health plan.[13]

The Clinton Administration Initiative

President Clinton made consumer protection a cornerstone of his health policy agenda in his second term. In 1997, he convened the President's Commission on Consumer Protection and Quality in the Health Care Industry to propose recommendations for reform and a consumer bill of rights with respect to health plans.[14] This commission proposed a "bill of rights and responsibilities" for health-care consumers that called for several reforms, including information disclosure, choice of providers and plans, access to emergency services, participation in treatment decisions, quality assessment and reporting on established quality indicators including patient satisfaction, and a fair and efficient appeal process that includes external review. These procedural recommendations were the basis of most Democratic patient protection bills in the 105th and 106th Congresses.[15]

In 1998, President Clinton also ordered responsible federal agencies to implement the commission's recommendations and the Patient's Bill of Rights in federally sponsored health insurance and services programs to the extent legally possible.[16] Major reforms included grievance-and-appeal procedures with expedited review in emergencies and mandated publication of information about plan benefits and coverage policy. Also required for federally sponsored health insurance programs is external medical review in patient appeal procedures. The Clinton executive order covered federally sponsored programs such as Medicare and Medicaid, the Federal Employee Health Benefit Plan, and health-care services programs for military personnel and their dependents, veterans, and Native Americans. In addition, the executive order required the Department of Labor to impose the Patient Bill of Rights to the extent possible on employer-sponsored health plans that it regulates under the Employee Retirement Income Security Act of 1974 (ERISA).[17] The extent of this executive order reform is substantial, reaching the 85 million Americans covered under federally sponsored health coverage programs as well as the millions more in ERISA-regulated employer-sponsored health plans.[18]

Congressional Legislative Proposals

Congress considered multiple patient protection bills in both the 105th and the 106th Congresses. Not surprisingly, the details of strategies to protect patients in managed care plans proved to be contentious political issues.

In the 105th Congress, patient protection legislation was tabled just before the 1998 election largely owing to failure to resolve the issue of access to state tort remedies against MCOs and also to the cost of consumer protections.[19] Similarly, the 106th Congress considered, but did not pass, bipartisan patient protection legislation just before the 2000 election.[20] In sum, the 105th and 106th Congresses were incapable of finding a middle ground for legislative success despite public concern and pressure. Nevertheless, the congressional debate did crystallize some consensus on appropriate measures for procedural reforms in managed care plans. The 107th Congress considered similar patient protection bills.[21] The contentious issues regarding these bills were the same as in prior congresses.

Nearly all the patient protection bills before both congresses would have imposed protections on employer-sponsored plans regulated under ERISA, and some bills would have extended protections to state-regulated plans. The Democratic bills tended to be the more inclusive. All bills contained similar procedural protections, such as enhanced grievance-and-appeal procedures and expedited review of coverage denials in emergency situations. With respect to grievance-and-appeal procedures, bills contained differing provisions for the scope and timing of review, control of reviewers, and availability of outside expert review. Most bills included more and better disclosure of information about the plan, including coverage of benefits, utilization review criteria, and quality performance measures. While most proposals called for disclosure of private policy that is the basis of plan coverage decisions and quality performance measurement, none addressed the processes by which health plans develop and/or obtain this policy. The existence of this policy is simply "a given" to be disclosed and/or used in a proper way.

In the 106th Congress, two separate bills were passed, one in the House and one in the Senate.[22] Both bills applied to ERISA and so-called self-insured plans that are not regulated under state law. However, the House bill applied to nearly all private health plans, including state-regulated health plans.

From a substantive perspective, both bills contained measures to assure protections in access to needed health-care services, including emergency and specialty care as well as approved clinical trials for experimental treatments. They also limited contractual provisions between plans and providers that compromise the quality of medical care or patient access to services outside of plans.

These bills contained procedural measures that were similar to those included in earlier bills described above. Both bills provided for reformed grievance-and-appeal procedures and external medical review for contested plan decisions involving medical issues as well as expanded civil liability against plans for tortious decisionmaking and other conduct. Regarding procedural protections, the House bill, in general, contained stricter provisions than did the Senate bill, particularly with respect to the authority and scope of external review and the extent of the civil liability of health plans.

In the 107th Congress, the patient protection debate continued after being a hotly contested issue in the 2000 presidential election. Early in 2001, Senator John McCain, with a bipartisan group of members of the House and Senate, introduced the Bipartisan Patient Protection Act of 2001.[23] There has been much political debate over patient protection in the 107th Congress, with both houses passing a patient protection bill.[24] The contentious issue, as before, but highlighted by Mr. Bush's threat to veto legislation with expanded liability in state court, is the extent of liability and the nature of remedies for HMOs and other health plans that contract with employee welfare benefit plans under ERISA. In the summer of 2001, Mr. Bush persuaded the Republican House to pass a bill with stricter limits on liability and damages than the bill that the Senate passed, thereby obviating the threat of a presidential veto.[25]

The Judicial Response

In addition, state and federal courts have weighed in on the issue of procedural protections for consumers of health care. Court decisions arise in the context of patient challenges against health plans for coverage denials and other conduct that patients perceive has injured their interests in health care. The judicial decisions tend to deal with three issues pertaining to state-regulated HMOs and MCOs that contract with employers to provide a health plan for an ERISA-regulated employee welfare benefit plan. The first issue is the degree to which HMOs and MCOs are liable under state law for tortious conduct in decisionmaking about coverage and other issues related to enrollees' medical care. The second is the degree to which remedies for violations of fiduciary obligations under ERISA apply to HMOs. The final issue is whether ERISA preempts provisions of recently enacted state patient protection legislation that apply directly to state-regulated HMOs and MCOS.

The oldest issue is the extent of the shield of state tort liability and other limitations on remedies and liabilities for employer-sponsored health plans and the HMOs and MCOs with which they contract to provide care for beneficiaries and participants of these plans. In a reticulated preemption provision, ERISA essentially preempts most conflicting state law.[26] As described in chapters 3 and 8, the Supreme Court has interpreted this preemption to bar common law tort claims against insurers contracting with ERISA-regulated plans. This preemption and associated litigation that it has spawned are discussed in greater detail in chapter 8. Nevertheless, this operation of the ERISA preemption to bar common law tort actions against health insurers and MCOs and also to frustrate state efforts to address health system problems generally has been troubling for many courts. Following three Supreme Court decisions in 1997 interpreting the ERISA preemption clause,[27] many lower federal courts and also state courts have exhibited concern about this shield of liability and its implications for leaving patients with limited damage remedies in the face of serious injury.[28]

Given the ERISA preemption clause and its arguably harmful effect on consumers in ERISA-regulated plans, court challenges have focused on how to extend ERISA fiduciary obligations on HMOs and MCOs that contract with employers to cover employees. The U.S. Supreme Court addressed this issue in *Pegram v. Herdrich*.[29] It overruled the Seventh Circuit's decision that HMOs were potentially liable as fiduciaries under ERISA when their payment methodologies encouraged physicians to limit care. In so doing, it was mindful of the complex nature of the U.S. health-care sector and the health plans within that system as grounds for determining that the Court should defer to the legislature to set policy in this area:

> But whatever the HMO, there must be rationing and inducement to ration. Since inducement to ration care goes to the very point of any HMO scheme, and rationing necessarily raises some risks while reducing others . . . , any legal principle purporting to draw a line between good and bad HMOs would embody, in effect, a judgment about socially acceptable medical risk. A valid conclusion of this sort would, however, necessarily turn on facts to which courts would probably not have ready access: correlations between malpractice rates and various HMO models, similar correlations involving fee-for-service models, and so on. And, of course, assuming such material could be obtained by courts in litigation like this, any standard defining the unacceptably risky HMO structure (and consequent vulnerability to claims like Herdrich's) would depend on a judgment about the appropriate level of expenditure for health care in light of the associated malpractice risk. But such complicated factfinding and such a debatable social judgment are not wisely required of courts unless for some reason resort cannot be had to the legislative process, with its preferable forum for comprehensive investigations and judgments of social value, such as optimum treatment levels and health-care expenditure.[30]

With this decision, the Supreme Court tossed the ball to Congress and state legislatures to delineate the contours of regulatory protections for patients in managed care plans—at least those regulated under ERISA. The Supreme Court also emphasized the availability of medical malpractice liability under state law as a remedy for the type of injury incurred in this case.

The third issue has emerged more recently and involves challenges from MCOs to state patient protection legislation as preempted by ERISA. The challenges have focused chiefly on two predominant state reforms—external review and express liability of HMOs for tortious medical decision-making. In *Corporate Health Insurance, Inc. v. Texas Department of Insurance,*[31] the U.S. Court of Appeals for the Fifth Circuit ruled that ERISA preempted the provisions of a Texas statute permitting external review of HMO medical necessity determinations but not the statutory provision imposing a tort liability on HMOs for failure to meet the statutory duty of ordinary care in making health-care treatment decisions for enrollees. In

Moran v. Rush Prudential HMO, Incorporated,[32] the U.S. Court of Appeals for the Seventh Circuit ruled that ERISA did not preempt external review of HMO medical necessity decisions mandated by Illinois's patient protection statute.[33] Both circuit court decisions have been appealed to the U.S. Supreme Court.

An important legal development is class action lawsuits against HMOs brought by expert trial attorneys seasoned in the tobacco litigation.[34] *Pegram v. Herdrich*, for example, was brought as a class action lawsuit. These lawsuits are based on a variety of theories, such as violation of the Racketeer-Influenced and Corrupt Practices Act[35] as well as the disclosure requirements of ERISA.[36] Many of these class actions have been dismissed or otherwise decided for the defendants.[37] Some, however, have been successful.[38] While most have been brought on behalf of plan members and consumers, some have been brought on behalf of providers.[39] To the extent that these class action lawsuits hold for the plaintiffs and conclude that HMOs have violated ERISA disclosure and other requirements, they have great potential for enhancing the forthrightness of advertising by HMOs and of HMOs' general treatment of consumers.

MAKING SENSE OF THE DEBATE

The patient protection debate has sounded several themes. One theme is the empowerment of consumers vis-à-vis health plans and providers. Attending to the special problems of the most vulnerable individuals is also an important concern with respect to consumer empowerment.[40] A second theme is the elimination of those aspects of the contractual relationship between managed care plans and providers that put consumers at risk for substandard or inaccessible care. A third theme is reform of processes that enable consumers to raise their concerns with health plans and providers. Then too a fourth and different theme is general skepticism about the need for or advisability of patient protection legislation.[41]

There are two general approaches in the proposals to enhance consumer empowerment. One approach is finding ways to strengthen consumers in their dealings with health-care professionals and health plans. Specifically, this approach would pursue strategies that give consumers greater voice in expressing concerns over health care.[42] One such strategy is to institute greater consumer involvement in the governance and policymaking of plans.[43] Another strategy is to teach consumers to be better purchasers of health plans and services[44] and also to make better health-care decisions generally.[45] Of note, many patient advocacy programs now exist to implement this strategy.[46] Providing consumers with more and better information about health plan policies and performance is an important strategy in this approach.

The second approach to greater consumer empowerment is to increase effective advocacy on behalf of consumers. Specifically, some propose enhancing legal advocacy on behalf of consumers[47] and also using class action lawsuits to press common consumer concerns.[48] Another idea is strengthening the role of labor unions in advocacy on behalf of health-care consumers—a traditional role of the American labor movement.[49] There has been some debate over creating a new profession of patient advocacy[50] or using nurses as patient advocates.[51] However, these ideas have generated concern about compromising the traditional role of the physician as the patient's advocate.[52]

Many have suggested that measures should enhance and strengthen the traditional role of the physician as the patient's advocate and mitigate the payment incentives and other factors in managed care arrangements that compromise this role.[53] Managed care has generated much concern about consumer protection largely because of the way MCOs employ and pay physicians and thereby encourage physicians to limit care.[54] Capitation pays physicians prospectively a fixed price per patient and is designed to encourage physicians to order fewer services and less intensive care.[55] Contracts with physicians and other providers contain provisions that create incentives for physicians unduly to limit care to plan members. At the very least, some observers maintain that physicians and health plans should disclose to patients financial arrangements that create these incentives.[56] However, others question the advisability of eliminating all incentives within physician payment methods to limit care in managed care plans.[57] The concern is fear of compromising a major force that makes managed care plans provide health-care services more cheaply and more efficiently.

The third theme is the improvement of processes for tapping and resolving consumer concerns with health plans and providers.[58] One approach is to accord patients more rights vis-à-vis health plans and providers. Rights, which by definition should be legally enforceable, have been the traditional legal vehicle for empowering individuals to protect their interests vis-à-vis governments and other private parties. Some congressional patient protection bills, as well as the work of President Clinton's Commission on Consumer Protection and Quality, have talked in terms of greater rights for patients to protect their interests in health care.

Most proposals have focused on reforms of existing grievance-and-appeal procedures in terms of making them simpler and more accessible to consumers as well as more efficient in terms of time and resources needed for final decisions. Many, particularly from the health plan and provider communities, which would seek to avoid the common law tort system, have promoted the use of contractual alternative dispute resolution (ADR).[59] For example, in a high profile reform proposal, the American Medical Association, the American Bar Association, and the American Arbitration Association called for more use of arbitration as the preferred means of resolving consumer disputes over health care.[60] In this regard, they have borrowed a page from the medical malpractice reform movement, which likewise has explored ADR as a way to reform medical liability litigation.[61]

Some final observations about the current patient protection debate are in order. Proposed reforms do not fully appreciate policies governing the content, quality, coverage, and price of health-care services. Often, policy made by private organizations is the basis of the information that must be made available to consumers, used in mandated quality assessment and improvement programs, or used to make utilization review and/or coverage determinations. Genuine consumer protection comes from a better understanding of how this policy is made and what procedural reforms can improve the policymaking processes.

Furthermore, with respect to the procedural reform of policymaking, it is important to appreciate that both public and private health plan sponsors use contract as the primary legal vehicle for establishing the relationship between the sponsor and the organizations that finance and/or provide health-care services to plan beneficiaries. Important policies governing the content, quality, coverage, and price of health-care services are often terms of these contracts or made pursuant to these contracts. Specifically, the terms of these contracts specify the details of the content and quality of health care available through the health plans as well as the price at which that care is to be offered. Contracts also govern the compensation of providers. Plan beneficiaries are not, as a general rule, parties to these contracts, nor are they involved in their drafting, negotiation, or implementation, although labor unions represent some employee groups in negotiations over these contracts.

It is noteworthy that recent evidence suggests that MCOs are becoming more sophisticated in the design and administration of capitated managed care plans with a view to pleasing consumers and attracting group purchasers on their behalf.[62] Research findings also suggest that the quality of care in capitated health plans is not generally compromised compared to care in other types of health plans and settings.[63] Specifically, MCOs are giving greater attention to quality of care and eliminating practices that constrain access to needed services among enrollees. It is clear that MCOs and those who purchase health plans are rethinking the design and management of managed care plans and are placing greater emphasis on quality and scientifically based medicine.[64] Proposed reforms should foster or at least not impede these most positive developments, which greatly benefit consumers in the long run.

Finally, the debate has not included procedural protections for those consumers of health care who are uninsured. This is an important gap, for, arguably, these consumers are most in need of protection. It is conceptually more difficult to think of procedural reform for a group of consumers who are not plugged into an institution, such as a health plan. For consumers who are covered by health plans have a predictable set of issues, and the organizations sponsoring health plans are in a position to implement systems for adjudicating disputes over these issues. Uninsured consumers do have important and unresolved concerns about health care that are not readily handled in existing dispute resolution institutions. The debate about health-care consumer protection should be expanded to include these uninsured consumers and their important concerns. Efforts should be made in conceptualizing theory and designing reform strategies to identify and address their concerns.

3 : Health Insurance Coverage in the United States

Insured Americans are enrolled in a mix of health plans with both public and private sponsors. The federal government and the states are the major sponsors of public health plans, while major private sponsors include employers, insurance companies, and managed care organizations (MCOs). Figures for health-care coverage in the United States today are displayed in table 1.[1]

For historical reasons, the regulation of health insurance coverage in the United States is distributed among multiple state and federal authorities.[2] This bifurcated regulation of the American private health insurance market has crucial implications for the structure of health insurance coverage in the United States and also for procedural protections for health-care consumers and patients. Consequently, current legal rules and arrangements for regulating health insurance coverage have failed to protect the coverage of health plan members or facilitate the extension of coverage to the uninsured. These failures have been a major force driving the call for more government regulation to protect the interests of Americans in their health care.

HISTORICAL DEVELOPMENT OF THE AMERICAN HEALTH INSURANCE SYSTEM

Several key developments dominate the history of health care in the United States. First is the idea that scientifically based medicine can actually cure or palliate disease. This idea has supported the enormous medical advances of the last century that continue today. Second is the fact that health care is expensive and beyond the resources of most people. To defray costs, consumers and providers use insurance to assure the availability of funds for needed care. Those unable to pay for or secure health insurance coverage are greatly disadvantaged. This chapter explains how this state of affairs evolved and the status of health insurance coverage in the United States today.

World War II was a watershed in the history of American medicine.[3] Tremendous scientific discoveries established modern medicine, a disci-

TABLE I. Health Insurance Table, 1999

Type of Health Insurance and Coverage Status	All People		Poor People	
	N	%	N	%
Total, covered and not covered	274,087	100.0	32,258	100.0
Total, covered	231,533	84.5	21,822	67.7
Private	194,599	71.0	8,310	25.8
Employment based	172,023	62.8	5,541	17.2
Public (government)	66,176	24.1	15,800	49.0
Medicare	36,066	13.2	4,251	13.2
Medicaid	27,890	10.2	12,884	39.9
Military	8,530	3.1	498	1.5
Not covered	42,554	15.5	10,436	32.4

Source: U.S. Census Bureau, Current Population Survey, March 1999 and 2000.
Note: The estimates by type of coverage are not mutually exclusive; people can be covered by more than one type of health insurance during the year. Figures are given in thousands.

pline firmly grounded in science. Antisepsis and anesthesia enabled modern surgery. Vaccinations and antibiotics enabled the prevention and cure of many infectious diseases. The discovery of insulin represented a unique victory in the effective treatment of a deadly chronic disease, diabetes. The discovery of DNA in the 1950s ushered in a new era promising even greater medical breakthroughs.

These developments fueled the ascendancy of academic medical centers, which conducted medical research, provided tertiary care, and trained medical specialists in addition to medical students. Also important was the 1910 Flexner Report on medical education, which called for academic training for physicians in clinical settings.[4] In the 1930s, the federal government expanded the National Institutes of Health to promote and support biomedical research. By the 1950s, there were multiple academic medical centers in the United States that had a great influence on the future course of American medicine.

At the close of World War II, American medicine indeed had much to offer consumers. The demand for services was great, as well as the demand for insurance to pay for services. Private coverage expanded dramatically in the postwar years in response to consumer demand led by the American labor movement. By the mid-1960s, the great majority of Americans had health insurance coverage, with similar patterns of coverage persisting today.[5]

This increased demand for health care and for health insurance coverage led to health-care cost inflation and more societal resources being devoted to health care. In 1929, health-care expenditures constituted 3.5 percent of the U.S. GNP and, by the end of the century, exceeded 14 percent.[6] Health-care expenditures rose from $73.2 billion in 1970 to over $1 trillion in 1996.[7]

This chapter provides some background on the developments that shaped the health-care sector in the United States.[8] Discussed are those factors that have influenced the current concerns of Americans about their health care as well as procedural reforms for addressing those concerns. The chapter closes with a description of health insurance coverage in the United States today.

Expanding Public and Private Health Insurance Coverage

There are four defining developments in the expansion of health insurance coverage in the United States: (1) the expansion of private health insurance coverage after World War II; (2) the establishment of the Medicare and Medicaid programs in 1965; (3) the expansion of public coverage for children from the 1980s through 1997; and (4) the enactment of the Employee Retirement Income Security Act of 1974 (ERISA).[9]

Expansion of Private Coverage. After World War II, employer-sponsored health insurance grew dramatically and became the predominant source of health insurance coverage for nonelderly Americans. With pressure from labor unions, private health insurance as a fringe benefit of employment expanded greatly when employers began providing health insurance to union workers in lieu of wages during a period of wage-price controls.[10]

Establishment of Medicare and Medicaid. In 1965, Congress enacted the Medicare and Medicaid programs to provide health insurance coverage for the elderly and some of the poor.[11] Congress added the seriously disabled to the Medicare program in the Social Security Amendments of 1972.[12] The advent of the Medicare and Medicaid programs was a seminal event in the history of American health care.[13] With these programs, the federal government and the states assumed a major responsibility for assuring access to health-care services for disadvantaged groups. Also, health-care costs, quality, and access moved from a private concern to a public policy issue.

In addition, the Medicare program's designers deliberately maintained the fee-for-service payment methods for all providers—and thereby seeding the cost inflation—to ensure the participation of reluctant providers. Indeed, the opening section of the Social Security Amendments of 1965 states: "Nothing in this title shall be construed to authorize any Federal officer or employee to exercise any supervision or control over the practice of medicine or the manner in which medical services are provided . . . or to exercise any supervision or control over the administration or operation of any such institution, agency, or person."[14] Wilber Cohen, the secretary of the Department of Health, Education, and Welfare at the time, observed that "the ideological and political issues between 1960 and 1965 were so dominating that they precluded consideration of issues such as reimbursement alternatives and efficiency options."[15] Immediately on implementation, these two programs greatly exacerbated the inflation of health-care costs.[16]

The Employee Retirement Income Security Act of 1974. In 1974, Congress enacted ERISA, which located the regulation of employer-sponsored health insurance—the predominant source of health insurance for the nonelderly— in the federal government instead of the state governments. The congressional debate over enactment focused on the security of employee pension benefits at a time of economic stagnation and movement toward a postindustrial workforce.[17] ERISA's legislative history suggests that Congress was only secondarily concerned with health benefits.[18]

Nevertheless, ERISA created a profound revolution in private health insurance coverage that has crucial implications for the precarious situation that health-care consumers face today and the consequent need for procedural protections for consumers in employer-sponsored health plans. ERISA located regulated employee welfare benefit plans (including health plans) outside the scope of state regulation. As a result, many employers designed their health plans to avoid state insurance code requirements by self-insuring their health plans.[19] The division of regulatory authority over health plans has thus inhibited state efforts to reform and expand health insurance coverage.[20] The legislative proposals for patient protection in recent congresses have sought to reform some of these problems with ERISA regulation.

Medicaid Expansions and the State Children's Health Insurance Program. Beginning in the 1980s with the expansion of Medicaid eligibility,[21] and culminating in 1997 with the enactment of the State Children's Health Insurance Program (SCHIP),[22] the federal government and the states expanded coverage for low income children. Now all children in families with incomes up to 200 percent of the federal poverty level have health insurance coverage through Medicaid or SCHIP.

The Battle against Health-Care Cost Inflation

The dominant health policy issue following the inauguration of widespread health insurance, and particularly Medicare and Medicaid, was health-care cost inflation and its amelioration. Of greatest concern were the rate of health-care cost inflation exceeding the inflation rate for the economy as a whole, increases in government expenditures for health insurance programs, and the increased proportion of the GNP commanded by the health-care sector. The Nixon and Carter administrations, which both had proposals for national health insurance,[23] considered control of costs a necessary step for implementation of national health insurance.

During this period, a consensus evolved recognizing that two major factors contributed to health-care cost inflation. First, the structure and financing of most health insurance plans contributed to excessive utilization of health-care services.[24] Specifically, health insurance insulated consumers from the financial consequences of their decisions to use health-care services, and provider payment methods based on costs and charges encouraged overutilization. The second factor was the increased utilization of costly medical technology.[25]

The Regulatory Attack on Costs. In the 1970s, the federal government and the states implemented a variety of regulatory strategies to control burgeoning health-care expenditures. The prominent strategies were hospital rate regulation[26] and capital expenditure review.[27] In the Social Security Amendments of 1972,[28] Congress adopted these strategies as well as utilization review for the Medicare and Medicaid programs. In 1974, Congress mandated capital expenditure review and health planning for all states.[29] In the late 1970s, the Carter administration unsuccessfully proposed global hospital rate expenditure controls as a necessary predicate to national health insurance.[30] With the Reagan administration came a policy sea change. The Reagan administration rejected regulatory approaches to addressing health-care cost inflation and supported competition among private health plans to control costs.

In the 1980s, the federal government reformed Medicare provider payment methods. In 1982, pressed by the need to reduce the growing federal budget deficit (estimated to be $107.2 billion in fiscal year 1983),[31] Congress imposed limits on hospital costs and established a strong peer review program to control increased Medicare utilization.[32] In the Social Security Amendments of 1983,[33] Congress adopted a prospective payment system for hospitals paying a price per case based on patient diagnosis.[34] With this payment reform, hospital cost inflation moderated.[35] In 1989, Congress enacted a revised payment system for physician services that paid physicians on the basis of the time and resources involved in treating specific conditions rather than on a charge basis.[36]

Health-care cost inflation was problematic for private payers as well. Following Medicare's leadership, most payers adopted payment reforms to control costs and utilization on a prospective basis, thus initiating the transition to managed care in the private health insurance market.[37] To curtail costs and enhance profits, private payers began contracting with so-called preferred provider organizations, which agreed to utilization management and other oversight in return for guaranteed groups of patients. Blue Cross and Blue Shield plans dropped their special nonprofit status with associated mandates for community rating and open enrollment to compete successfully with commercial insurance companies.[38] With the enactment of ERISA, many employers adopted self-insured plans to avoid state regulation with its costly mandates on benefits and other regulatory requirements.[39] Private payers also gave greater attention to coverage policy and utilization review in order to curtail costs.[40]

The Movement toward Prepaid, Managed Care. The 1980s and 1990s witnessed a profound change in the financing and delivery of health care to insured Americans with the movement to prepaid capitated health plans and so-called managed care (a term that surfaced in the early 1990s to describe payer strategies for curtailing cost and utilization in health plans).[41] The basic concept of managed care is managing the cost and utilization of health-care services offered through health-care plans. The theoretical policy heritage of managed care is the proposals for competitive approaches to the delivery of care in the early 1980s and the promotion of health maintenance organizations (HMOs) in the 1970s.[42]

In the early 1970s, the Nixon administration championed HMOs as its major health reform initiative in the Federal Health Maintenance Organization Act of 1973.[43] This statute authorized federal financial and other support for HMOs meeting federal requirements to promote the development of HMOs and their adoption by employer-sponsored health-care plans. One by-product of this federal effort was the development of national HMOs that were not subject to state regulation.[44] A second by-product was that the foundation for the managed care revolution of the 1990s was laid.

By the 1980s, health policy was embracing private, competitive approaches to controlling costs and expanding coverage and rejecting regulatory approaches to cost containment.[45] The theory of competitive approaches was to enable employers and other major group purchasers to select among competing managed care plans on the basis of quality and price and make consumers more cost-conscious users of health-care services through reductions in tax and other subsidies. HMOs gained stature as the ideal health plan to compete efficiently in the new medical marketplace and even become a model for Medicare and Medicaid. In 1981, Congress accorded the states greater flexibility to use prepaid health-care plans in state Medicaid programs.[46] The federal government eased regulatory requirements on HMO participation in the Medicare program.[47]

The rhetoric of competition continued throughout the 1990s with proposals for "managed competition" emerging.[48] Managed competition called for competition among prepaid health plans within a regulatory framework to control expenditures and protect consumers from the predatory practices of competing health plans. The movement toward prepaid managed care got a boost when President Clinton adopted managed competition as the approach for his health reform initiative in the early 1990s.[49] This decision signaled to the health insurance industry and the provider community that they needed to organize into integrated delivery networks with member hospitals, physicians, and other professionals providing comprehensive care.[50] Despite the failure of the president's health reform initiative in 1994, the movement toward prepaid managed care in integrated delivery networks continued.[51]

By 2000, 29 percent of nonelderly Americans with employer-sponsored health insurance coverage were in HMOs, 35 percent were in a preferred provider plan, 24 percent were in a point-of-service plan (which covers out-of-plan services with greater cost sharing by the plan member) and only 14 percent were in a conventional plan.[52] Of interest, between 1996 and 2000, the proportion of covered workers in conventional plans decreased from 27 to 14 percent, and the proportion in point-of-service plans increased from 14 to 24 percent.[53] For public health insurance programs, the proportion enrolled in managed care plans has also increased, although not as dramatically for Medicare as for Medicaid.[54] Recent evidence suggests that the move toward prepaid managed care has abated as consumers in a tight labor market have signaled their displeasure with prepaid managed care to employers.[55] Nevertheless, while managed care has generated considerable concerns among health-care consumers, it is here to stay despite its problems. The challenge is how to design managed care in ways that will protect consumers and ensure their access to high quality care.

THE UNIVERSE OF PRIVATE HEALTH INSURANCE COVERAGE

Most Americans—71 percent—have private health insurance coverage (see table 1). Most privately insured Americans have coverage through an employer. Employers include private corporations with ERISA-regulated employee benefit plans as well as federal, state, and local governments, which offer, in general, private health-care plans to public employees.[56] The largest public employer program is the Federal Employees Health Benefit Plan, which purchases private health insurance coverage for federal employees through a variety of private health plans, including prepaid plans, to accommodate consumer preferences.[57]

No employer is required to provide health insurance coverage to employees. Employers are motivated to do so as employee health insurance is a deductible business expense under federal and state income tax codes.[58] The tax expenditure for employer-sponsored health insurance coverage was estimated to be $111 billion in 1998.[59] Yet only 17.2 percent of the population with incomes below the federal poverty level have employer-sponsored health insurance coverage (see table 1). Further, all employers have great flexibility in the design of health plans within applicable regulatory constraints.

Private insurance companies and MCOs sell health plans to private and public employer health plan sponsors or administer health plans as "third party administrators" for ERISA regulated employers that want self insured plans. They also sell health insurance coverage directly to individuals. As discussed below, states regulate private insurance companies and MCOs, including HMOs.

Private health plans vary greatly in terms of benefits, coverage, and other features. In general, private health plans cover hospitalization for acute illnesses, including mental illness, and physicians' services and associated laboratory and other services on an outpatient basis. Many cover prescription drugs as well. A few cover home health care for acute illness and dental care.

Private health plans often require some "cost sharing," such as the payment of deductibles or coinsurance, or impose annual caps on expenditures (often on a disease-specific basis) in a given time period. They have limited authority to impose coverage limitations on preexisting conditions. Commercial health plan sponsors often offer a more limited plan with greater cost sharing to make coverage more affordable, especially to individual purchasers.

There is significant evidence that cost sharing for individuals has been increasing in the 1980s and 1990s, thus increasing the likelihood that those with private health insurance will have inadequate coverage.[60] Acording to a major study of health insurance, as many as 16–19 percent of insured individuals are inadequately insured, with coverage that could leave them exposed to large out-of-pocket expenses (exceeding 10 percent of their annual family income) in the event of a serious illness.[61] The major reasons for inadequate coverage among the privately insured are cost-sharing provisions and limits on benefits and coverage in private health plans.

State Regulation of Health Insurance

States have historically regulated insurance and continue to do so under the unique allocation of federal and state supervision of the insurance industry that Congress established in the McCarren-Ferguson Act in 1945.[62] State insurance regulation addresses insurer solvency and market conduct with respect to consumers.[63] The National Association of Insurance Commissioners (NAIC), a nonprofit organization composed of state insurance commissioners, effectively coordinates insurance regulation among the states through model laws and regulations.[64] The NAIC also provides common services and technical assistance to state insurance departments. This dominance of state regulators coordinating their regulatory programs through a private organization is unique. In virtually all other areas where national uniformity is perceived as necessary, Congress has established a federal regulatory program.

As with other types of insurance, state regulation of health insurance companies, MCOs, and HMOs has focused on solvency, rate regulation with a view toward preventing insolvency, and nondiscrimination in underwriting practices.[65] States license and regulate all commercial health insurers, MCOs, and HMOs. The NAIC's Model HMO Act is the basis of most state HMO statutes.[66] In addition to solvency regulation, state insurance regulation also addresses grievance procedures and other consumer issues. Recent state legislation, discussed in chapter 2, has established greater protections for enrollees in managed care plans.

Historically, state regulation unique to health care has focused on two efforts. The first has been to improve the benefit packages of health insurance plans through mandating specific benefits for health insurance plans.[67] This regulatory effort has been controversial as it arguably curtails the flexibility of health plan sponsors in designing affordable health plans. State benefit mandates are a major reason employers elect to self-insure.[68]

The second effort has been the reform of underwriting and pricing practices that discriminate against seriously ill people in individual and small group health plans.[69] Since the 1980s and that decade's highly competitive health insurance market, state-regulated health insurance companies engaged in underwriting practices that threatened the availability and affordability of health insurance for many.[70] State reforms generally prohibit restrictive underwriting practices and also mandate portability of health insurance coverage.[71] These efforts have been severely hampered by ERISA, which, as discussed below, has not regulated these practices until recently.

The NAIC has become quite active in the regulation of managed care plans, including the new risk-bearing entities that have emerged in recent years. The NAIC has proposed model legislation to strengthen the state regulation of health insurance and managed care in its "Consolidated Licensure for Entities Assuming Risk" initiative.[72] This initiative endeavors to promote uniform regulation of health plans across states through common definitions and regulatory requirements.[73] This initiative includes several model statutes addressing the several types of health plans: the Managed Care Plan Network Adequacy Model Act; the Health Carrier Grievance Procedure Model Act; the Utilization Review Model Act; and the Health Care Professional Credentialing Verification Model Act.[74] The NAIC has also focused on the treatment of provider-sponsored networks that have developed in response to corporate managed care and HMO expansion in many states.[75]

The Employee Retirement Income Security Act

Congress enacted ERISA in 1974 to provide greater security for employee benefits, especially pensions.[76] ERISA regulates pension plans and also employee welfare benefit plans, which include life, health, and disability insurance plans for employees.[77]

Key Statutory Provisions. ERISA establishes requirements for employee benefit plans that are eligible for favorable federal tax treatment. ERISA establishes the plan's administrator as a "fiduciary" with associated duties and liabilities to plan participants and beneficiaries (dependents of employees).[78] ERISA requires that plan fiduciaries act solely in the interest of plan participants and beneficiaries and imposes sanctions and limited liability for failure to so. Key requirements include the disclosure of plan characteristics to plan participants and beneficiaries and other reporting requirements.[79] Specifically, plan administrators must provide plan participants and beneficiaries with a summary plan description that is both comprehensive and comprehensible.[80]

ERISA has very specific enforcement provisions.[81] Section 503 requires that all plans must maintain internal review procedures.[82] Section 502(a) authorizes civil actions against plan fiduciaries for any breach of ERISA requirements, including plan fiduciary determinations under section 503.[83] ERISA authorizes equitable relief as well as damages, although damage awards are limited essentially to the recovery of lost benefits only.[84] In *Pilot Life Insurance v. Dedeaux*,[85] the Supreme Court ruled that ERISA's enforcement remedies preempted state tort law remedies.

For qualified plans,[86] ERISA preempts state laws that would otherwise relate to the plans.[87] However, ERISA explicitly excludes state insurance codes when regulating the business of insurance.[88] However, it then provides that ERISA plans will not be deemed insurers for purposes of state insurance regulation.[89] Consequently, a self-insured employee health plan clearly falls under the ERISA preemption and is subject only to ERISA requirements. If the employer purchases health insurance from a commercial insurance company or MCO, aspects of the health plan that relate to the business of insurance may be regulated by state insurance laws.[90]

The jurisprudence on the ERISA preemption is convoluted. Courts have historically interpreted the ERISA preemption broadly.[91] In *Pilot Life Insurance Co. v. Dedeaux*,[92] the Supreme Court ruled that ERISA preempted state causes of action in tort for bad faith breach against employee welfare benefit plans and the commercial insurers that funded these plans.[93] The effect of this decision has been to limit greatly the tort liability of HMOs to members of employer-sponsored plans. After three 1997 decisions in which the Supreme Court articulated the boundaries of the ERISA preemption more precisely,[94] many lower federal courts and state courts have sought to limit the shield of liability for HMOs that leaves many patients with limited remedies in the face of serious injury.[95]

The Effect of ERISA Preemption on State Health Reform. The ERISA preemption provision and its interpretation by the federal courts have caused considerable dislocation in the private health insurance market. ERISA creates a bifurcated structure for the regulation of insurance that is easily manipulated by employers to circumvent state insurance regulation, especially when such regulation raises the cost of commercial insurance. Consequently, state insurance regulators are unable to implement insurance market reforms effectively.[96] Of note, the NAIC has strongly condemned ERISA and its effect on state insurance regulation.[97]

Not surprisingly, many employers—in the quest for cheaper employee benefits—have become self-insured and thus exempt from state regulation. In 1995, about 40 percent of all Americans insured through employment were in self-insured, employer-sponsored health plans, and evidence suggests that more employers are self-insuring their health plans to escape state insurance regulation.[98] In addition, to protect themselves from undue risk, employers with self-insured plans purchase stop-loss insurance to pay for losses for a particular patient above a specific dollar amount, which is often set as low as $5,000.[99] One fallout of ERISA preemption is the development of provider-sponsored networks that contract directly with employee welfare benefit plans and thereby escape insurance regulation altogether.[100]

Two recent cases exemplify the problem with ERISA-regulated plans and the operation of the ERISA preemption provisions. In *McGann v. H and H Music Co.,*[101] the U.S. Court of Appeals for the Fifth Circuit upheld the district court's summary judgment against an AIDS victim in an employer-sponsored health plan that had limited coverage for AIDS to $5,000 in the year following diagnosis.[102] In *American Medical Security, Inc. v. Bartlett,*[103] the U.S. Court of Appeals for the Fourth Circuit rejected the effort of Maryland's insurance regulators to require employee welfare benefit plans that purchased state-regulated stop-loss insurance to comply with state-mandated benefit provisions for the primary plan.[104]

With greater appreciation of the problems posed by the division in the regulation of private health insurance, Congress has enacted health insurance reforms with amendments to ERISA and the federal tax laws as well as mandates to states. The Consolidated Omnibus Budget Reconciliation Act of 1985 mandated that employer-sponsored health plans make coverage available to employees and their dependents who would lose benefits because of termination or other change in employment.[105] In 1996, Congress mandated two benefits pertaining to mental health and obstetric coverage for all, including ERISA-regulated health plans.[106]

Also in 1996, Congress enacted the Health Insurance Portability and Accountability Act of 1996.[107] This statute regulates the portability of all private health insurance coverage through limits on preexisting exclusions and other underwriting practices that limit job mobility and otherwise threaten health insurance coverage. It also prohibits employers from basing eligibility decisions on health status, disability, claims experience, or other similar factors and from charging higher premiums for comparable coverage on the basis of these factors.[108]

THE UNIVERSE OF PUBLIC HEALTH INSURANCE PROGRAMS

Public health insurance programs are quite varied. They include such programs for vulnerable groups as Medicare, Medicaid, and SCHIP. The federal government also provides coverage to military personnel directly, to the dependents of military personnel through the Civilian Health and Medical Program of the Uniformed Services (CHAMPUS), and to veterans through its system of veterans medical centers. In addition, the federal government has a direct services program for Native Americans as part of treaty obligations with tribes.

The Medicare Program

Medicare, a federal program, provides comprehensive health insurance for the elderly, the severely disabled, and people with end-stage renal disease.[109] As shown in table 1, 36 million Americans (13.2 percent of the population) had insurance through Medicare in 1999. Nearly all the elderly and the severely disabled are eligible for Medicare,[110] as are individuals with end-stage renal disease.[111] Medicare benefits include hospital and related benefits for acute illness and injury as well as physician and other outpatient services that are "reasonable and necessary for the diagnosis and treatment of illness or injury."[112]

Medicare actually consists of three programs. Traditional fee-for-service Medicare is composed of two programs—the Hospital Insurance program (Part A)[113] and the Supplementary Medical Insurance program (Part B).[114] Part B is funded through enrollees' premiums and congressional appropriations.[115] Part A is funded through the mandatory social security payroll tax on all wage earners.[116] Part A covers hospital care and related home health and skilled nursing home care, and Part B covers physician and other outpatient services. Part C of the Medicare program is the Medicare+Choice program (Part C), which offers prepaid managed care plans for both Part A and Part B benefits and replaces the previous Medicare HMO program.[117] The Medicare+Choice program has had some trouble getting off the ground, with many MCOs pulling out of the program and enrollee dissatisfaction.[118]

For Parts A and B, the Medicare program contracts with private organizations, including private health insurers and professional peer review organizations, to administer the Medicare program, including implementation of Medicare coverage and payment policy.[119] Further, Medicare contracts with health-care institutions to serve Medicare beneficiaries and often deems private accreditation of health-care institutions as compliance with Medicare requirements for participating in the Medicare program.[120] For the Medicare+Choice program (Part C), Medicare contracts directly with MCOs to provide health plans for Medicare beneficiaries.[121]

The Medicaid Program

Medicaid, a joint federal-state program, provides health and long term care insurance for recipients of assistance programs as well as for some other poor children, pregnant mothers, the disabled, and the aged.[122] In 1999, as shown in table 1, Medicaid served 27.8 million recipients.[123] Medicaid covers about 10 percent of the population but almost 40 percent of the poor. To participate in Medicaid, states submit to the federal government a "state plan" describing the state program and giving assurances on how they will meet federal requirements.[124] The federal government matches state dollars at different rates depending on the state's per capita income.[125]

Historically, Medicaid eligibility has been linked to eligibility for the two major cash assistance programs under the Social Security Act—Aid to Families with Dependent Children (AFDC) and Supplemental Security Income.[126] In the 1980s, following sharp cuts in all programs for the poor under the Reagan administration,[127] Congress incrementally expanded Medicaid eligibility for infants, children, and pregnant mothers.[128] As of 2002, all poor children whose family's income is under 133 percent of the federal poverty level will be eligible for Medicaid.[129] States may also cover children and pregnant women with incomes under 185 percent of the federal poverty level.[130] In the Personal Responsibility and Work Opportunity Reconciliation Act of 1996,[131] Congress fundamentally changed the cash assistance program for low income mothers and children and their access to the Medicaid program. Although the Temporary Assistance to Needy Families program requires recipients to return to work after two years of benefits,[132] states must provide Medicaid coverage to children and parents who would otherwise be eligible for the former AFDC program—children and pregnant women in families with incomes under 133 percent of poverty.[133]

States may also aid the "medically needy"—individuals who, but for income, meet the other eligibility requirements for cash assistance programs under the Social Security Act.[134] The medically needy program also provides coverage for lower income people who must "spend down" their income and resources to obtain Medicaid eligibility. Seventy percent of states have a medically needy program.[135]

States must cover some specified services and may cover specific additional benefits for which the federal match is available.[136] States have greater flexibility in structuring the benefit package for their medically needy programs.[137] For all programs, coverage of services must be "sufficient in amount, duration and scope to reasonably achieve their purpose."[138] To assure that states do not unduly favor one group of Medicaid eligibles over another, there are limits on the degree to which they can provide coverage of benefits for some groups of Medicaid eligibles and not for others.[139] In addition, states cannot discriminate in the coverage of mandatory services on the basis of diagnosis, type of illness, or condition.[140] Nevertheless, there is considerable variation among states as to coverage of both mandated and optional Medicaid benefits.[141]

Medicaid has been moving to prepaid managed care—particularly for children and pregnant women—since 1981. The enactment in that year of the primary care case management waiver authority has enabled states to enroll Medicaid eligibles in prepaid managed care plans.[142] In 1997, Congress authorized the states to serve Medicaid beneficiaries through prepaid managed care plans without getting a waiver of program requirements.[143] Further, the Clinton administration permitted states to use the waiver authority under Section 1115 of the Social Security Act[144] to expand coverage in prepaid managed care plans for the low income uninsured who do not otherwise meet Medicaid eligibility requirements, and almost a third of the states have elected to use this waiver to expand coverage.[145]

The State Children's Health Insurance Program

The Balanced Budget Act of 1997 established SCHIP to expand health insurance coverage for children.[146] Specifically, states can establish programs for children whose family's income is under 200 percent of the federal poverty level.[147] Under the SCHIP program, states can expand their Medicaid programs to include covered children, or they can establish an independent program.[148]

Within federal guidelines, states have great flexibility in designing benefit packages under their SCHIP programs. They can proceed with the state's Medicaid benefit package and align their program with Medicaid. Or they can offer independent managed care plans that are comparable to a so-called benchmark plan within the state, including the standard Blue Cross and Blue Shield plan for federal employees, the state's health plan for state employees, or the commercial HMO having the largest enrollment in the state.[149] States also have the option—within certain constraints—of covering the families of poor children.[150]

Other Federal Programs

The federal government and the states provide health insurance coverage to other groups as well. The most important group is government employees. However, as coverage for government employees is often purchased through the private market and functions much like employer-sponsored health insurance coverage, it is described below in the section on private health insurance. The federal government also provides coverage for specific groups to which it has special obligations. For example, it provides a direct services program to Native Americans pursuant to treaty obligations with tribes.[151]

The U.S. Department of Defense (DOD) provides direct services to active duty personnel in military facilities and to military dependents and retirees through CHAMPUS.[152] As shown in table 1, DOD provides health insurance coverage to 8.5 million military personnel, dependents, and retirees. CHAMPUS has inaugurated a managed care program, TRICARE, for CHAMPUS beneficiaries.[153]

The U.S. Department of Veterans Affairs operates a substantial direct services program for military veterans and some dependents in special cases through the VA Health-Care Network.[154] This network includes VA hospital and clinic care and also dental care, long term care, and alcohol and drug treatment. VA medical centers and outpatient clinics are competing with each other to become the primary care provider of choice for all veterans and to enroll veterans in comprehensive care plans. All veterans are eligible for care, although free care is available only to certain veterans with service-related injuries and other specified needs.[155]

Other State Programs

In recent years, the states have been active in extending health insurance coverage for the uninsured poor. At least seven states have enacted comprehensive health reform and major coverage expansions, although these efforts have not always succeeded, even in big states with large tax bases and sophisticated bureaucracies to finance and manage comprehensive programs.[156] Many other states have made less ambitious efforts, generally through Medicaid expansions, to expand coverage and/or access to care for the low income uninsured.[157] Since 1992, some states have expanded Medicaid coverage pursuant to Section 1115 waivers under the Social Security Act for the uninsured poor. Further, as mentioned above, SCHIP enables states to expand coverage for families of uninsured children and thereby makes available an additional source of federal funding to support state health insurance programs for the poor.

Of critical importance, as revealed in table 1, 42.5 million Americans (15.5 percent) have no health insurance coverage. The percentage of the uninsured population increased dramatically in the last decade, from 13.9 percent in 1990 to 15.5 percent in 1999. This upward trend is remarkable and disturbing. In 1990, the economy was in recession, while, later in the decade, it experienced a period of unsurpassed and sustained growth and prosperity.[158] The uninsured are in a particularly precarious position when it comes to protecting their interests in health care.

Who is uninsured and how long people remain uninsured have been studied extensively in recent years.[159] Clearly, as revealed in table 1, the largest group of uninsured are low income workers. In a December 1997 poll, more than half of adults in low income working families (those whose annual income is under $35,000) reported having been uninsured at some time during the previous two years.[160]

There is also evidence that health insurance coverage—particularly for the poor—is unstable, that sponsors of health insurance coverage cut back benefits or fail to provide affordable coverage at all. For example, in the early 1990s, the proportion of those covered by employer-sponsored health insurance declined, particularly among families.[161] Cost sharing and benefit limits in private health plans have increased in recent years, and thus many employees decline coverage when it is offered because of the cost.[162] Some question the future ability of employers to assure affordable health insurance coverage to the nonelderly population.[163]

4 : Relevant Law and Theory

Several sources of law and theory have shaped the current debate about procedural protections for the interests of individuals in their health care. This chapter presents these sources of law and theory and explains how they shape both the debate and visions of reform. In many respects, current law and theory have dictated reform options and perhaps have hindered the collective imagination of more innovative procedural protections for health-care consumers.

The law is organized in theoretically artificial but practically workable categories. The areas of law that are most pertinent to procedural protections for health-care interests are (1) regulatory law, (2) corporate and associated tax law, (3) administrative law, (4) contract law, and (5) tort law. While other areas of law relate to procedural protections for health-care interests, these particular areas shape current procedural protections and are most directly implicated in their reform.

Further, three important dichotomies pervade the law governing procedural protections for the interests of Americans in health care. These three dichotomies and their associated legal and political arrangements play a crucial role in the conception and reform of procedural protections for health-care interests.

The first dichotomy is the distinction between public and private in modern Western law that relegates the same function to different legal subject areas depending on the ownership characteristics of the organization performing the function. This dichotomy has especially crucial implications for procedural protections for American consumers of health care. Specifically, private organizations make the bulk of relevant policies governing the content, quality, and cost of and access to health-care services in private policymaking processes that are poorly understood. Further, these policies are also made in contracts between health plan sponsors, health-care providers, and managed care organizations (MCOs) that establish the arrangements for the financing and delivery of health-care services for consumers in public and private health plans.

The second dichotomy is the division in American federalism between state and federal, in which different governing authorities have legal and regulatory jurisdiction over various procedural protections for health-care consumers. States have historically regulated health insurance and health-care providers under their police power. Thus, states have played a key role in conceiving and implementing procedural protection for health-care consumers. The role of the federal government derives from its role as the sponsor and financier of health insurance and health-care services programs for the elderly and some of the poor as well as the regulator of employee welfare benefit plans under the Employee Retirement Income Security Act of 1974 (ERISA).[1] However, the broad scope of these federal responsibilities accords the federal government a major role in defining the content, quality, and cost of consumers' health care and implementing procedural protections to protect consumers' interests.

The third dichotomy, which has proved to be a defining construct of the current patient protection debate, is the distinction between the legislating and the adjudicating functions that pervades modern administrative law and theory. This dichotomy describes two fundamental functions of the legal process. While a valid conception of process, this dichotomy has served to channel thinking about procedural protections into two separate tracts and perhaps stifled more innovative procedural reforms that reflect the fundamental connection between these two functions in protecting the interests of health-care consumers.

REGULATORY LAW

When government addresses public concerns about private activity, it does so mainly through regulation. In regulation, a public statute establishes a regulatory program, which is assigned to an administrative agency, to address an identified problem. The problem is generally some failure of the private market to fulfill economic or social needs. The statute for the regulatory program establishes requirements and standards with which affected parties must comply and also mechanisms to enforce their compliance. Under regulatory programs, different techniques are used to achieve conformity with regulatory requirements. Regulatory techniques include licensure, audited self-regulation, and ratemaking.

In modern liberal political theory, the purpose of regulatory programs and regulatory agencies is to protect and represent the public.[2] However, modern legal and political science scholarship has undermined this liberal theoretical position.[3] This scholarship analyzes how interest groups influence regulatory programs and agencies using principles of economics.[4] Building on this scholarship as well as on scholarship in the law and economics movement, public choice theory deliniates how interest groups advance their objectives in legislative and regulatory processes, often at the expense of the public.[5]

Described below are the major regulatory programs governing health-care professionals, institutional health-care providers, and private health insurers that most directly affect procedural protections for American consumers of health care. Of great current interest is whether these protections are adequate for protecting the interests of health-care consumers in affordable and high quality health care.

Regulation of Physicians and Health-Care Professionals

State licensure is the dominant method of regulating the medical profession and other health-care professions. Licensure is a grant of official permission to an individual or a business to engage in a particular activity. Through statutes, states define the scope of practice and discipline practitioners that fail to comport with regulatory requirements in their practice.[6] Licensure and discipline provide great protection to health-care consumers as state licensure authorities monitor the professional performance of health-care professionals. Recently, many licensure authorities have, for the benefit of consumers, begun publishing data on the practice patterns and disciplinary records of physicians and other practitioners.[7]

But the medical profession is also self-regulated. Physicians sit on state medical boards that implement state licensure and discipline programs. In addition, physicians are subject to ethical norms developed by medical professional associations, such as the American Medical Association, that govern the practice of medicine.[8] Self-regulation is important for patient protection. For example, the critical role of physicians as advocates for patients is predicated on the assumption that physicians will be subject to ethical norms imposed by the profession rather than just regulatory requirements of government.

Regulation of Hospitals and Health-Care Facilities

States also license and regulate health-care facilities, including hospitals, extended care facilities, and home health agencies.[9] States use accreditation, a form of audited self-regulation, in the licensure and regulation of hospitals and some other health-care institutions.[10]

Accreditation is a voluntary process by which an organization demonstrates that it meets the standards established by its professional peers. Accreditation serves two important functions. First, it establishes standards against which to measure the quality of an organization. Second, it determines whether institutions have complied with established standards and have therefore earned the imprimatur of accreditation. Customarily, accreditation is the responsibility of private organizations that have expertise establishing standards for and measuring the quality of services offered by the institutions seeking accreditation.

Similarly, states license health maintenance organizations (HMOs) that provide services within the state. State statutes regulating HMOs, many of which are based on the Model HMO Act of the National Association of Insurance Commissioners,[11] set forth requirements for the operation of HMOs that are similar to requirements for other health-care facilities.[12] State insurance regulatory authorities also license HMOs as risk-bearing insurers.

Private accreditation often serves as evidence that state institutional licensure requirements have been met.[13] Further, for hospitals, home health agencies, and some other health-care institutions, private accreditation also serves to demonstrate compliance with participation requirements for the Medicare and Medicaid programs and private health plans.[14] Nursing homes, historically, have not been able to use private accreditation in this manner because of concerns about the quality of care and patient safety.[15]

The most important—from the perspective of consumers at least—of the licensure and accreditation standards for hospitals and other health-care institutions are the mandates that institutions engage in quality assurance and improvement activities.[16] Both state licensure laws and private accreditation standards have such mandates, mandates that include credentialing physicians and other practitioners and monitoring clinical services through peer review.[17] These quality assurance activities play a major role in the identification of individuals' concerns about their health care that do not surface in patient complaints.

Regulation of Health Insurance

The regulation of private health insurers, HMOs, and employer-sponsored health insurance has been described in chapter 3. In brief, state insurance codes regulate commercial health insurers and HMOs, and ERISA regulates employer-sponsored health plans. Both state insurance codes and ERISA mandate procedural protections for enrollees in health plans. Most state health insurance codes also regulate the rates and underwriting practices of commercial health insurers and HMOs.

Further, publication of policies and other information about the regulated parties is an important regulatory strategy under state insurance codes and ERISA.[18] With enhanced concerns about consumer protection in managed care plans, states are becoming more aggressive in their regulation of HMOs and MCOs. Recent state legislation, discussed in chapter 2, includes requirements for publication of policies used in defining coverage, utilization review, and quality. Publication of policy has been an important feature of proposed patient protection legislation before Congress in recent years.

CORPORATE AND TAX LAW

Corporate law establishes requirements for the formation and operation of private corporations. State corporation laws authorize both for-profit and not-for-profit corporations. For-profit corporations are established to make profits for shareholders, while not-for-profit corporations cannot issue stock to raise capital or distribute profits to shareholders.[19] Not-for-profit corporations must engage in a charitable or public-oriented enterprise that, in theory, for-profit enterprises cannot readily perform.[20] State not-for-profit corporation laws impose requirements on corporate membership and governance.[21] For example, not-for-profit corporations must have governing boards that are representative of the community in which the corporations are located, particularly if they are tax exempt organizations.

For-profit corporations are subject to federal, state, and local taxation. Not-for-profit corporations can be exempt from federal taxation if they meet the requirements of Section 501 of the Internal Revenue Code.[22] To retain their tax exemption, these private organizations must be organized and conduct business within certain constraints.[23] They are also eligible for various tax exemptions from state and local law.[24]

Regarding procedural requirements, state corporation laws require corporations to have bylaws stating general policies as to governance and operations.[25] These bylaws and amendments thereto are legally enforceable policy. Corporate bylaws and associated internal corporate policies generally promote the business objectives of the corporation or implement regulatory mandates. Otherwise, corporate and tax law does not affect the content of policy of private organizations and, except for governance requirements, does not specifically address procedures for making policy or processes for resolving consumer disputes with corporations.

Most health insurance companies, MCOs, and HMOs are for-profit corporations. Since the 1980s, payers have increasingly selected the for-profit corporate form in part because of the strict requirements for tax exempt status for HMOs and the loss of tax exempt status for Blue Cross plans during this period.[26] The fact that these payers, especially HMOs, are for profit has been a major factor in the patient protection debate and fueled the perspective that for-profit health plan sponsors design capitated health plans to limit care for patients and maximize profits.[27]

The types of corporate control for American hospitals are public, private not for profit, and private for profit. Different types of corporate control have critical implications for access to hospital services for the uninsured and poor. Public hospitals often are required to serve the uninsured poor as a matter of statute and receive state and local tax relief and government subsidies to do so.[28] Some private, not-for-profit hospitals, particularly those established by religious organizations, often are required by their charters or even foundational charitable trust documents to provide care for the poor and the uninsured who are unable to pay.[29] Most not-for-profit hospitals are exempt from federal taxation as charitable organizations under Section 501(c)(3) of the Internal Revenue Code[30] and enjoy comparable tax exemptions under state and local law.

The obligations of not-for-profit hospitals with charitable missions have been hotly debated with the conversion of many hospitals into for-profit networks.[31] Further, use of the not-for-profit corporate form of business as well as of associated charitable tax exemption has been a controversial issue as well.[32] Since the advent of third party payment, all hospitals became more profitable and downplayed their charitable mission or even adopted the for-profit corporate form. Many maintain that special treatment of not-for-profit hospitals, especially with respect to taxation, does not make sense any more, especially when most not-for-profit hospitals do not have policies mandating the provision of services to all the poor in need of care.[33] Others lament the resulting decline of the tradition of voluntary health-care delivery.[34]

Private organizations that make health-care policies have assumed a variety of corporate forms. Many medical professional associations, voluntary health organizations, and private accrediting bodies are organized as not-for-profit corporations under state law. In general, they are exempt from federal taxation under Section 501(c)(6) of the Internal Revenue Code as trade associations.[35] Voluntary health organizations are usually tax exempt as charitable organizations under Section 501(c)(3),[36] as are private accrediting bodies.[37]

ADMINISTRATIVE LAW

Administrative law establishes and governs the procedures by which government agencies conduct their business and, in particular, make policy and adjudicate disputes. Administrative law is important in the health-care sector because of the major role that federal, state, and even local government agencies play in the financing and delivery of health-care services. Further, as public procedural law, administrative law also offers many models for procedural protections of health-care consumers.

The two procedural functions of rule or policymaking and adjudication predominate in American administrative law.[38] For example, these two processes are the organizing principle of the federal Administrative Procedure Act of 1946 (APA)[39] and the Model State Administrative Procedure Act of the Uniform State Law Commission.[40] Agencies legislate, as do legislatures, when they make policies and rules that have general application and future effect. Agencies adjudicate, as do courts, when they make decisions by applying legal rules to specific cases. The distinction between these two functions is reflected in the types of facts at issue in each type of proceeding. Specifically, legislative proceedings deal with "legislative facts," such as the findings of social science research, necessary to determine policy, and adjudicative proceedings deal with "adjudicative facts," which generally involve circumstances and events at issue in a dispute.[41]

A major theme in modern administrative law has been a vision of the state—that is, government agencies—representing the public interest in the sound administration of public programs as opposed to promoting the rights of individuals vis-à-vis the state with enhanced opportunities for participation in agency proceedings.[42] In the 1960s, there was a great push to accord rights of participation in agency processes as well as rights to force agency accountability for adverse actions against private interests—as a means of legitimizing the administrative process.[43] Since then, as Jerry Mashaw observes, administrative law jurisprudence has moved from a model of recognizing and protecting beneficiaries' rights to benefits to a more "statist" model that focuses on facilitation of state administration and the general welfare over individual rights.[44]

In the 1960s and 1970s, administrative law began addressing the procedural issues faced by beneficiaries of government benefit programs. In the late 1940s, benefits in government programs had the status of privileges with no constitutional protection under the due process clause of the U.S. Constitution.[45] The federal APA has provided little guidance on procedural protections for government benefit programs or, for that matter, more informal agency hearings in general.[46] Further, the APA reflects the vision of government benefits at the time as less in need of procedural protections in its exemption of government benefit programs from its rulemaking requirements.[47] In 1970, the U.S. Supreme Court recognized a constitutionally protected property interest in government benefit programs in the seminal decision of *Goldberg v. Kelly* and established requirements for hearings regarding the newly protected interests.[48]

Rulemaking

As government agencies, public sponsors are subject to the general principles of administrative law regarding rule and policymaking.[49] The procedural due process clause in the Fifth and Fourteenth Amendments to the U.S. Constitution governs public policymaking at the state and federal level, although procedural requirements are fairly minimal.[50] States have comparable due process provisions that they have generally, but not always, interpreted in the same manner.[51]

Legislative Rulemaking. The preferred model of legislative rulemaking in modern American administrative law is the "notice-and-comment" or informal rulemaking model under Section 553 of the federal APA. For legislative rules, the federal APA requires that agencies provide the public notice of the proposed rule and an opportunity to comment.[52] This model is predicated on the assumption that an open process that solicits opinions and other information from the interested public will result in a better rule from a policy perspective. This process ideally ferrets out legitimate adverse comments that can be accommodated before final promulgation. While state rulemaking procedures vary, they are similar to federal models, and at least twenty-one states have moved toward the notice-and-comment model.[53]

Until the 1960s and 1970s and the advent of new and extensive federal regulation designed to prevent discrimination and reduce risks to health and safety in the workplace, the environment, and other sectors, federal agencies did not use legislative rulemaking extensively.[54] With greater use of rulemaking by federal agencies, administrative law scholarship has, not surprisingly, been concentrated on sorting out the issues and problems with and implications of this relatively new phenomenon of widespread legislative rulemaking by federal regulatory agencies.

Most scholarship on federal rulemaking addressed problems posed by the use of notice-and-comment rulemaking under Section 553 of the federal APA.[55] An early problem addressed was the appropriate scope of judicial review as the federal courts struggled to sort out the relation between courts and agencies in the rulemaking process.[56] As notice-and-comment rulemaking became more accepted, scholarship focused on the practical problems of rulemaking[57] and new rulemaking techniques such as negotiated rulemaking.[58] Reacting to concerns about the social regulation of the 1960s and 1970s, rulemaking scholarship focused on the nature and extent of regulatory reform,[59] deregulation and its implications for rulemaking,[60] and efforts of the legislative and executive branches to control federal agency rulemaking.[61]

Courts and scholars have wrestled with the issue of what processes best achieve accuracy in the content of agency rules, particularly those involving highly technical scientific and/or controversial matters.[62] One particular issue has been the ability of notice-and-comment rulemaking procedures to assure the validity of policy on technical and scientific issues. It is implicitly assumed that a wide open process in which all interested parties have a meaningful opportunity to present their views will result in accurate and thus valid and credible policy. In *Vermont Yankee Nuclear Power Corp. v. Natural Resources Defense Council, Inc.,*[63] the Supreme Court emphatically ruled that courts could not impose additional requirements on agencies' rulemaking proceedings to assure better development of highly technical scientific facts and issues.[64]

But are more rigorous procedures, such as cross-examination, necessary or effective in eliciting accuracy and validity in scientific policy? For there is a "disconnect" between the submission of information and the ultimate decision on policy content that is not addressed in the notice-and-comment process. Some rulemaking reforms, such as hybrid rulemaking adding procedures beyond notice and comment, assume that more rigorous procedures will assure better consideration of technical issues underlying legislative rules.[65] The prevailing view in administrative law scholarship is that such trial type procedures are neither necessary nor appropriate given the types of policy decisions based on legislative facts usually at issue.[66] Interestingly, the medical models for health-care policymaking address this gap explicitly and, as discussed in chapter 7, craft processes that better and much more directly assure more accurate policy content than do these more legally oriented models of policymaking.

Nonlegislative Rule and Policymaking. For nonlegislative rules, such as interpretative rules and general statements of policy, government agencies (including public health plan sponsors) have more flexibility. They are not bound by legal requirements except when specified in their enabling statute or prior regulation.[67] In most administrative agencies, there are generally designated processes for making nonlegislative rules.

Further, the federal APA expressly exempts government benefit programs from rulemaking requirements.[68] As government benefit programs expanded in the 1950s and 1960s, widespread criticism of this exemption emerged, and the Administrative Conference of the United States called for its elimination.[69] Agencies responded by voluntarily using notice-and-comment rulemaking rules of major government benefit programs.

Processes for making interpretive and nonlegislative rules for government health insurance and health-care services programs have received less scholarly attention. The major issues addressed are the circumstances for properly invoking interpretative rulemaking and the legal effect of nonlegislative rules.[70] Other than concerns about facilitating public participation and publication described below, scholarship has not really addressed the procedures for making nonlegislative rules.

Publication of Rules and Policy. In administrative law, publication is an important procedural element in a sound policymaking process. The federal Freedom of Information Act embodies this value in its mandates for publication of government policy whenever possible, including regarding federal health insurance and health-care benefit programs.[71] Most states have comparable so-called sunshine laws that require state agencies, including those that administer health insurance and health-care services programs, to publicize relevant policy.[72] With respect to nonlegislative rules, prevailing scholarship and theory emphasize publicizing policy and facilitating public input in policymaking processes as key strategies for protecting the interests of the public.[73]

Adjudication

In government benefit programs, including public health insurance and health-care services programs, the law of adjudication has been driven by the mandates of the constitutional procedural due process doctrine.[74] Modern procedural due process jurisprudence evolved after *Goldberg v. Kelly*.[75] In this case, the U.S. Supreme Court confirmed that government benefits are protected property interests under the procedural due process doctrine and required administrative agencies to provide notice and an opportunity to be heard before adversely affecting an individual's government entitlement. The Court also ruled that the requisite procedures for termination of welfare benefits included the right to confront witnesses, an unbiased decisionmaker, and a decision on the record, among other protections.

Following *Goldberg,* there was a great expansion in the number and type of government benefits accorded property status and due process protection.[76] The *Goldberg* decision precipitated a fierce debate over the appropriate elements of hearings for government entitlement programs that generate an enormous volume of cases involving relatively small amounts of money.[77]

In a 1976 decision, *Mathews v. Eldridge,*[78] the Supreme Court articulated the formula for analyzing the constitutionality of specific procedures in procedural due process challenges. Specifically, this formula calls for a balancing of the private and the public interests at stake and an analysis of the procedures in terms of their potential for resulting in an erroneous deprivation of the private rights as well as the probable value of additional procedures. Subsequent Supreme Court decisions, involving diverse and hardly comparable fact patterns, have been markedly more circumspect than the *Goldberg* decision was about hearing requirements, particularly with respect to trial type procedures.[79]

Since the 1970s, some scholars have criticized the *Mathews v. Eldridge* decision as a somewhat bloodless cost-benefit approach to constitutional jurisprudence.[80] Some scholars assert that required proceedings should emphasize the dignity of the individual involved whatever the outcome.[81] Other scholars have criticized the current due process jurisprudence from a more conservative perspective and even the recognition of a property interest in government benefits altogether.[82]

An important vein of scholarship following *Goldberg* has been empirical research from social psychology.[83] Empirical theorists in law and social psychology identified characteristics of fair process through empirical experiments with simulated or actual adjudicative models that report perceptions of research subjects as to the fairness of various adjudicative models.[84] The findings of this research have been helpful in conceptualizing fair processes for dispute resolution.

The constitutional due process protections for beneficiaries of public programs are by no means static or secure. There has been significant erosion in due process protections since the 1970s.[85] In *American Manufacturers Mutual Insurance Company v. Sullivan,*[86] the U.S. Supreme Court sharply limited constitutional protections for consumers in public health insurance programs. This case involved workers' compensation benefits that the state purchased for beneficiaries through a private insurance company. The Court held that the private insurer's decision to withhold payment for a medical treatment over which there was a coverage dispute was not state action for purposes of the procedural due process doctrine. Further, the Court concluded, claimants have no property interest in having insurers pay for medical treatment prior to the insurer's determination that treatments are reasonable and necessary—in other words, after the insurer's coverage determination. This decision has crucial implications for the accountability of publicly sponsored health plans in making coverage and other decisions about the care of plan members. One critical implication is that, now, contrary to prior case law,[87] private health plans are not public actors for the purposes of the procedural due process clause, nor are their coverage decisions subject to procedural due process review.

Another threat to procedural due process is the judicial sanction of the diminished status of benefits in government entitlement programs through their statutory definition. For example, in *Colson v. Sillman,*[88] the Second Circuit ruled that a program client had no constitutionally protected entitlement interest in program benefits because the enabling legislation accorded discretion to the state in determining need for benefits and limited benefits to those funded from fiscal appropriations.

A recent and quite remarkable federal district court decision, *Westside Mothers v. Haveman*,[89] ruled that plaintiff Medicaid recipients could not sue Medicaid officials for failure to provide statutorily mandated Medicaid benefits under 42 U.S.C. Section 1983[90] (which authorizes suits against state employees for violations of federal constitutional provisions). The court's basis was that the Medicaid statute, enacted under the spending clause of the federal constitution, established an option program. Therefore, the relation between the states and the federal government was contractual, and the Medicaid statute was not the supreme law of the land for purposes of Section 1983. If this decision gains currency in other higher court decisions, it could greatly limit the ability of recipients of needs-based government health insurance programs such as Medicaid and the State Children's Health Insurance Program (SCHIP) from seeking judicial remedies to protect their interests in these programs.

This combination of statutory denial of entitlement and thus property status with subsequent judicial approval and justification spells potential doom for the protection of vulnerable beneficiaries in existing and new public health insurance programs. In recent legislation for the new welfare reform program and the SCHIP, Congress affirmatively stated that program benefits are not entitlements, thus eliminating open-ended obligations to actual and potential program clients.[91] With judicial sanction of these arrangements, the constitutional protection of benefits is greatly diminished.

In addition, alternative dispute resolution (ADR) methods have become widely utilized in courts, administrative agencies, and other dispute resolution institutions.[92] With federal legislation explicitly authorizing the use of ADR,[93] federal agencies have increasingly used it in federal agency adjudications,[94] although not much in the mass justice context involving disputes with individuals over government benefits.

CONTRACT LAW

Contracts are the predominant way in which individuals and organizations make legally binding policy that governs their relationships. Contract law outlines the requirements for making private, legally binding agreements between and among individuals, private organizations, and, increasingly, government agencies. To the extent that these agreements establish courses of present and future action, they are establishing legally enforceable policy. Contracts are generally enforceable in court provided that they meet specified criteria in common law.

Contractual relationships have always pervaded the health-care sector, beginning with the physician-patient relationship. With widespread third party payment after World War II, both private and public health plan sponsors entered contracts with group purchasers and individuals for health-care coverage. They also contracted with physicians and other providers that serve covered beneficiaries. In addition, public health plan sponsors, such as Medicare, contracted with private health insurance companies and other organizations to administer public health insurance programs.

With the expansion of managed care, both public and private health plan sponsors used contract in a new way in their capitated health plans.[95] Specifically, both public health plan sponsors (e.g., administrative agencies) and private health plan sponsors (e.g., employers) contracted with private MCOs to cover their beneficiary groups. In addition to establishing formal relations to provide care to health plan members, MCOs also use contracts with providers to achieve efficiencies and cost savings.

Key Contractual Relationships in the Health-Care Sector

There are five sets of important contractual relationships in the health-care sector that govern the provision of health-care services to health-care consumers and are implicated in procedural protections for the interests of consumers of health care. These relationships are the following:

—contracts between *patients* and *providers,* including contracts between patients and (*a*) physicians and (*b*) institutional providers;

—contracts between *individuals* and *employers or commercial health plan sponsors,* including contracts between consumers and (*a*) employers offering health plans, (*b*) health insurance companies offering conventional health plans, (*c*) HMOs and MCOs offering prepaid managed care plans, and (*d*) non-risk-bearing provider-sponsored networks offering prepaid health plans;

—contracts between *employers* and *commercial health plan sponsors* regarding group health insurance coverage for employees, including contracts between employers and (*a*) health insurance companies offering traditional health plans, (*b*) HMOs and MCOs offering prepaid health plans, (*c*) health insurance companies serving as third party administrators for employer self-insured plans, and (*d*) non-risk-bearing provider-sponsored networks offering health plans;

—contracts between *government agencies* as public health plan sponsors and *commercial health plan sponsors* offering prepaid health plans for the entitled beneficiaries of government health insurance programs; and

—contracts between *commercial health plan sponsors* and *health-care providers,* including contracts between sponsors and (*a*) physicians and (*b*) institutional providers.

All these different contractual relationships impose legal obligations on participating parties. However, whether or not individual consumers are parties to the contracts, the contract terms often have a critical effect on their interests in health care. In what follows, each of these contractual relationships is examined in detail and the implications for procedural protections for consumers clarified. To the extent that the uninsured obtain care from physicians, hospitals, and other providers, the obligations in these relationships are generally derived from tort law, statutory law, or ethics in addition to contract. These sources of obligation for the care of the uninsured are described below.

Contracts between Patients and Providers. The contractual relationship between patients and their health-care providers, especially physicians, is the foundational relationship in health care. It is a voluntary relationship for both parties and, absent the involvement of third party payers, involves an agreement to provide a service for a fee. The relationship is also governed by professional ethics, including the command that the physician hold the patient's needs above any other competing concerns.[96] From this ethical precept has evolved the ideal of the physician as advocate for the patient in grappling with both the complexities of medical treatment and, more recently, the financing of that treatment.[97] The fact that third party payers pay for most of the health care of American consumers has changed this contractual relationship dramatically and has given rise to many of the concerns addressed in this book.

The contract between a patient and an institutional provider is also ostensibly voluntary and similar to that between patient and physician. However, because of third party financing and public law obligations, the relationship is markedly different. Specifically, institutional providers have extensive obligations to patients, especially the uninsured poor, established through a variety of state and federal laws as well as their own corporate charters and policies. Some of the more important of these obligations are described in greater detail below.

Contracts between Individuals and Commercial Health Plan Sponsors. For the small percentage of the American population who purchase health insurance coverage independently through a health insurance company, an HMO, or an MCO, there is a direct contractual relationship between the consumer and the payer. The content of these contracts, in terms of rates, benefits, and nondiscrimination against like purchasers, is regulated under state insurance codes. In addition, these contracts are subject to several judicially created doctrines regarding the interpretation of insurance contracts that generally favor consumers, such as construing ambiguous contract terms in favor of the consumer and honoring the reasonable expectations of the insured.[98]

Contracts between Employers and Commercial Health Plan Sponsors. The majority of insured Americans under age sixty-five have health insurance through their employer or the employer of a family member and are members of a group health plan. There are a variety of contractual relationships that employers have with commercial health plan sponsors that offer health plans. The crucial distinctions between these relationships are whether the employer bears the risk of paying for care and thus is self-insured and whether the health plan is prepaid. Basically, there are four types of contractual arrangements. Employers may transfer the risk and purchase traditional health plans from insurance companies, or they can purchase prepaid health plans from MCOs and HMOs. If they retain the risk, they may contract with a health insurance company to serve as the third party administrator of their self-insured plans. A self-insured employer plan may also contract directly with non-risk-bearing provider-sponsored networks offering health plans.[99]

In all these contractual arrangements, the relationship between the health plan and individual plan members is more indirect. Under the principles of insurance law, when the employer purchases group coverage from an insurance company or even an HMO, it is only an intermediary that facilitates the purchase of health insurance coverage by individual enrollees.[100] In many respects, the health plan sponsor serves as an agent of the insurer in arranging the group health insurance coverage, and the contractual relationship exists between the insurer and the consumer.[101] One advantage of group coverage—and a major reason that it is cheaper than individual coverage—is that the insurer does not need to work through an agent. Rather, the insurer can work through the sponsor of a group to reach individuals to insure.

Indeed, the relationship between an enrollee in an employer-sponsored health plan and the health insurer, MCO, or HMO that sponsors the plan is quite indirect and hardly equal. The employer provides health insurance to employees and their family members as compensation for work. The employer then contracts with a health plan sponsor to provide health insurance coverage for the employees on its terms, and the health plan sponsor then contracts with providers—either individually or through networks—to provide care. The employees, unless represented by a union, generally have little input in the selection of the health plan, the health plan sponsors, or features of the health plan. To the extent that they have choice in the terms of health plans, it is only because an employer offers a choice of health plans to its employees. In 1999, only 35 percent of covered employees had a choice of more than one plan.[102]

Contracts between Government Agencies as Public Health Plan Sponsors and Commercial Health Plan Sponsors. Increasingly, federal and state government agencies responsible for public health insurance programs are contracting with MCOs and HMOs to provide prepaid health plans to program beneficiaries. The Medicare+Choice program contracts with MCOs and HMOs for prepaid health plans for Medicare beneficiaries. States now have the authority to do likewise for Medicaid beneficiaries. The Department of Defense also contracts with payers to offer prepaid managed care plans through the Civilian Health and Medical Program of the Uniformed Services (CHAMPUS).

While statutes, regulations, and other agency policies may govern the content of the contract in a general sense, there is much latitude for agencies and commercial health plan sponsors to delineate critical policies pertaining to the content, quality, and cost of health-care services in the contract. The contracting process is regulated under government procurement procedures that are generally designed to protect the private contractor.[103] These procurement procedures do not generally provide extensive opportunities for public participation by or even comment from consumers.[104]

The Supreme Court decision in *American Manufacturers Mutual Insurance Company v. Sullivan*[105] may have a detrimental effect on beneficiaries of government programs enrolled in private health plans pursuant to contract with sponsoring government agencies. Specifically, the coverage decisions of these health plans may be insulated from challenge under the procedural due process clause. Not only are beneficiaries of state and federal public programs affected, but so are enrollees in health plans sponsored by the Federal Employees Health Benefit Plan and state governments for government employees.

Contracts between Providers and Health Plan Sponsors. MCOs or other commercial health plan sponsors contract with certain providers or networks of providers to participate in their health plans. Often they require providers or provider networks to bid competitively for these contracts.[106] Such selective contracting has been an effective means of managing healthcare costs and is now commonly used by public and private health plan sponsors to establish relationships with the networks of physicians and hospitals that care for their enrollees.[107] In the selective contracting process, there is concern that contract terms, especially for capitated payment levels, place too much of the risk of expensive care on providers and encourage providers to curtail needed care for patients in need.

The terms of the contract between providers and health plans have, as explained above, been a highly controversial issue in the current patient protection debate. Of major concern are specific contract terms that require or encourage providers to limit care for patients.[108] Many contract terms specifically encourage physicians, who are paid prospectively a fixed price per patient on a capitated basis, to order fewer services for patients.[109] Also, in prepaid managed care plans, primary care physicians control access to specialty care, and physician compensation methods penalize primary care physicians for referring patients to more costly specialists.[110] Many state managed care reform laws as well as the patient protection bills before recent congresses have sought to preclude or otherwise regulate such contract terms between public and private health plan sponsors and the physicians and other providers with which those sponsors contract.

Pertinent Developments in Contract Law and Theory

From the perspective of health-care consumers, contract law does not contemplate the public effect of the myriad policies defining the content, quality, coverage, and price of health-care services established and embedded in many health plan contracts. In general, contracting parties do not have to provide notice of the content of a proposed contract in a public process, nor do they have to publish the contract on its completion. Health plan contracts often do not specify the details of relevant quality or coverage policies or even require that health plans or provider networks make and implement such policies. Furthermore, many health plan contracts are standard form contracts developed by the health insurer, MCO, or HMO.[111] Even the public and private health plan sponsors that purchase coverage through the contract may have little to say about the actual terms of the contract.

These characteristics of the contracting process further insulate the policymaking process from public view and limit the ability of providers, patients, and other interested parties to influence the content of relevant policy. Policymaking thus becomes more remote and inaccessible to affected parties. Although, as described in chapter 7, federal and state disclosure and publication laws under ERISA and state insurance codes do require disclosure of the terms of the health plan contract, consumers still have little or no access to the contracting process that actually determines policy. In addition, private health plan sponsors and also health-care providers often include required use of ADR for resolving all kinds of consumer disputes, including medical malpractice claims against plan providers and coverage disputes. Consumers are not always aware of these provisions when they enroll in a health plan. They have little power to object to these provisions in any event.

Because of the private nature of ADR, concerns exist about its use to adjudicate consumers' contract disputes with health plans and providers. This use of ADR has generated considerable criticism. One criticism is that ADR is unfair whenever vulnerable parties with unequal bargaining power are involved.[112] Many have raised this concern with respect to the elderly and the poor in health plans.[113] Some have recommended that ADR not be used when there is an imbalance of power existing between the parties.[114] The use of ADR to settle contract disputes with health plans, providers, and patients has also been sharply criticized for taking the adjudication of important legal issues out of the public domain.[115]

Of note, health plan contracts have been conceived as important vehicles for health-care reform. Specifically, contracts enable consumers, and especially those who represent consumers in purchasing health care, to bargain with providers to obtain a good price for services and define the content and quality of purchased health care. In addition, contracts permit parties to opt out of some legal requirements, particularly those imposed in tort, that parties may view as onerous or otherwise undesirable for their contractual relationship.[116] Clark C. Havighurst has been the most articulate advocate of the use of contract as a vehicle for health-care reform.[117] The basic thrust of Havighurst's argument is as follows: "Private contracts could help make the efficient microdecisions about health care spending: that is, in making the myriad clinical choices concerning resource use that cumulatively determine how much of the national wealth is spent on health care. Contracts . . . have an unappreciated potential for transmitting signals from cost-conscious consumers on the demand side of the market, through health plan middlemen, to health care providers on the supply side. Contracts can also simultaneously supply the legal authority that health plans and providers need before they can safely respond to economizing signals thus received."[118]

However, in the real world, consumers have little input into the content of health plan contracts between employers and commercial health plan sponsors. They are in a weak bargaining position vis-à-vis all of these parties in negotiating contract terms.[119] On reading proposed contract provisions on coverage, a consumer might well respond: "I would never choose such a contract for myself or my family; the deck is stacked too heavily in favor of the plan's cost-containment efforts." On reading the contract provisions calling for the use of medical practice guidelines to set the standard of care, the response might well be: "Why would I voluntarily consent to a standard of care for my family and me that I know is not the best?" The contractual commitment to use ADR procedures could well provoke the response: "Why would I surrender my right to sue for harms I might suffer unless I absolutely have to?" Especially troublesome—to those sophisticated enough to understand them, at least—would be the provisions that forfeit the protections afforded by established principles of insurance law that construe ambiguities in insurance contracts against the insurer on the theory that the insurance company was the party that drafted, and thus effectively dictated, the contract terms. One might well conclude: "What's in this contract for me and my family? The only way in which I would sign such a contract is if health insurance coverage were not offered to me, regardless of price, on any other terms"—the classic context for a contract of adhesion.

The vitality of the use of contract as a vehicle for health reform is further vitiated by the fact that consumers who obtain health insurance coverage through public or private heath plan sponsors do not, in fact, have much choice in the selection of their health plans.[120] Consequently, the degree to which their interests are represented in the negotiations between employers or government agencies and commercial health plan sponsors over the content, cost, and quality of the health plans in which they enroll is suspect. Clearly, both public and private health plan sponsors, faced with rising health-care costs and competing priorities for funds devoted to financing health care for sponsored groups, are unlikely to put consumer interests paramount in negotiations with commercial health plan sponsors such as insurance companies or MCOs. At least one prominent ardent supporter of the idea of using contract to accomplish reform has decried its lack of progress.[121]

Nevertheless, with increased capitated managed care organized and delivered through prepaid health plans designed by MCOs, the dominant role of a contract in defining health care for American consumers is here to stay. Contract theorists, and especially the advocates of contract as a vehicle for health reform, simply have more work to do to figure out how contracts can assure the protection of consumers when, in fact, most consumers have little control over the content of health plan contracts, let alone choice of health plan. This need is especially pressing given the Supreme Court's decision in *American Manufacturers Mutual Insurance Company v. Sullivan*.[122] This case limits the accountability of health plan sponsors to plan enrollees especially with respect to coverage decisionmaking.

TORT LAW

Tort law outlines the obligations of private individuals, corporations, and government agencies to other private individuals and organizations that neither arise in contract nor are imposed by criminal or regulatory statutes.[123] The major duty in tort that governs important relationships involving the interests of individuals in health care is the duty in negligence law not to expose others to a reasonably foreseeable risk of injury.[124] To recover damages in negligence, three elements must be present: the plaintiff must be damaged; the defendant must be at fault; and the defendant's fault must be the legal cause of the plaintiff's damage. To show fault, the plaintiff must prove that the defendant breached the legal duty not to expose the plaintiff to a reasonably foreseeable risk of injury.[125] For the most part, tort, like contract, is governed by state law, and tort claims are adjudicated in state court. Chapter 8 describes the state court causes of actions in tort that individuals have against both providers and health plan sponsors.

Key Tort Relationships in the Health-Care Sector

Tort, like contract, pervades the relationships in the health-care sector and imposes obligations on patients, providers, health plans, and their sponsors. There are several relationships in the health-care sector that are shaped by important obligations in tort. These include the following:

—relationships between *patients* and *providers,* including (*a*) physicians and (*b*) hospitals and other institutional providers;

—relationships between *consumers* and *health plan sponsors,* including (*a*) health insurers, (*b*) HMOs and MCOs, and (*c*) employers (in the case of self-insured plans); and

—relationships between *beneficiaries of government entitlement programs* and *government agencies* sponsoring the public health insurance programs.

Relationships between Patients and Providers. There are three major expressions of the tort of negligence in the relationship between patients and providers. First is the tort of medical malpractice or professional negligence between patients and their physicians and other health-care professionals. Second is the general tort of negligence between patients and hospitals and other health-care institutions. These two expressions of the tort of negligence involve only patients who have entered into a consensual relationship, which situation generally occurs when, by virtue of wealth or insurance, patients are able to pay for their care. The common law does not require physicians, hospitals, or other providers to care for any patient who requests care.[126] Medical ethics uphold the right of physicians to choose whom they serve, although it imposes additional obligations on physicians in emergencies and when dealing with the poor.[127] Hospitals are not required to treat nonpaying patients unless, by virtue of their corporate structure and tax status, they are required to do so under state and/or federal law.[128]

The third expression of the tort of negligence in the relationship between patients and providers pertains to patients who are unable to pay for care and thus are unable to enter a straightforward contractual relationship with a provider. In these cases, patients must establish a relationship with the provider that then invokes tort duties through a variety of tort theories.[129] Establishing such a relationship is not easy, and, even once the relationship is established, the attaching tort duties impose only limited obligations on providers.

Relationships between Consumers and Health Plan Sponsors. The second most important relationship in tort is that between consumers and all kinds of health plan sponsors. The tort of bad faith breach allows for recovery in disputes between an insured and an MCO, HMO, or other insurer for bad faith coverage denials and other misconduct.[130] This theory provides tort along with contract remedies for the insured when MCOs, HMSs, and other insurers act in bad faith in rejecting a claim. In several states, the cause of action has developed as essentially a contract action with contract damages and associated tort damages for emotional injury and other noncontract injuries arising from the breach of contract.[131]

With the confluence of providing and paying for services, the liability of commercial health plan sponsors has expanded to include the ramifications of clinical decisions made by plan physicians. Further, the clinical decisions of plan physicians are influenced by plan coverage policies and, allegedly, the plan's payment terms with physicians. These realities have inspired many scholars to reconceive the medical liability rules for health plans and their providers.[132] This confluence has become particularly tricky in recent years because ERISA and other federal statutes establishing federally sponsored health plans preempt state tort causes of actions for bad faith breach against health insurers, HMOs, and MCOs that contract with employers or the federal government to fund health plans for employees or other designated beneficiaries.

Relationships between Public Beneficiaries and Government Agencies. Beneficiaries of public health insurance programs, as discussed in chapter 8, have some tort remedies against government agencies that are responsible for public health insurance programs.[133] They also have claims against government officials for so-called constitutional torts, which involve violations of federal constitutional rights that do not otherwise involve conventionally tortious conduct.[134] The recent remarkable decision in *Westside Mothers v. Haveman* (discussed above) would limit such liability and, if widely followed in the future, could have serious implications for Medicaid and SCHIP recipients who would use 42 U.S.C. Section 1983 to address problems with sponsoring state agencies.

Regarding the federal government, beneficiaries have a cause of action against federal officials for intentional torts and other tortious conduct under the Federal Tort Claims Act.[135] However, the Federal Tort Claims Act expressly excludes claims "based upon the exercise or performance or the failure to exercise or perform a discretionary function or duty" on the part of the government.[136] The U.S. Supreme Court has also permitted so-called claims for constitutional torts against federal officers for violations of constitutional rights.

Pertinent Developments in Tort Law and Theory

Since the 1950s, there has been a tremendous explosion in tort liability. One consequence of this explosion in tort law has been calls for the reform of the common law tort system and curtailment of expanding liability. Tort reform has been a serious policy initiative of the business community for the last twenty years, with many proponents arguing that tort law is irrational and inefficient.[137] Thus, most so-called tort reform efforts have focused on controlling the frequency and severity of tort claims by making it more difficult for injured individuals to recover large damage awards from tortfeasors. In some areas of tort, such as product liability, courts have responded to these concerns with some retrenchment from expanding tort liability.[138]

However, other tort reformers are concerned about the degree to which they address the two fundamental objectives of tort law: adequate compensation for injury and deterrence of conduct that causes medical injury.[139] Tort scholars have persistently questioned whether the common law negligence system compensates injured parties adequately and deters unsafe conduct efficiently or fairly.[140] Others have suggested that tort reforms that aim to limit the frequency and severity of claims are contrary to consumer interests and unwarranted.[141]

The expansion in tort liability after 1960 also touched the health-care sector with increased liability for institutional providers, medical malpractice against professional providers, and the tort of bad faith breach against health insurers, HMOs, and MCOs. As with business generally, there has been much pressure, particularly from physicians and other providers, for tort reform in the health-care sector since the 1970s. Following periodic "crises" in the availability and affordability of medical liability insurance beginning in the mid-1970s, a situation that was precipitated by sharp increases in the frequency and severity of malpractice claims, health-care providers and medical liability insurers have pressed for malpractice reform.[142] Most of the early reforms sought to change the behavior of litigants chiefly by making it more difficult for claimants to sue or trying to control the frequency or severity of claims through modifications of legal doctrines or process and the medical liability insurance market.[143]

Since the 1970s, particularly in academic circles, there has been considerable interest in and a plethora of proposals for medical malpractice reform.[144] These proposals explicitly try to improve the malpractice adjudication or compensation system from the perspective of claimants and to address negligent medical practice more directly. Some proposals, such as those for enterprise liability, endeavor to tailor tort liability rules to the realities of managed care.[145]

One aspect of tort reform has been to allow parties to use contract to define rules governing liability that are different than other common law tort rules. An important aspect of tort reform through contract is contracts to use ADR methods to resolve claims outside the judicial system—an appropriate use of ADR provided that parties have adequate bargaining power to influence the terms of the contract.[146] Indeed, the use of ADR is one of the few proposed malpractice reforms to be widely adopted.[147] Many promote ADR as an important cost-saving innovation in lieu of the common law tort system, provided that parties have adequate bargaining power to influence the terms of the contract.[148] The basic idea of ADR is to give parties more authority to contract on the procedural design of dispute resolution procedures as well as their outcome.

ADR theory has also made important contributions to the theory of process elements that result in fair proceedings. Much of the work in ADR theory has focused on ways to simplify and expedite discovery and other aspects of the process as well as how parties can tailor ADR processes through contracts to accommodate special needs and concerns of the parties in the process.[149] Well-designed dispute resolution processes permit parties to negotiate discovery parameters as well as other characteristics of the process.[150] Historically, ADR has been used most successfully in situations in which the bargaining power of the disputants is relatively equal, as is the case in most commercial arbitration or highly structured and strong religious or ethnic communities.[151] However, there are real questions about its use for the adjudication of malpractice and coverage disputes because of the unequal power relationship between individuals and health plans and providers in disputes over health care.

In the 1980s and 1990s, with the movement to managed care, there has been great interest in and concern about tort liability of health plans, particularly those that are regulated under ERISA and subject to the ERISA preemption of state bad faith breach actions in tort. This preemption of the tort of bad faith breach is described and explained in greater detail later.

The issue of preemption of state tort causes of action to enable enrollees in ERISA and other federally sponsored health plans to sue HMOs and other health plans for tortious coverage denials has been an exceptionally explosive issue. Indeed, tort liability of managed care plans has proved to be a most contentious issue in recent years, particularly in the debate over patient protection legislation in recent congresses.

Tort law, however, despite its alleged flaws and the trauma inflicted on those who are sued, is a powerful vehicle to enhance the accountability of health plans and providers to individuals enrolled in health plans or receiving care from providers. Health plans and providers play the dispositive role in the generation of consumer concerns about health care. Tort law is a legal resource that has served American civilization well in terms of greater safety for individuals in most areas of modern life. It should not be lightly discarded if one seeks to assure the availability of true procedural protections of the interests of individuals in their health care.

5 : The Universe of Consumer Concerns about Health Care

This chapter describes the universe of consumer concerns about health care and how these concerns are manifested. Consumer concerns about health care vary greatly in subject matter and degree of importance to the consumer, provider, and plan. Nevertheless, consumer concerns about health care generally pertain primarily to three concepts—quality, cost, and access. These three concepts provide a useful framework for organizing consumer concerns about health care and creating a typology of consumer concerns that facilitates analysis and understanding.

A TYPOLOGY OF CONSUMER CONCERNS

Table 2 presents a typology of the different types of consumer concerns about health care and the current methods for their identification and resolution.[1] Chapter 4 describes the sources of law and theory that govern consumers' health-care concerns, and chapter 8 describes the informal and formal legal processes and institutions currently in place to resolve these concerns.

Concerns about the Quality of Care

A typology of quality concerns should proceed from the work of Avedis Donabedian, a leading scholar on health-care quality who conceptualized the vocabulary used to define health-care quality today.[2] The management of an episode of health care can be divided into a technical domain and an interpersonal domain. The technical domain involves "the application of science and technology of medicine, and of other health sciences, to the management of a personal health problem."[3] The interpersonal domain involves "the management of the social and psychological interaction between client and practitioner."[4]

Thus, the two major elements of quality are, according to Donabedian, *technical competence* and *interpersonal competence*.[5] Technical competence goes to the actual performance of medical procedures and services and relates to the appropriate application of professional knowledge, training,

TABLE 2. Typology of Consumer Concerns about Health Care

Type of Concern	Method of Identification	Informal Process for Resolution	Legal Process for Resolution	Optimal Resolution
Quality concerns: breaches of technical competence				
No injuries	—Complaint —CS survey —Incident report —Lawsuit	—Internal discussion —Ombudsman program —Contractual ADR —Insurance claim adjustment	—Lawsuit with or without court-sponsored ADR or medical malpractice review system	—Explanation —Apology
Negligent injuries	—Complaint —CS survey —Incident report —Lawsuit	—Internal discussion —Ombudsman program —Contractual ADR —Insurance claim adjustment	—Lawsuit with or without court-sponsored ADR or medical malpractice review system	—Explanation —Apology —Insurance settlement —Court judgment
Nonnegligent injuries	—Complaint —CS survey —Incident report —Lawsuit	—Internal discussion —Ombudsman program —Contractual ADR —Insurance claim adjustment	—Lawsuit with or without court-sponsored ADR or medical malpractice review system	—Explanation —Apology —Insurance settlement —Court judgment
Quality concerns: breaches of interpersonal competence				
Communication failures	—Complaint —CS survey —Incident report —Lawsuit	—Internal discussion —Ombudsman program —Grievance procedure	—Lawsuit with or without court-sponsored ADR or medical malpractice review system	—Explanation —Apology —Insurance settlement —Court judgment
Bioethical concerns	—Consumer —CS survey	—Informal discussion	—Lawsuit with or without court-	—Explanation —Apology

TABLE 2. *continued*

Type of Concern	Method of Identification	Informal Process for Resolution	Legal Process for Resolution	Optimal Resolution
	—Incident report —Lawsuit	—Ethics committee —Grievance procedure —Ombudsman program	sponsored ADR or medical malpractice review system —Statutory actions for discrimination or access denials	—Treatment change —Insurance settlement —Court judgment
Quality concerns: breaches of personal preferences				
Denial of amenities and other breaches of personal preferences	—Complaint —CS survey —Incident report —Lawsuit	—Internal discussion —Grievance procedure —Ombudsman program	—Lawsuit with or without court-sponsored ADR or medical malpractice review system	—Explanation —Apology —Insurance settlement —Court judgment
Access concerns				
Coverage denials	—Consumer complaint —CS survey —Lawsuit	—Internal discussion —Grievance procedure in health plans —Ombudsman program	—Administrative review in publicly sponsored plans with judicial review —Lawsuit or court-sponsored ADR for private plans	—Explanations —Apology —Access to treatment —Insurance settlement —Court judgment
Wrongful denials of care	—Consumer complaint —Incident report —Lawsuit	—Internal discussion —Ethics committee —Ombudsman program	—Statutory actions for discrimination or access denials —Lawsuit with or without court-sponsored ADR or medical malpractice review system	—Explanation —Apology —Access to treatment —Insurance settlement —Court judgment

TABLE 2. *continued*

Type of Concern	Method of Identification	Informal Process for Resolution	Legal Process for Resolution	Optimal Resolution
Denials due to discrimination	—Consumer complaint —Lawsuit	—Internal discussion —Ethics committee —Ombudsman program	—Statutory actions for discrimination or access denials —Lawsuit with or without court-sponsored ADR	—Explanation —Apology —Access to treatment —Insurance settlement —Court judgment
Cost concerns				
Bill disputes	—Consumer complaint —Counter-claim to col-lection suit	—Internal discussion —Ombudsman program —Contractual ADR	—Collection suit	—Explanation —Apology —Bill adjustment —Judgment

Note: CS = consumer satisfaction. ADR = alternative dispute resolution.

and skill. As Donabedian explains: "The quality of technical care consists in the application of medical science and technology in a manner that maximizes its benefits to health without correspondingly increasing its risks. The degree of quality is, therefore, the extent to which the care provided is expected to achieve the most favorable balance of risks and benefits."[6] Interpersonal competence addresses the relationship between the physician and the patient and includes other aspects of care. As Donabedian explains: "The management of the interpersonal relationship must meet socially defined values and norms that govern the interaction of individuals in general and in particular situations. These norms are reinforced in part by the ethical dicta of health professions, and by the expectations and aspirations of individual patients."[7]

A separate dimension of quality is personal preferences regarding health care and amenities. This dimension of quality is arguably less substantive than the dimensions of technical competence and interpersonal competence. However, this dimension is important to health-care consumers and a source of many of their concerns about health care.

At the heart of the debate over the definition of quality since the 1970s has been whether and to what degree the societal costs of health care should be considered in defining quality in the care of individual patients. Again, Donabedian provides guidance on the different standards for the definition of quality in different contexts.[8] In an "absolutist" definition of quality, all care that affords some benefit should be provided regardless of cost. Donabedian prefers a patient-centered definition that considers patient concerns and preferences but excludes external factors. One could argue that some malpractice and coverage disputes may reflect the fact that patients view quality from an absolutist standpoint and therefore believe that providers or plans inappropriately applied a societal standard in their particular case.[9] Indeed, several commentators have analyzed how resource constraints accounted for in a "societal" definition of quality are affecting the legal standard of care in tort litigation.[10] Interestingly, empirical studies suggest that prepaid managed care has not demonstrably compromised the quality of health-care services for enrollees.[11]

Breaches of Technical Competence. Breaches of technical competence are determined by ascertaining whether medical injury has occurred and, if so, whether the medical injury is the result of medical malpractice. However, the fact of injury itself does not necessarily mean that a breach of technical competence has occurred since many medical procedures involve some degree of risk of injury to the patient irrespective of the physician's skill and the care that he or she takes. Breaches of technical competence constitute medical malpractice when treatment departs from the legal standard of care of how a practitioner would assess the potential risk of injury to the patient. Medical malpractice is the tort of negligence committed by physicians and other health-care professionals.

Breaches of technical competence, especially if they result in an injury that the patient or family member recognizes, are more likely to surface in existing systems for recognizing consumer concerns. Specifically, reports of patient injuries are generally part of provider risk management programs. Further, when more serious incidents are involved, and especially when injury is involved, the patient or the patient's family may bring a malpractice claim.

Because of the importance of medical malpractice to the medical profession and the sharp increases in the frequency and severity of malpractice claims in the mid-1970s and again in the mid-1980s,[12] there has been considerable empirical research on medical malpractice claims and medical injury in recent years.[13] Much research has focused on who sues for malpractice and why.[14] A 1984 study of the incidence of adverse events and negligence in New York hospitals found that about 4 percent of hospital patients suffer iatrogenic injury, of which injuries half are preventable and 1 percent are due to actionable negligence.[15] Another study estimates that about 1.3 million iatrogenic injuries occur annually, of which 180,000 result in death.[16] A more recent study indicates that number and type of claims vary if the tort regime is no-fault or traditional negligence.[17] In another study of patient complaints about health care, 30 percent of complaints were found to focus on care and treatment.[18]

In its important study *To Err Is Human,* the Institute of Medicine examined these and other studies.[19] Extrapolating death rates from medical error from two prior studies to all hospital admissions in 1997, the Institute of Medicine estimated that from forty-four to ninety-eight thousand Americans die as a result of medical error annually—more than in motor vehicle accidents, from breast cancer, or from AIDS.[20]

Breaches of Interpersonal Competence. There are a wide variety of diverse situations that fall into the category of breaches of interpersonal competence. Indeed, almost any concern that arises in the context of the treatment relationship and does not involve a breach of technical competence constitutes a breach of interpersonal competence. There are two major types of breaches of interpersonal competence: (1) communication failures and (2) bioethical concerns.

Communication failures occur when the provider and the patient have endeavored unsuccessfully to convey information and feelings to one another. Communication failures generate bad feelings between patients and providers. They also generate failures by patients to understand and comply with treatment regimens. In this respect, communication failures can contribute to breaches in quality that lead to medical injury to the same extent as breaches in technical competence do. Indeed, problems with physician-patient communication are an acknowledged factor in medical injury and the generation of malpractice claims.[21]

It would be virtually impossible to estimate the number of communication failures between health-care professionals and consumers that occur each year. However, an important quality improvement effort is tapping consumer satisfaction with care through systematic surveys. A recent study reported that 18 percent of patient complaints about care concerned communication problems with physicians and that 7 percent pertained to the provider's "humaneness."[22] Another study of malpractice suits over prenatal injuries found that nearly a quarter of subjects (24 percent) sued because the physician did not tell the truth about the injury and that another fifth (20 percent) sued because they could not find out what had happened.[23]

These breaches of interpersonal competence are not generally identified in a systematic fashion. They may be made known to providers only at a very decentralized level—through complaints at the time of the infraction and, possibly, through a provider's risk management and quality assurance surveillance activities. In general, however, breaches of interpersonal competence do not surface in courts of law or other legal institutions for resolution unless they precipitate a malpractice claim.

Another important type of breach of interpersonal competence is concerns and disputes that arise in those circumstances, such as end-of-life decisionmaking, that fall within the realm of medical ethics.[24] These disputes generally involve differences between patients and their families and providers about what to do about the initial provision of care or the continuation of care in ethically charged contexts. In general, these disputes over ethics involve communication failures because the parties involved have not reached a mutually satisfactory decision about how to handle the ethically complex situation.[25] It is noteworthy that the Robert Wood Johnson Foundation's major study of end-of-life care found that treating physicians were often uninformed about patient preferences with regard to end-of-life treatment despite having been advised of such preferences.[26]

Concerns about and disputes over differences in the treatment of ethically charged issues, such as the denial of services or aggressive treatment for terminally ill patients or patients for whom treatment is futile, also generate claims against health plans for coverage denials, suits for bad faith breach and medical malpractice, and suits for denials of statutorily mandated emergency services. These causes of action are discussed below. When these disputes arise in the context of hospital care, hospital ethics committees are often consulted about the appropriate course of action to take.

Breaches of Personal Preferences. The third dimension of quality is breaches of personal preferences, including the denial of amenities. "Amenities," according to Donabedian, are "properties of the more intimate aspects of the settings in which care is provided" but can also be "properties of the care itself."[27] This overlap is evident when amenities are described "in the abstract form as comfort, promptness, privacy, courtesy, acceptability, and the like."[28] Breaches of personal preferences is really a residual category and includes characteristics of health-care services that, for whatever reason, are contrary to the taste or desires of the consumer. They can range from truly trivial concerns about styles of health-care delivery to more serious concerns about dimensions of health-care delivery that are contrary to the legitimate expectations of the consumer.

Likewise, breaches of personal preferences are often not expressed or identified in provider or payer quality assurance surveillance efforts or even in low level complaint processes. They might be raised in contract action over an unpaid bill. In extremely egregious cases, they might also surface as a lawsuit for a dignitary tort such as negligent or intentional infliction of emotional distress.[29] Often, violations of personal preferences and denial of amenities motivate consumers to take steps such as switching plans or providers in lieu of making a complaint.

Concerns about Access to Care

Access to care is of crucial concern to consumers. Access issues are manifested in two types of wrongful denials of care: (1) when a payer has improperly denied coverage of a service and (2) when a provider has improperly denied a service to an individual for any reason, including lack of health insurance coverage or inability to pay for services otherwise.

Coverage Denials by Payers. Coverage is an insurance concept that, in the context of health insurance, pertains to the amount, duration, and scope of items or services that are benefits under a health insurance plan. A coverage denial is technically a decision of the insurer or MCO that a particular item or service does not meet the contractual definitions of coverage under the plan contract. In traditional indemnity insurance plans, which pay insureds and/or providers after services have been provided, coverage disputes are easy to distinguish as they arise only in connection with a claim for payment or a request for prior authorization. Also, if a decision about a particular medical treatment requires the plan's prior authorization or otherwise comes to the attention of the plan's utilization review apparatus, coverage denials are explicit.

When care is paid for by prepaid managed care plans, this distinct separation between a payer's coverage decision and a provider's denial of care blurs. Coverage decisions are made in the context of care and are often indistinguishable from clinical judgments about care.[30] They surface only when the physician recommends or the consumer requests a service that the plan then decides not to provide or pay for. Insidious coverage denials may occur when patients are not referred to needed specialty care or are offered only less expensive treatment options when other treatment options are available. Many of the reforms of managed care have sought to make coverage decisionmaking by plans more fair by requiring publication of coverage policy used in utilization review as well as by using grievance-and-appeal procedures to contest denials of health care.

Coverage disputes have always been a major source of contention between health plans and health-care consumers.[31] They constitute a major category of consumer concerns raised in the internal grievance procedures of managed care plans. Often, they are presented to state insurance regulators in the form of complaints against MCOs, HMOs, and insurance companies. They also constitute the basis for most tort claims for bad faith breach against MCOs, HMOs, and insurance companies.

There is little empirical data on the prevalence and nature of coverage denials, especially at the plan level. Some empirical evidence on the coverage decisionmaking practices of MCOs and other decisionmakers suggests that considerable variation exists depending on the type of procedure involved.[32] One U.S. General Accounting Office (GAO) study of selected HMOs found that grievance-and-appeal procedures varied among HMOs and that complaint and appeal data are neither comparable nor accessible.[33] In the HMOs studied, the GAO reported that complaints ranged from 0.5 to 98.2 per 1,000 enrollees while the number of appeals ranged from 0.07 to 69.4 per 1,000 enrollees.[34] The most common complaints and appeals concerned denials of emergency room care and disputes over benefits and referrals.[35] The Health Care Dispute Resolution Center, which handles all Medicare HMO external appeals, reported that, in 1998, the rates of external review remained near or below 2 cases per 1,000 enrollees.[36] State-mandated external review programs have a much lower rate of review.[37] Medicare requires external review for all final determinations made by Medicare HMOs in a grievance-and-appeal process, while state programs operate differently.

A more recent qualitative but thorough study conducted by the American Bar Association's Commission on Legal Problems for the Elderly examined dispute resolution in fifty health plans.[38] This study found that coverage issues predominate the concerns that consumers raise with their health plans. Specifically, types of concerns, in order of frequency, were as follows: emergency room coverage, pharmacy issues, coverage for referrals that were not authorized, out-of-network coverage questions, contractual interpretations of benefit coverage, needed benefits excluded in plan contracts, billing problems (which is not a coverage issue), and coverage for durable medical equipment.[39]

There has also been some empirical work analyzing appellate opinions in bad faith breach claims involving insurer coverage denials.[40] Reconsiderations and, especially, reported appellate opinions provide only a limited picture of consumer concerns about coverage denials given that few coverage denials actually proceed to appealed lawsuits or even reconsiderations.[41]

Care Denials by Providers. Wrongful denials of care by providers occur when a provider denies care for an inappropriate reason unrelated to the consumer's need for medical care. Such denials can arise in three contexts: (1) a consumer is unable to pay for services; (2) a provider illegally fails to provide a service through proscribed discrimination on the basis of race, ethnic origin, religion, sex, or disability; and (3) the provider, who is also the payer, denies coverage of a service. This third category is addressed in the discussions of coverage denials in chapter 7.

The first category of wrongful denials of care occurs when a consumer is unable to pay for a service that a provider is obligated by law to provide. Unless required by law, providers have no obligation to provide care without compensation.[42] However, there is a significant body of statutory and common law that imposes obligations on institutional providers in particular to provide care without proof of payment especially in emergency situations. Providers, unless constrained by internal corporate policies, may still bill for emergency care subseqeuntly.

There is considerable evidence that many Americans are denied the health-care services that they need because they have no insurance and are unable to pay.[43] Occasional media stories highlight egregious access problems.[44] Litigation regarding access to care has been extensive over the years.[45] This litigation suggests that denials of care do occur with some frequency and are an important category of consumer concern about health care. A study of consumer complaints registered with a medical practice group reported that 2 percent of patient concerns about care involved refusals to provide care.[46]

Wrongful denials of care for inability to pay exemplify an important problem with the current methods of identifying and resolving consumer concerns about health care. They are not easily identified unless the denied party presses a claim. Yet it is not easy to press such a claim since there are only a few statutory actions for access denials and most claims must be brought in court under common law tort theories. Unlike members of public and private health plans, the uninsured simply do not have access to most nonjudicial legal institutions for the resolution of their disputes.

Concerns about the Cost of Care

The cost of health-care services is also an important concern for many consumers despite the fact that most consumers have health insurance to defray most of the costs of their health care. Concerns about the cost of health-care services exist, not only among the uninsured and underinsured, but also among the insured. The Center for Medicare and Medicaid Services (formerly the Health Care Financing Administration) reports that 17.1 percent of all health-care expenditures are paid by individuals.[47] Another indication of consumer concern is recent evidence that consumers are declining employer-sponsored insurance because of cost, particularly when the cost of the associated coinsurance is high.[48] Notably, the generally low level of cost sharing in prepaid managed care plans rose sharply in 1996, compared to other types of health plans.[49] Occasionally, media stories highlight consumers' problems with the cost of care.[50]

Consumers have raised concerns about costs generally in disputes over noncovered medical bills. There is little empirical evidence about the extent of consumer concerns about health-care costs. Research suggests that bills are a particularly serious problem for those with serious illnesses.[51] Indeed, some research suggests that 38 percent of the chronically ill cannot afford needed care.[52] Another study reports that three of four Americans who have trouble paying medical bills do have health insurance.[53] Further, a study of consumer complaints with a large medical practice group found that complaints about billing and payment constituted 35 percent of all consumer complaints—the single largest group of consumer complaints.[54]

Disputes over medical bills do end up in litigation. Some evidence suggests that disputes over health-care bills make up a substantial portion of the docket of small claims courts.[55] For example, findings from a study of small claims courts in Ohio showed those seeking payment for medical services to be the second largest category of plaintiffs in that forum.[56]

Unfortunately, the research on small claims courts is dated and limited. The Ohio finding has not been replicated in other studies that did not look specifically at claims for medical bills.[57]

Claimants' concerns over the cost of care arise in two contexts primarily. First is cost-sharing arrangements and their application. Second is when health plan payment levels are insufficient to pay the provider bills for services. This latter situation is a grave one for people with serious illness, who generate the greatest proportion of health-care costs.[58] For many seriously ill people, tangling with health insurers over payment for services is a difficult problem.[59]

TAPPING AND RESOLVING CONSUMER CONCERNS ABOUT HEALTH CARE

The process of tapping and resolving a consumer's concern about some aspect of his or her health care is not straightforward. In analyzing consumer concerns about health care, it must be appreciated that not all concerns are voiced or presented as complaints or grievances to responsible parties. Even fewer are presented to legal institutions for adjudication. Many factors go into consumers' decision to lodge a complaint about their health care or, more especially, to initiate legal action.

In "The Emergence and Transformation of Disputes,"[60] William Felstiner and his colleagues review the law and society literature on the generation of disputes that are presented for resolution in legal institutions.[61] These authors posit three transformations. The first occurs when individuals perceive that they have been harmed. The second occurs when individuals recognize that a perceived injurious experience forms the basis of a grievance and attribute blame for the injury to a specific party. The third occurs when the individual with a grievance presents that grievance to the responsible party and seeks a remedy. The authors describe how this transformation process of "naming, blaming, and claiming" is influenced by many factors, including the socioeconomic and psychological characteristics of the affected individual: "Transformations reflect social structural variables, as well as personality traits. People do—or do not—perceive an experience as an injury, blame someone else, claim redress, or get their claims accepted because of their *social position* as well as their individual characteristics."[62]

The insight that multiple socioeconomic and psychological factors determine whether consumers will present claims to legal institutions for resolution is crucial. Particularly disturbing is the fact that people of lower socioeconomic status are far less likely to press claims—a finding confirmed by other empirical research.[63] It is this group that is expressly disadvantaged in the health-care sector and its systems for identifying and resolving consumer concerns.

Also, not all consumer concerns reach the stage at which a complaint, grievance, or appeal is filed. Often, a consumer determines not to press a concern about his or her health care in any process for which some kind of acknowledgment by the responsible party or relief is available. Such concerns may be picked up through other provider- or plan-initiated measures such as the consumer satisfaction surveys described below. Or a consumer may simply not recognize that he or she had an experience about which concern is warranted. Such occurrences are identified, not by soliciting information from consumers, but by means of other quality assurance efforts of responsible parties.

Further, how to resolve an identified concern is also not straightforward. Solutions are neither easy nor uniform. They involve asking essentially two questions: (1) what is the nature of the action or decision needed to resolve the concern; and (2) what are the types of issues and underlying facts that must be decided to accomplish the action or decision? This first question is critical given the range of matters that can give rise to consumer concerns about health care. Not all concerns are matters that health-care providers, health plans, public policy makers, or other responsible parties can do much about. For example, concerns about the withdrawal of medical treatment at the end of life often raise ethical or religious issues that are not appropriately brought before or adjudicated by legal institutions. Other issues, such as violations of personal preferences, have to do with cultural norms for which there is no legal recourse except in egregious cases. Some of these issues are simply not justiciable because they raise moral, philosophical, or cultural concerns for which legal relief is not available.

In designing systems to identify and resolve consumer concerns about health care, it is critical to account for the differences among types of consumer concerns and also to appreciate both that the ability of the legal system to resolve consumer concerns about health care is greatly limited and that not all concerns are amenable to legal resolution. Those that are amenable to legal resolution are usually governed by a variety of health-care policies pertaining to quality, access (generally coverage), and cost that are established in a variety of policymaking processes.

For example, breaches of technical competence, as well as wrongful denials of care by providers, are often determined by reference to some standard of medical practice developed within the medical profession. These standards of care can be the professional norms for clinical practice taught in medical education and training. In medical malpractice suits, in which breaches of technical competence and wrongful denials of care are often raised (as discussed below), they are articulated and accorded status as the legal standard of care in tort when presented in expert testimony. They may even apply in breaches of interpersonal competence, although, with the exception of bioethical disputes, these concerns generally implicate moral, philosophical, religious, or cultural norms and values.

Policies also play a major, if not dispositive, role in the adjudication of coverage concerns. Ostensibly, coverage decisions in individual cases are based on policies of a health plan or health plan sponsor. The universe of various types of coverage policies for public and private health plans is described in greater detail in chapter 6. These policies, along with the medical standards of care that also govern medical practice and physicians' decisions, are at the basis of many consumer concerns about coverage.

Two categories of policies are most often implicated. The first is medical standards of care developed by the medical profession and their organizations, private accrediting bodies, and government agencies. The second is the wide array of coverage policies that all health plans use to define available health-care benefits and implement coverage decisions. Consequently, real consumer protection in many situations lies, not in the processes for adjudicating disputes, but in the processes for making the policies that govern adjudicative proceedings.

Given the critical role of policies in the generation and ultimate resolution of individuals' concerns about their health care, the fact that other avenues than legal action exist for individuals to express and resolve concerns about their health care is important.[64] Individuals can raise concerns in "political" contexts in which they endeavor to reform or otherwise influence the conditions that give rise to those concerns. Many observers have called for ways to empower consumers vis-à-vis health plans and even give consumers greater political power in the design and management of managed care plans.[65] It is unclear whether these reform strategies are sufficient to give individuals effective procedural opportunities to influence the myriad policies that affect their health care.

A major theme of this book is the importance of processes and procedural protections that permit consumers to influence policies that affect the quality and cost of as well as access to health care. At present, such processes do not really exist, especially with respect to policies made by private organizations—arguably the most important policies affecting the health care of individuals. The lack of such processes is a serious deficiency in the arsenal of procedural protections for American consumers of health care. Suggestions for procedural reforms are presented in chapters 9 and 10.

INSTITUTIONAL MECHANISM FOR TAPPING CONSUMER CONCERNS

Providers and plans do get notice of individuals' concerns about health care through a variety of means and also have different programs for the immediate resolution of concerns. Specifically, quality assurance programs mandated by state and federal law as well as private accreditation tap consumer concerns about all aspects of health care. Provider and plan risk management programs endeavor to identify and resolve individuals' concerns that might involve medical liability on the part of the provider or plan. Provider ethics committees offer consultation and advice on patients' concerns about bioethical issues. Finally, as discussed in chapter 8, most providers and plans have consumer relations programs, including ombudsmen, to clear up identified consumer concerns immediately and informally.

Quality Assurance and Improvement Programs

Institutional health-care providers are required by state licensure laws to have processes in place to assess and improve the quality of their services. Specifically, health-care institutions have quality assurance programs as a condition of state licensure,[66] private accreditation,[67] or conditions of participation in the Medicare program.[68] As explained in chapter 4, private accreditation generally serves as compliance with Medicare conditions of participation for most health-care facilities, except nursing homes.[69] Increasingly, the regulation of health-care professionals has been directed at quality performance.[70] The Medicare program also requires quality review of care provided to program beneficiaries by independent peer review organizations.[71]

HMOs are also required to engage in quality assurance activities under state and federal law. State HMO licensure statutes require HMOs to have quality improvement programs comparable to those of other institutional providers.[72] For federally qualified HMOs, the Health Maintenance Organization Act of 1973 requires quality assurance programs as well.[73] These mandates do not detail the content of the programs very specifically. The major private accrediting body for HMOs, the National Committee for Quality Assurance (NCQA), also requires HMOs to engage in extensive quality assurance and improvement activities.[74]

In the 1980s and 1990s, as described in chapter 6, health-care quality scientists made great advances in the theory and measurement of quality, with intensified focus on performance measured in outcomes, including consumer satisfaction.[75] By the end of the 1980s, a consensus emerged that consumer satisfaction is an important outcome of care and an important measure of health-care quality. Although certainly not a new concept,[76] consumer satisfaction was viewed as an important measure of quality and as crucial information for purchasers when selecting among competing health plans.[77] Providers, health plans, accrediting bodies, and regulators now have incorporated consumer satisfaction as an integral part of quality measurement and improvement.[78] Now, with the NCQA's Health Plan Employer Data and Information Set (HEDIS),[79] a standardized set of measures to compare the performance of both private and public managed care plans that taps consumer satisfaction, it is possible to obtain standardized data on consumer satisfaction with health care that is comparable across health plans. The collection of consumer satisfaction data holds great potential for improving methodologies for identifying, preventing, and even resolving consumer concerns about health care.[80]

Risk Management Programs

Further, most institutional providers, including some HMOs, have established claims management programs that seek to identify and resolve potential malpractice claims arising from adverse events in treatment, for example, breaches of technical competence.[81] These adverse events are generally recorded in incident reports or reports of various provider and plan committees with official quality assurance and risk management responsibilities. The information about these events is used to manage potential future litigation as well as to improve quality prospectively.

Apparently, the information gleaned in risk management programs is rarely used to inform a patient that he or she has been injured and may have an actionable complaint against the provider or plan. However, where a breach of technical competence is particularly egregious or a very serious injury has occurred irrespective of the breach, a provider or plan may inform a malpractice insurance carrier. The malpractice insurance carrier and/or the provider may actually contact a consumer and attempt to compensate for associated damages in order to avoid the filing of a malpractice claim.[82] Some institutional providers even have informal grievance procedures as part of their risk management programs.[83] Many complaints and disputes are resolved informally before proceeding to established dispute resolution procedures. Indeed, the early identification and resolution of disputes is a cardinal principle of good risk management.[84]

Many liability insurers seek out early settlement to save costs associated with the claim.[85] It should be noted that such efforts are not without risk of harm to the consumer, who may be settling a serious medical injury without adequate legal advice or judicial supervision, as would be provided in conventional malpractice suits that proceed to court. Settlement of disputes even under judicial supervision in a lawsuit can result in oppressive settlements that are damaging to consumers.[86] Consumers should never be called on to settle cases unless they are accorded a full understanding of the relevant medical facts and an opportunity to retain counsel or obtain other expert advice.

Several scholars have examined how to integrate risk management and quality assurance to facilitate the prevention and early resolution of medical malpractice claims and other consumer concerns.[87] Hickson and his colleagues have proposed a patient complaint analysis system for physician multispecialty groups to generate data that then is used through peer review to improve physician behavior toward patients.[88] Dauer and Marcus have proposed a system for the use of mediation in a risk management program to resolve medical malpractice claims immediately on their discovery.[89] The theory behind this approach is that most malpractice claimants are motivated primarily by a "search for understanding, communication, and correction" rather than compensation and thus that their claims are amenable to early resolution through immediate mediation.[90] In another empirical study comparing the formal and informal resolution of medical malpractice disputes in one hospital, Farber and White found that cases initiated by incident reports in risk management programs were more likely to be dropped than were cases initiated by consumer complaints or a lawsuit.[91]

Provider Ethics Committees

Hospitals and HMOs also have ethics committees to adjudicate disputes over bioethical issues with consumers. These committees serve in an advisory capacity only and have no authority to decide a disputed issue.[92] There has been considerable criticism of the role of these committees in assisting in the resolution of consumer concerns about care.[93] A review of the empirical literature about ethics committees found that ethics committees were often dominated by providers and did not always promote the interests of patients and families, especially when those interests conflicted with institutional interests.[94] Some have suggested mediation and other alternative dispute resolution approaches to adjudicate disputed ethical issues associated with the care of specific patients.[95]

6 : The Universe of Medical Standards and Other Policies

Regarding Health Care

Today, medical standards of all types define the content and quality of health-care services in a variety of contexts.[1] Despite an ongoing debate about the degree to which standards of care actually affect practice,[2] medical standards of care inform the treatment decisions of health-care professionals and the processes of care of institutional providers. They inform contract terms in public and private health plan contracts. They inform the content of coverage policy for health plans. Purchasers use published quality measures to compare health plans and providers. Finally, medical standards of care form the basis for the legal standard of care used to adjudicate disputes over health care between consumers and health-care providers or plans.

This chapter first traces the history of medical standard setting in the United States, including the importation of modern industrial quality science in the health-care sector in the 1980s. It then describes and classifies the many kinds of health-care policies that are available. This chapter also describes the role that these policies play in the generation and disposition of the concerns of individual patients and consumers about health care. How these private medical organizations develop and publish medical practice guidelines and other standards of care affecting an ever increasing range of medical practice is described in chapter 7.

THE HEALTH-CARE QUALITY REVOLUTION AND MEDICAL STANDARDSETTING

As American medicine advanced scientifically, so did the interest within the medical profession in the quality of medical services. In the early 1950s, the American College of Surgeons joined with the American College of Physicians, the American Medical Association (AMA), and the American Hospital Association to establish the Joint Commission on the Accreditation of Hospitals (now called the Joint Commission on the Accreditation of Healthcare Organizations (JCAHO)).[3] In part, this effort resulted from mandates that hospitals be licensed to participate in public and private health insurance programs as well as the Hill-Burton health-care facility construction program.[4] Providers sought private accreditation to retain control over the definition and regulation of quality in hospitals and, later, other health-care organizations.

Health maintenance organization (HMO) accreditation came later, in part due to the role of the Health Maintenance Act of 1973.[5] This statute established federal standards that HMOs must meet if they are to qualify for federal financial assistance and other benefits under the act. The National Committee for Quality Assurance (NCQA) developed an accreditation program for HMOs and managed care plans in the 1980s.[6] The NCQA program is now the dominant HMO accreditation program in the country.

In the 1950s and 1960s, the National Institutes of Health (NIH) poured millions of dollars into biomedical research conducted chiefly by specialists in academic medical centers.[7] These medical specialists in academic medical centers—who dominated medical specialty societies and some voluntary health organizations—were interested in improving the quality of clinical practice and its scientific base. As described below, they directed the attention of medical specialty societies and voluntary health organizations to developing standards of care to improve the clinical practice of medicine. It is not coincidental that, during this period, the standard of care in medical malpractice cases moved from a local standard of general practitioners to a national standard of medical specialists.[8]

In 1967, Avedis Donabedian, an academic specialist, published his classic "Evaluating the Quality of Medical Care,"[9] which, with later works, delineated the prevailing definition of health-care quality and the taxonomy of quality criteria, that is, *structure, process,* and *outcome* of care.[10] *Structure* criteria pertain to organizational characteristics of institutions insofar as those characteristics affect the delivery of quality care. *Process* criteria address the actual delivery of care, for example, whether it is appropriate and how well it is performed. *Outcome* criteria pertain to whether the care results in a positive outcome, such as the improvement of the patient's medical condition, or other clinical endpoints, such as death, that result from care. Another important outcome measure is patient satisfaction, which addresses patients' perception of care and their quality of life following care.[11] This taxonomy now organizes the discussion of quality indicators and measures.

Health Services Research and the Development
of Standards of Care

Beginning in the early 1970s, the federal government began funding the relatively new field of health services research to develop strategies to understand better the problems with health-care delivery and financing in the United States.[12] The newly established National Center for Health Services Research and National Center for Technology Assessment within the Department of Health and Human Services spearheaded a federal effort to attain a better understanding of the issues of the cost and quality of and access to health-care services. Much of this research focused on the content and quality of ever more expensive health-care services. The field of health services research soon became an important influence in the making of both public and private policy in the American health-care sector.

The findings of this new field of health services research were remarkable and had an important impact on policy.[13] In particular, research identifying wide geographic variations in medical practices[14] was exceptionally influential as it fundamentally questioned the objectivity of physicians' decisions about the content of health-care services. Other health services research focused on the outcomes of specific procedures and suggested that many medical procedures did not, in fact, have the anticipated effect on patients.[15] As a result of this research, the leaders of the medical profession, along with leading health services researchers, called for greater attention to "outcomes" of medical care. They called for more research to demonstrate scientifically the outcomes that could be obtained from specific and often costly medical procedures.[16] Reporting of the outcome of care to potential purchasers of health plan services has become a definitive feature of the movement to make the delivery of health care more competitive that evolved in the 1980s and 1990s.[17]

Starting in the 1960s, and picking up steam in the 1970s and 1980s, the medical profession, in its professional associations, specialty societies, and voluntary health organizations, became more involved in developing standards of care, including medical practice guidelines, through processes designed to elicit a wide range of expert opinion and forge consensus.[18] The medical specialties recognized that the quality of health care could be elevated with systematic development of standards of care. As discussed in chapter 7, scientific training and research experience informed the medical specialties' approach to standardsetting activities and also the processes utilized in developing standards. In 1987, the American Council of Medical Specialty Societies, while appreciating the potential risk of liability inherent in medical standards, announced that the American medical profession and American specialty societies should set standards to define quality medical care.[19]

Of note, the pursuit of quality among medical specialties and the leadership of the medical profession continues. In March 2001, the Institute of Medicine published a major report, *Crossing the Quality Chasm,*[20] decrying the quality of medical care in the American health-care system and calling for major reforms.

Increased Payer Interest in Quality and Medical Standard Setting

When health insurance became widespread in the second half of the twentieth century, the health insurers and their sponsors left the determination of the content and quality of health-care services primarily up to the medical profession. Specifically, health insurers did not define the benefits in their plans specifically, nor did they supervise the selection of services in individual cases.[21] Further, health insurers did not attempt to define the quality of specific medical services. Rather, they required only that providers be licensed under state law or accredited.[22] Quality of care was primarily a concern of the medical profession and other providers, which focused specifically on quality of medical practice with no reference to costs of care or concerns of third party payers.

This quest for better cost-containment strategies—beginning in the 1970s—changed this paradigm fundamentally. With escalating costs, both public and private payers turned to coverage policy as a means of both controlling costs and setting prices for care. This turn of events inevitably led both public and private third party payers to become increasingly interested in the definition of quality and an enhanced role for third party payers in determining that definition. Further, health plan sponsors and healthcare providers, along with or at the direction of accrediting bodies, sought to implement standards of quality by establishing concrete performance measures and other strategies. Inevitably, because of cost pressures, health plans and their sponsors became increasingly interested in the use of coverage policy to contain costs and also to assure quality of care.

At the same time, third party payers became increasingly interested in developing medical review criteria to assess the utilization and medical necessity of health-care services. They perceived that medical practice guidelines and other standards that promoted good outcomes of care were a useful mechanism for identifying and defining more specifically inappropriate medical care currently provided on a widespread basis and that great savings could be realized if such guidelines were followed. For example, in the late 1970s, the Blue Cross and Blue Shield Association became actively involved with the American College of Physicians and other medical specialty societies in assessing the medical necessity of routine tests and procedures.[23] Public and private health insurers used these quality standards as the basis of utilization review criteria and sometimes even incorporated them in a computerized claims review process. The Medicare program and its contractors developed and used medical review criteria for utilization review and, in some cases, incorporated medical practice guidelines and other standards of care explicitly into its coverage determinations.[24]

The Health Care Financing Administration (HCFA)—now the Centers for Medicare and Medicaid Services (CMS)—became very interested in the use of standards of care, including medical practice guidelines, as a means to make better Medicare coverage policy and thereby achieve better value for Medicare expenditures.[25] The Physician Payment Review Commission, a congressional agency charged with advising Congress on physician payment methodologies, articulated the potential of guidelines in formulating physician payment policy for the Medicare program, stating: "Practice guidelines may be unique among available methods to contain costs in that they can increase the quality and efficiency of care in the process of slowing increases in expenditures."[26] In 1988, the HCFA, with the Public Health Service, sponsored an initiative to evaluate and improve the effectiveness of health care in the United States.[27] This initiative spent millions of dollars on clinical research comparing different treatments to determine their effectiveness in terms of cost savings and patient outcomes. This research provided the empirical evidence for future medical standards of care.

In 1989, building on these developments, Congress established the Agency for Health Care Policy and Research (AHCPR) to enhance the quality, appropriateness, and effectiveness of health-care services through research and the promotion of improvements in clinical practice.[28] Within the AHCPR, Congress established the Forum for Quality and Effectiveness in Health Care to foster the development of clinically relevant practice guidelines and standards of quality, performance measures, and medical review criteria. The forum sought to facilitate guideline development through the convocation of expert panels and the formal recognition of guidelines developed by other appropriate groups.[29]

The standard setting activities of the AHCPR became controversial because they inevitably took on strong medical specialty groups with economic interests in certain procedures and the guidelines that affected them.[30] In the 1990s, AHCPR guideline setting activities generated considerable and powerful political opposition from affected medical specialists.[31] The Republican Congress responded with support for the concerns of some medical specialty groups and gave sharp attention to the standard setting and other activities of the AHCPR. While the AHCPR continues to promote and facilitate the development of medical practice guidelines, its efforts are now focused on fostering the development of medical quality standards.[32] In December 1999, Congress changed the name and mission of the AHCPR.[33] The new agency, called the Agency for Healthcare Quality and Research (AHQR), now coordinates all federal quality improvement efforts and health-care services research and no longer supports the development of clinical practice guidelines.

Industrial Quality Science and the Revolution in Quality Management

Early in the 1980s, medical care quality assurance theory focused on the reduction of errors in the technical aspects of care in individual cases as well as the identification of ideal processes and the comparison of actual practice with the ideal.[34] Most quality assurance activities within the health-care sector focused primarily on determining whether health-care institutions met required structural and process criteria.[35] However, advances in health services research on medical outcomes had a dramatic impact on quality assessment in the health-care sector in the late 1980s and early 1990s. There was greater emphasis on outcomes of care as the paramount quality indicator that health services researchers promoted. Also quality assessment borrowed extensively from modern industrial quality science, which emphasized outcomes measures among other features.

Beginning in the 1980s, the principles *total quality management* and *continuous quality improvement* (TQM/CQI), developed by W. Edward Deming, Joseph Juran, and Walter Shewhart,[36] caught the attention of leading researchers in health-care quality.[37] The theory of TQM/CQI focuses on the reduction of variation in the production process and continuous improvements in outcomes, including customer satisfaction, rather than on identification and elimination of defects.[38] Health services researchers, armed with better scientific information about outcomes and effectiveness of care, explored the application of TQM/CQI theory to the health-care services.[39] Many provider organizations then adopted TQM/CQI approaches in their quality assurance programs.[40] The JCAHO and other private accrediting bodies moved from traditional assessment methods in their quality regulation procedures and embraced TQM/CQI as an important methodology for quality assurance and improvement in health-care institutions.[41]

These developments also coincided with the movement to infuse the delivery of health care with more competition, which called for publishing information on the quality of services of competing health plans. Proponents of managed competition, including President Clinton's health reform proposal,[42] placed great emphasis on requiring health-care plans to provide consumers with reports of their performance on selected quality measures.[43] For example, the federal government sought to improve quality measurement in the Medicare program in ways that promoted use of outcome measurements.[44] HMOs and other managed care organizations (MCOs) also pursued more sophisticated quality assessment and improvement methods.[45] In the 1990s, the JCAHO began accrediting HMOs and MCOs as well as health-care networks. In the early 1990s, the newly founded NCQA became the premier accrediting body for prepaid health plans, HMOs, and MCOs and developed the prevailing system of quality performance measures for health plans.[46] Indeed, in developing performance measures for managed care plans, private efforts soon surpassed government efforts to develop universal measures for the comparison of health plans.[47] These developments greatly accelerated the move to the private regulation of health care and, in particular, private policymaking for quality standards and measures.[48]

The Computerization of Medical Standards

In recent years, there has been great progress in the computerization of medical standards in a variety of contexts. The most widespread use of computerized medical standards has been by payers and third party administrators who have used computerized medical review criteria to review claims data on the utilization of services by covered beneficiaries for payment purposes. These computerized medical review criteria—often referred to as *screens*—have become an important tool in the management of care for purposes of achieving cost savings and greater efficiency in the delivery of care.[49] Such use of computerized screens by the Medicare program, managed care organizations, and other private payers has also generated concerns from consumers as they often define noncovered services more restrictively than published coverage policy does.[50] As discussed in chapter 2, many congressional patient protection bills addressed this problem in calling for publication of all types of medical review criteria that health plans use for utilization review and care management strategies that influence coverage of services for patients.

A most exciting advance is the incorporation of medical standards of care into computerized medical records—an advance that holds great promise for better clinical care and more accurate quality measurement and reporting. Efforts to computerize medical records are widespread and have been implemented with varying degrees of success.[51] This effort is exemplified by the groundbreaking work of the Regenstrief Medical Records System, developed and implemented at the Indiana University School of Medicine and the Regenstrief Institute for Health Care.[52] The Veterans Administration (VA) health system also has a well-developed computerized medical records system.[53]

There are two purposes for incorporating medical standards of care into the computerized medical record. First is to facilitate the collection of data on quality measures for quality assessment and improvement activities and mandated reports on quality reporting. In this regard, data for purposes of quality performance, such as that collected under the HEDIS system (see below), can be aggregated from all patient records and incorporated into required reports without independent data entry. Many managed care plans and integrated delivery networks are moving toward computerized medical records systems with these capabilities.[54]

The second, and arguably more important, capability of computerized medical records is the incorporation of medical standards directly into the computerized medical records system to facilitate adherence to these standards in clinical settings. For example, the VA health system, by virtue of the bar coding of administered drugs and medical standards embedded within the VA system, is able, on the basis of lab reports and other patient data, to advise caregivers at the point of clinical decisionmaking whether drugs are indicated.[55] Many computerized medical records systems incorporate algorithms that remind physicians and caregivers that certain steps in the treatment process might be indicated or contraindicated—reminders based on embedded medical records.[56] These computer reminders at the point of clinical decisionmaking in the delivery of care are designed to bring the content of medical standards of care immediately to bear on the medical treatment of individual patients.

There are also computer programs with embedded medical practice guidelines and other standards of care that guide physicians in the treatment of a particular condition.[57] These programs permit physicians to manage the care of patients more effectively and facilitate the collection of data for quality monitoring and reporting efforts. For example, research has demonstrated that use of such a comprehensive computer program in the treatment of diabetes patients in managed care plans can have a significant impact on the quality of care as measured by recognized quality performance measures and can also improve patient satisfaction with care.[58] The potential for the use of standards of care in this manner is great and promises to transform the delivery of care in the future and the role of medical standards of care in health-care delivery.

ORGANIZATIONS THAT MAKE HEALTH-CARE POLICIES

Health-care policies are made by a variety of organizations in the health-care sector. Private medical organizations and accrediting bodies make most medical standards of care that define the content and quality of care. Individual providers also make policy regarding the quality and cost of the care that they provide as well as when they will provide care for the poor on an uncompensated basis. It should be emphasized that state corporation law (as well as the federal, state, and local tax laws that govern these organizations) does not dictate the specific content of corporate policy and would not control the content of either health-care policy or the processes by which that policy is made.

Public and private sponsors of health plans also make policy regarding the content and quality of their services. However, in doing so, they rely heavily on the standards of care developed by private medical organizations and accrediting bodies. Health plan sponsors also set policies as to the cost of the care provided through health plans. MCOs, pursuant to contract with health plan sponsors, also make policies affecting the coverage, quality, and pricing of health plan benefits.

Private Medical Organizations

Two major types of private organizations make medical standards of care: medical professional associations and voluntary health organizations. The organizations make all kinds of medical standards of care through established procedures described in chapter 7.

Medical Professional Organizations. Medical professional associations include organizations such as the AMA that represent predominantly primary care physicians. Medical specialty societies represent physicians who have advanced specialty training and credentials in a particular area of medicine. According to the AMA, there are at least 315 private medical organizations in the United States.[59]

Medical professional associations have long been engaged in medical standard setting. Most of these organizations make a variety of standards of care defining the content and quality of medical care, especially medical quality standards and medical practice guidelines. For example, in 1989, the AMA established the Practice Parameters Partnership and the Practice Parameters Forum, in which over sixty-five medical specialty societies and other physician organizations are actively involved in developing and evaluating medical standards of care.[60] Similarly, medical specialty societies develop medical practice guidelines and medical quality standards in their field of specialization.[61] Today, building on this history, the medical standard setting of medical professional associations is extensive.

Medical professional associations and medical specialty societies have varied corporate structures and policymaking processes. Most professional associations and medical specialty societies are not-for-profit organizations and therefore enjoy special taxation rules under state and federal law. Most organizations have some type of formal policymaking processes for medical standards of care of various types. Some organizations, particularly medical professional associations, have constituent assemblies that may also become involved in the process of determining medical standards of care. Almost all medical professional organizations and medical specialty societies use a process in which committees composed of experts make medical standards of care (see below).

Voluntary Health Organizations. Voluntary health organizations are devoted to the improvement of the health of individuals afflicted with a particular disease. They differ from medical professional associations in that they are composed primarily of non–medical professionals. Voluntary health organizations, while generally not-for-profit, tax exempt organizations, vary widely in their organizational structure. Some have a very democratic structure with constituent assemblies and more open policymaking processes, while others have a more traditional structure that does not include formal procedural institutions such as constituent assemblies to garner the input of members on policy matters.

The membership of voluntary health organizations is constituted mainly of persons with the subject illness and their families as well as physicians, including medical specialists, and other professionals working with the subject disease. Some voluntary health organizations also have a strong professional component in which physicians and other health professionals who specialize in the care of patients or who conduct research on the care and cure of the disease are also actively involved. Through their professional sections, such voluntary health organizations engage in developing medical standards of care. The American Diabetes Association is an excellent example of a voluntary health organization that includes professional sections engaged in standard setting activities.

Voluntary health organizations with strong physician and health practitioner memberships also engage in setting medical standards of care for their disease of interest. Because they have patient members, they have enhanced opportunities for patient involvement in the policymaking process, although voluntary health organizations vary in the degree to which they capitalize on this opportunity. Some voluntary health organizations have constituent assemblies, although, given that these assemblies are composed predominantly of non–medical professionals, they do not generally get involved in medical standard setting. However, like medical professional associations and medical specialty societies, voluntary health organizations with an organized professional membership generally utilize a professional committee process of the type described in chapter 7.

Private Accrediting Bodies

Private accrediting bodies accredit health-care institutions and, more recently, health plans of MCOs and HMOs. As part of their accrediting function, they engage in establishing medical quality standards and performance measures. The major private accrediting organizations in the health-care sector are the JCAHO and the NCQA. Both accredit most health plans in the United States. However, there are numerous other bodies that accredit other types of health-care institutions, such as hospitals and nursing homes. Private accrediting bodies establish standards for determining whether the entity in question meets the qualifications for accreditation. Often they base their medical quality standards on medical quality standards established by medical organizations or adopt medical quality standards and quality performance measures that providers and/or health-care plans must adopt and implement as a condition of accreditation.

Private accrediting bodies are generally not-for-profit corporations with boards, designed as commissions or committees in some cases, that make most accrediting decisions and supervise and approve the formulation of the organization's medical quality standards and performance measures. Often, the governing boards of private accrediting bodies have representatives from the providers or health-care plans that they accredit as well as members that represent the public. Private accrediting bodies also utilize a professional committee process for making medical quality standards and performance measures with varying degrees of board participation.

Finally, it should be emphasized that health-care plans and their sponsors are also actively involved in the determination of performance measures by which the quality of the plan's health care will be assessed. For example, the NCQA developed the Health Plan Employer Data and Information Set (HEDIS), a standardized set of measures against which the performance of managed care plans can be compared, which is widely used by both private and public health plan sponsors.[62] If the plan is accredited, the plan's performance measures will be those of a private accrediting body or governed by criteria of a private accrediting body. Generally, plan performance measures—even those from HEDIS—are based on standards of quality promulgated by private medical organizations and/or private accrediting bodies.

Providers as Health-Care Policymakers

Professional and institutional providers are important players in making health-care policy. Physicians make cost and quality policy, usually implicitly, in the course of running their practices. They also participate in the policymaking activities of medical professional associations, voluntary health organizations, and private accrediting bodies. Institutional providers, especially not-for-profit hospitals, are especially important policymakers, particularly with respect to the uninsured.

There are a variety of not-for-profit institutional providers that serve the poor as a matter of corporate mission. Such providers include some public hospitals, generally municipal corporations, that are required by law to serve the uninsured poor and are supported in this endeavor by local property tax subsidies. Some private, not-for-profit hospitals, often founded and operated by religious and/or educational organizations, also have the mission to serve the uninsured poor. These private organizations may have corporate charters that specify their obligations in this regard. Additionally, there are publicly funded community health centers and other not-for-profit clinics that serve the uninsured poor. These hospital and outpatient organizations—often referred to as *safety net providers*—are programmatically committed to serving this population and design their services to implement this mission.

All hospitals and other institutional providers, especially not-for-profit hospitals, are governed by a variety of state and federal statutes that specify their obligations to the poor. These complex sources of legal obligation are found in the following areas of law: (1) state corporate and charitable trust law; (2) federal, state, and local tax law; (3) federal and state statutes requiring hospitals to serve the poor and uninsured in emergency and other situations; and (4) state tort law, which imposes obligations on these institutions to provide care for the poor on the basis of a variety of tort theories. The legal obligations and the legal remedies thus created to enable the uninsured poor to achieve access to care in these institutions are explained in greater detail later.

The affected health-care providers are required by law to develop internal policies on how they will implement these obligations. However, these policies are generally made in internal institutional processes as there are no legal mandates for public input in their formation or, for the most part, for their publication. In reality, the protection of the uninsured poor derives from legal mandates and not from internal policies that institutions might establish to implement these mandates. Consequently, this book does not address the content of these policies or the processes for making them. Rather, the legal obligations are discussed in chapter 3, which describes primarily judicial remedies for their enforcement.

Health Plan Sponsors as Policymakers

Public and private health plan sponsors are major policymakers with respect to health care. Health plan sponsors, such as government agencies and employers, determine the benefits and other features of health plans that are offered to specified groups of beneficiaries. There are three major categories of health plan sponsors in the United States: (1) government agencies; (2) employers; and (3) insurance companies and MCOs that offer health plans for sale either to government or employer health plan sponsors or directly to individuals. The most important policies that health plan sponsors make are coverage policies, which effectively define access to health-care services for plan beneficiaries. Health plan sponsors use medical practice guidelines and other standards of care in the delineation of coverage policy and, in particular, the common coverage policy that care be a medical necessity.[63] Health plan sponsors also make policy regarding the cost of health plans for health plan sponsors and beneficiaries, which also has great influence on the accessibility of services to plan beneficiaries.

The Role of Federal Agencies in Developing Health-Care Policies

Several agencies of the federal government, such as the U.S. Department of Veterans Affairs (VA) and agencies within the U.S. Department of Health and Human Services, are involved in setting medical standards of care. Their activities in this regard are closely coordinated with the work of medical professional associations, medical specialty societies, voluntary health organizations, and private accrediting bodies.

The NIH, along with the VA, funds biomedical and health services research on the causes and treatment of disease and injury and improvements in the delivery of health-care services. Advances in research are often the basis of new medical standards of care. The Centers for Disease Control is actively involved in the "translation" of medical research for health-care practitioners to improve the quality of health care. The Food and Drug Administration (FDA) approves most drugs, devices, and biologics used in medical care. Thus, FDA regulatory decisions have a tremendous impact on the content of medical standards of care and, in particular, whether extant medical standards of care remain current and valid. Federal agencies have also been more directly involved in the development of medical standards of care. The NIH continued funding the biomedical research that has generated the medical breakthroughs that lead to new medical treatments for disease. Regarding these research findings, the NIH holds consensus conferences of medical and other experts about appropriate medical care to resolve disparate views of treatment methods and also translate research findings into clinical practice.[64] The former AHCPR sponsored the development of medical practice guidelines and medical quality standards in the past and facilitated the development of all types of medical standards of care.[65] Its successor, the AHQR, continues to play a crucial role in setting priorities for health services research and facilitating the development of medical quality standards and quality performance measures by private medical organizations and accrediting bodies. The Centers for Medicare and Medicaid Services (CMS; formerly the HCFA) also funds health services research with the ostensible purpose of developing medical standards to define, not only the content and quality of health-care services, but also coverage policy for Medicare and other public health insurance programs.[66]

The role of federal agencies is important. First, they have funds to pay for the research that informs credible quality standards. Second, they have the status, authority, and resources to convene experts to facilitate the professional dialogue needed for developing consensus on the content of standards. Federal agencies have two motives for involvement in standard setting activities. As sponsors of public health insurance and service delivery programs, they are vitally concerned that their program beneficiaries get high quality, cost-effective care. Second, as funders of biomedical and health services research, they are interested in translating research findings into better clinical practice. Private medical organizations, voluntary health organizations, and private accrediting bodies work closely with federal agencies in the various activities that affect the development of medical standards of care through participation on advisory boards, direct consultation, and other methods.

The upshot of these developments is a great capacity within the American health-care sector to define and measure the quality of health-care services. This capacity has great potential for the protection of patients who receive health care and also consumers as they select among health plans.

This section identifies and classifies the multiple, varying policies about health care in ways that facilitate an understanding of their role in the generation and disposition of consumer concerns about health care. Most policies of interest to consumers address the issues of the quality of, access to, and the cost of health-care services for health plans. For the uninsured, the major policies regarding access are those corporate bylaws and internal policies of providers, often mandated by law, regarding the provision of care for the poor. For uninsured consumers, provider policies on the price of health-care services are critical as well. Table 3 presents a taxonomy that organizes and describes the universe of different types of policies governing health-care services and the standards of care that inform these policies in health plans and among providers today.

Policies Pertaining to Quality

The definition of quality of health-care services is illusive and has been a major subject of scientific analysis and discussion among the medical profession, payers, and policymakers since World War II. Avedis Donabedian, the leading scholar on health-care quality, who conceptualized the vocabulary for describing health-care quality,[67] has defined quality as follows: "The degree of quality is . . . the extent to which the care provided is expected to achieve the most favorable balance of risks and benefits."[68] The application of this principle as well as the determination of quality in specific treatment contexts is complex and problematic. There are virtually thousands of standards of care that address, define, and affect health-care services in the United States today.[69]

A useful point of departure for developing a taxonomy of quality policy is the Institute of Medicine's classification scheme for standards of care in medicine. Specifically, in 1990, the Institute of Medicine (IOM) divided the universe of standards of care into four categories: (1) medical practice guidelines; (2) medical review criteria; (3) standards of quality; and (4) performance measures.[70] These standards of care are defined as follows:

—*Standards of quality* are authoritative statements of (*a*) minimum levels of acceptable performance or results, (*b*) excellent levels of performance or results, or (*c*) the range of acceptable performance or results.

—*Medical (or clinical) practice guidelines* are systematically developed statements that assist practitioner and patient decisions about appropriate health care for specific clinical circumstances.

—*Medical review criteria* are systematically developed statements that can be used to assess the appropriateness of specific health-care decisions, services, and outcomes.

—*Performance measures* are methods or instruments that estimate or monitor the extent to which the actions of a health-care practitioner or provider conform to practice guidelines, medical review criteria, or standards of quality.

There are numerous examples of these four types of quality policies. Most of these standards of care are made by medical specialty societies, voluntary health organizations, and private accrediting bodies in processes described in chapter 7. Except with respect to medical review criteria, they are not coverage policies but serve as the basis of most coverage policy that is conscientiously conceived.

Standards of quality, which pertain to levels of performance or results, are generally made by medical specialty societies and medical professional organizations. They establish the definitive characteristics of quality with respect to different medical treatments and procedures and other aspects of medical care. Performance measures are related to medical quality standards and are specific measures of a quantitative nature that estimate or monitor provider compliance with quality standards. These performance measures are often made by accrediting bodies, health plan sponsors, and health-care providers that are directly responsible for quality assurance and improvement either in the direct provision of health-care services or in determining compliance with accreditation standards.

Medical practice guidelines are systematically developed statements that assist practitioners of secondary care in specific clinical settings. They are conceptually different from other types of standards of care. Medical specialty societies and medical professional organizations usually make these guidelines to assist practitioners in maintaining high quality standards. One objective of these guidelines is to assist practitioners to meet medical quality standards in the delivery of clinical care.

Medical review criteria—statements used to assess the appropriateness of specific decisions, services, and outcomes—are of two types. First are criteria developed by peer review organizations and similar bodies charged with monitoring the quality of care in an institution. For example, peer

TABLE 3. Taxonomy of Policy Governing Consumer Concerns about Health Care

Type of Policy	Definition	Sponsor	Promulgation Process
Quality policies			
Standards of quality	Standards of quality are authoritative statements of minimum to excellent levels of performance or results	Medical professional organizations and specialty societies Voluntary health organizations Private accrediting bodies, e.g., NCQA and JCAHO NIH AHQR (facilitator)	Private policymaking processes of medical professional organizations, voluntary health organizations, & private accrediting bodies NIH, AHQR, & CMS non-legislative rulemaking processes
Medical-practice guidelines	Medical (or clinical) practice guidelines are systematically developed statements to assist practitioner and patient decisions about appropriate health care for specific clinical circumstances	Medical professional organizations Medical specialty societies Voluntary health organizations	Private policymaking processes of medical professional organizations & voluntary health organizations
Performance measures	Performance measures are methods or instruments to estimate or monitor the extent to which the actions of a health-care practitioner or provider conform to practice guidelines, medical review critieria,[a] or standards of quality	Private accrediting bodies, e.g., NCQA and JCAHO CMS Other federal agencies sponsoring health plans State Medicaid agencies Other state agencies sponsoring health plans HMOs, MCOs, and private insurers	Private policymaking processes of medical professional organizations, voluntary health organizations, & private accrediting bodies Internal, unspecified processes of private payers, e.g., health insurers, HMOs, MCOs, & employers NIH, AHQR, & CMS through nonlegislative rulemaking processes

TABLE 3. *continued*

Type of Policy	Definition	Sponsor	Promulgation Process
Access policies			
Formal statements of coverage	Statements in plan contracts and other documents defining the amount, duration, and scope of covered plan benefits, including medical devices and durable medical equipment and new medical technologies and procedures	CMS Medicare contractors Other federal agencies sponsoring health plans State Medicaid agencies Other state agencies sponsoring health plans HMOs, MCOs, and private health insurers	CMS through (1) the Medicare national coverage policy process for medical devices, durable medical equipment, and new medical technologies and procedures and (2) nonlegislative rulemaking processes for all items and services Medicare contractors through local coverage policymaking processes State agency nonlegislative rulemaking processes HMOs, MCOs, and health insurers through (1) contract negotiations with public and private health plan sponsors and (2) internal, unspecified processes Corporate policymaking processes of private payers, including employers
Medical-review criteria	Medical review criteria are systematically developed statements that can be	CMS Medicare contractors Other federal agencies sponsoring health plans	Medicare contractors through private, unspecified processes State agency nonlegisla-

TABLE 3. *continued*

Type of Policy	Definition	Sponsor	Promulgation Process
Medical-review criteria	used to assess the appropriateness of specific health-care decisions, services, and outcomes	State Medicaid agencies Other state agencies sponsoring health plans HMOs, MCOs, and private health insurers	tive rulemaking processes HMOs, MCOs, and health insurers through contract negotiations with public and private health plan sponsors Corporate policymaking processes of private payers, including employers
Provider policies on treatment of uninsured poor	Corporate bylaws, trust documents, and policies thereunder stating the obligations of some public and private, not-for-profit institutional providers on care for the uninsured poor Statutes establishing public hospitals	Some public and private, not-for-profit hospitals and other institutional providers State and local governments	Corporate policymaking processes of hospitals and institutional providers State and local legislative and policymaking processes
Cost policies			
Provider-payment methods of public programs	Payment methodologies for providers for public health insurance and health-care services programs	CMS Medicare contractors Other federal agencies sponsoring health plans State Medicaid agencies Other state agencies sponsoring health plans	Nonlegislative rulemaking processes
Payment policies in contracts between public and private sponsors of health-care plans	Payment methodologies specified in contracts for the provision of health-care services to	CMS Medicare contractors Other federal agencies State Medicaid agencies	Contract negotiations between public health plan sponsors and HMOs, MCOs, and health insurers

TABLE 3. *continued*

Type of Policy	Definition	Sponsor	Promulgation Process
	specified groups of beneficiaries	Other state agencies sponsoring health plans Employers Private health insurers, HMOs, and MCOs	
Pricing policies of health insurance and prepaid health plans	Payment methodologies specified in contracts for the provision of health-care services to specified groups of beneficiaries	Private health insurers, HMOs, and MCOs Employers	Internal, unspecified process
Pricing policies of health-care providers	Prices for services set by providers	Hospitals, physicians, and other providers	Internal, unspecified process

ᵃ Medical review criteria are set forth under "access policy."

review organizations for Medicare use medical review criteria for this purpose. Similarly, health-care institutions and health plans use such criteria for internal utilization review for quality purposes.

Policies Pertaining to Access

As a practical matter, the major type of policy affecting access for insured consumers is coverage policy for public and private health plans. The policies that affect access for uninsured consumers are fundamentally different, and they include internal policies of various institutional providers, which are often mandated by corporate, tax, and trust law, depending on the organization's type of corporate control. These internal policies dictate whether and under what circumstances the organization will provide health-care services to individuals who have no insurance and who are otherwise unable to pay for care.

Coverage Policy. Coverage is clearly the most important type of policy affecting access to and the cost of health-care services from the perspective of insured consumers of health care. Coverage is an insurance concept that defines the amount and characteristics of the risk that an insurer underwrites.[71] All health plans, regardless of sponsorship, require specification of plan benefits and their coverage. Benefits are simply a list of health-care services that the plan will pay for or provide. Coverage pertains to the amount, duration, and scope of the services. In general, the definition of coverage necessarily reflects a judgment on the part of the health plan sponsor as to what amount, duration, and scope of benefits are required for services of acceptable quality.

However, coverage policy is also influenced by the pricing of health plans. If a health plan sponsor wants to offer the plan to consumers or purchasers on behalf of a group of consumers, the health plan sponsor is likely to include fewer benefits, more cost sharing, and more restrictive coverage policy. For example, health plan sponsors often exclude or limit mental health and substance abuse services to make health-care plans more affordable. These services, in the parlance of insurers, are more likely to be the subject of "moral hazard" as insureds and the providers who direct their care have greater control over the utilization of these services and thus the occurrence of the insured loss.

Coverage restrictions generally target two types of services. First are low cost, high volume items or services such as home health care or outpatient laboratory services. Increasingly, the problem of expensive excess in the delivery of these items or services is addressed in prospective or capitated methods of paying providers that shift the financial risk of excess care to providers. Second are extremely expensive services, such as autologous bone marrow transplantation for breast cancer, that are needed by few of the catastrophically ill. Such services are often denied coverage on the grounds that they are experimental—a common coverage exclusion in both public and private health plans.

There are basically two types of coverage policy. The first category of coverage policy is a formal statement that a specific medical procedure, item, or service is a covered benefit. In general, these formal statements or rules address three categories of benefits: (1) the amount and duration of conventional services, such as hospital days or physician services; (2) medical devices and durable medical equipment; and (3) medical technologies and procedures. These formal statements of coverage are most likely to be based on standards of care and medical practice guidelines developed by private medical organizations.

The second category of coverage policy encompasses a wide variety of medical review criteria that are used by health plans and their sponsors to make coverage decisions in individual cases. The Institute of Medicine's standard of care, "medical review criteria," pertains to this type of coverage policy. Often, these medical review criteria take the form of computerized "screens" that identify cases in which services exceed expected norms regarding amount and duration in reviewing data on claims. There is some evidence that some MCOs use medical review criteria that are based on factors other than medical standards of care developed by the medical profession, such as assessments of impact of diagnosis and treatment options on financial performance and the medical-legal risk of more conservative diagnosis and treatment approaches.[72]

Provider Policies on Care for the Uninsured Poor. As indicated above, the major category of policy affecting access to care for the uninsured is internal policies of providers as to whether and under what circumstances the organization will provide health-care services to individuals who are without insurance and who are otherwise unable to pay for care.

Policies Pertaining to Costs

There are two kinds of payment policy of interest to health-care consumers. The first is the price that providers charge for their services. The importance of this type of policy cannot be overestimated given the large percentage of health-care expenditures that are paid directly by individuals without third party reimbursement (described above). For the most part, providers have control over the prices that they charge patients for their services. Public ratesetting programs may constrain what affected providers can charge for services. Similarly, payment policy requirements of the Medicare and Medicaid programs also affect whether and what providers can charge individuals for care.

Public and private health plan payers make policies to set payment levels for covered services. These range from prices to be paid for specific services on a retrospective basis to global capitated payment rates for groups of patients. Policies governing the cost of health care are, of course, also important for consumers as they often have a critical effect on the content and quality of health-care services that consumers receive and thus may be a factor in creating situations from which consumers' concerns about health care emerge.

Another type of payment policy of health plan sponsors that directly affects consumers is coinsurance for health coverage. Specifically, cost-sharing policies include deductibles, coinsurance, and copayments as well as benefit limits. These cost-sharing policies have become widespread in the private health insurance market in recent years.[73] They are also a major factor in the problem of inadequate health insurance coverage among the privately insured.

It should be emphasized that, in prepaid managed care plans, the concepts of coverage and payment converge—hence their prominence in the consumer protection debate. In fee-for-service health care with insurance that pays on a retrospective basis, a coverage determination is a straightforward decision as to whether the services provided meet the contractual terms for coverage. When services are paid on a prepaid basis, there is no opportunity for payers to make independent decisions about coverage of specific services. Rather, a decision about coverage is often made implicitly by the health plan's provider in the context of providing clinical care out of concerns to contain costs within payment rates. Coverage becomes an issue only when the consumer and/or the attending physician makes a clinical judgment that a service is needed and the consumers' plan concludes that that service is not covered.

Nevertheless, the effect of payment policy on particular consumer concerns is generally more indirect. Insured consumers rarely pay for the major part of their health-care expenses and thus are rarely concerned with how and by what methods payers pay providers. Uninsured consumers are not directly affected by the payment policies of payers except for the crucial fact that the widespread availability of health insurance has clearly raised the cost of health-care services for which they must pay directly.[74] Because they indirectly affect consumers and are of primary interest to providers, they have not been included in the analysis of health-care policy and policymaking in this book.

7 : Processes for Making Policies

Regarding Health Care

There are multiple and varied public and private processes in the American health-care sector for making policies affecting the content, quality, and cost of as well as access to health-care services. Two dispositive factors govern the procedures to be followed in making policy. First is the type of policy that is being made. Second is the character—public or private—of the sponsor of the policymaker.

This chapter describes the processes for making policies pertaining to the content and quality of health care, access to and the coverage provided by health care, and the cost of health care. It reviews how policy is made by government agencies that sponsor health-care plans and bear other responsibilities regarding health care. Also reviewed is how private organizations make policy. By way of illustration to explain the interrelation between health-care policies of different types and the effect of those policies on the interests of health-care consumers and patients, the chapter closes with a description of how policy is made for the care and treatment of diabetes.[1]

PROCESSES FOR MAKING POLICIES REGARDING THE CONTENT AND QUALITY OF HEALTH CARE

The makers of the policies that define the content and quality of health care in the United States are primarily private medical organizations and private accrediting bodies for providers. Private payers and government agencies as stewards of public health insurance programs also make such policy. The processes for making these policies are virtually unregulated. This phenomenal unregulated character of private policymaking is due in large part to the power and prestige of the medical profession and historical deference to its expertise. As a practical matter, only the medical profession has the requisite expertise to define the content and quality of good medical care.

Because policymaking regarding the general quality of medical standards of care occurs primarily in private rather than public processes, it is not subject to the same kinds of administrative law requirements, such as notice, opportunities for public comment, and publication, that attend policymaking by government agencies. Consequently, opportunities for input from individual patients and consumers is limited.

It is also important to appreciate that government agencies rely extensively on standards made by private organizations for public regulatory programs.[2] They often delegate the actual function of regulation to private organizations, such as private accrediting bodies in the health-care sector.[3] The rationale for such delegation in both instances is that private bodies have unique expertise in setting standards and also in determining whether standards are in fact being met. As explained in chapter 4, state and federal agencies use private accrediting bodies in this manner to regulate quality in health-care institutions.

One important result of the unregulated character of policymaking for medical standards of care has been the evolution of markedly different models. With respect to policies pertaining to the content and quality of medical care, the medical profession and the health services research community have asserted leadership in designing processes for making quality policy. Specifically, as described below, a "health services research" model of process has evolved for making medical standards of care that focuses on assuring the scientific accuracy of policy. This private policymaking is much different than the administrative law model of providing opportunities for public comment and participation.

For the most part, medical standards of care defining the content and quality of health-care services are set by private medical organizations, voluntary health organizations, and private accrediting bodies in a committee process. Generally, a committee of professionals will develop a standard of care in a process that involves consulting relevant scientific literature and garnering other medical and clinical expertise. Committees vary in the degree of formality with which they solicit comments from within relevant medical specialties and, more especially, from outside the organization. The committee process usually considers research findings on outcomes of a particular medical treatment or procedure that has been developed by a federally funded biomedical research program. In general—except perhaps in voluntary health organizations—non–medical professionals, including people with the relevant disease, are not involved in the committee process. Usually a draft of the standard of care is made available for comment from other association members and sometimes the public. In some cases, although not frequently, major policies might be submitted to a constituent assembly for debate and approval. All medical professional associations, medical specialty societies, and voluntary health organizations generally publish their medical standards of care in the professional journals published by their organizations.

The committee process of the National Committee for Quality Assurance (NCQA) for the development of Health Plan Employer Data and Information Set (HEDIS), a standardized set of measures with which to compare the performance of managed care plans, is representative of the committee processes used by private organizations to develop medical standards of care. Specifically, the NCQA's Committee on Performance Measurement is charged with developing HEDIS. The composition of this committee reflects public and private purchasers of health care, such as organized labor, medical providers, and public health officials, including policymakers for government health insurance programs. The work on specific performance measures is conducted by Measurement Advisory Panels, composed primarily of experts in relevant fields. The NCQA then formally acts on the committee recommendations.

The process by which medical standards of care are formulated has garnered considerable attention among health services researchers. The focus of this attention is on designing policymaking processes that ensure the validity and credibility of standards of care. In the 1980s, medical quality theorists argued that the process by which guidelines were developed was important especially to the credibility and validity of the guidelines.[4] For example, some have argued for a process in which all professionals with relevant experience participate in structured deliberations, using the delphi technique to yield consistency in the recommended standards irrespective of the particular professionals involved.[5] Others argued that medical practice guidelines and other standards of care must generally be based on the findings of prospective comparative studies of the outcomes of specific medical procedures and treatments.[6]

Several organizations have specifically addressed the design of processes for setting medical standards of care. For example, in the mid-1980s, when medical practice guidelines were being developed on a widespread basis, the American Medical Association established basic principles to ensure that practice parameters are scientifically sound and clinically relevant.[7] In 1990, the Institute of Medicine (IOM) convened a blue ribbon panel of experts that specified the ideal characteristics of sound medical practice guidelines and their use in support of the establishment of the Agency for Health Care Policy and Research and in support of its responsibilities with respect to developing standards of care.[8]

The IOM recommendations were consistent with the process recommendations of leading health services researchers discussed above.[9] Specifically, the IOM stressed that the "credibility of the development process, the participants, and the scientific grounding of guidelines must be clear" and also reflect a "truly multidisciplinary approach." The guidelines, according to the IOM, should be "specific, comprehensive, and flexible enough to be useful in the varied settings and circumstances of everyday medical practice and in the evolving programs to assess the appropriateness of care provided in these settings." The guidelines should also specify what information about the clinical problem, the patient's circumstances and preferences, and the delivery setting should be recorded to permit later evaluation of the appropriateness of care (judged against criteria generated in the guidelines). Finally, the language, logic, and symbols of guidelines should be easy to follow and unambiguous "so that movement from guidelines statements to educational tools, review criteria, and other instruments is unimpeded."

More recently, the Joint Commission on the Accreditation of Healthcare Organizations (JCAHO) has proposed standards related to the use of clinical practice guidelines for inclusion in its accreditation manuals for ambulatory care, health-care networks' hospitals, and preferred provider organizations.[10] While not mandating that leaders of these organizations use medical practice guidelines, the JCAHO outlines a "framework" to guide organization leaders in selecting and implementing guidelines for their organizations. These proposed standards reflect the prevailing view of guideline adoption and development in their emphasis on evaluating outcomes of care, insistence on a scientific basis for standards, and validation through evaluation.

One important dimension of the debate over process within the medical profession reflects the underlying concern of many physicians that standards of care developed by medical specialists in academic medical centers cannot be implemented in practice settings outside tertiary care institutions. Specifically, these physicians were concerned that the standards imposed would be unattainable and would increase their exposure to medical liability.

Nevertheless, the result of these deliberations within the medical profession was the evolution of a different model of process for assuring the validity and accuracy of medical standards of care, a model informed by the methodologies of scientific research. According to this health services research model, the policymaking process should focus on obtaining the latest and best scientific information. It should also be designed to achieve a genuine consensus on the content of a standard that is specific to a given medical problem, will lead to improved patient outcomes, and can be feasibly implemented in realistic practice settings. Another crucial feature of process according to the health services research model is some assurance that another group of similarly trained experts will arrive at essentially the same standard. Further, the health services research model calls for an ongoing process beyond promulgation. Specifically, there should be an evaluation of the implementation of the standards of care in terms of practitioner behavior and patient outcomes, with an opportunity for revision of standards of care based on evaluation findings.

Unlike the legal "notice-and-comment" model, the medical health services research model does not address the traditional process values in legal theory of notice to all interested parties, opportunity to comment on the content of the proposed policy, and subsequent publication. The theoretical purpose of the health services research model is assuring the scientific accuracy and validity of the standards of care, not just at promulgation, but also on a continuing basis through evaluation. The health services research model focuses on the content of the policy directly and in great detail. This focus is not characteristic of the underlying theory of the notice-and-comment model of administrative law.

POLICYMAKING REGARDING ACCESS TO HEALTH-CARE SERVICES

Processes for making coverage policy for public and private health plans greatly affect access to health-care services for insured individuals. For uninsured consumers, important policymaking processess—to the extent that they exist—are those of institutional providers mandated by law to provide services to the poor.

Sponsors of public and private health plans make coverage policy for their plans. The coverage policymaking processes and activities of health plan sponsors vary greatly. Specifically, health plan sponsors are not uniformly involved to the same degree in the formulation of policy for their health plans. At one end of the continuum is Medicare, for which national coverage decisions are made in a formal public process. At the other end of the continuum, coverage policy may be a negotiated term of a contract for group coverage or an internal corporate decision. At best, coverage policy is based on the findings of medical research and the standards of care and medical practice guidelines developed by medical professional organizations. It is also informed by the quality performance measures developed by private accrediting organizations.

There are essentially three models for making coverage policy in American health plans: (1) an administrative law model, which is sometimes used by public health plan sponsors; (2) a corporate policymaking model, used by private health plan sponsors; and (3) a contract model, used by both private and public health plan sponsors. Use of this third model for making coverage, payment, and other pertinent policies for health plans is a definitive characteristic of managed care plans. It should be noted, however, that these policymaking processes are not mutually exclusive.

Policymaking by Public Health Plan Sponsors—the Administrative Law Model. Responsible government agencies make coverage policy for their health plans in conventional as well as unique public policymaking processes. The formality of the policymaking process depends on the public importance of the policy, although, in general, the statutory rulemaking procedures for legislative rules described in chapter 3 are rarely invoked at either the federal or the state level. Further, all government sponsors of public health plans rely extensively on private quality policy developed by medical specialty societies, voluntary health organizations, and private accrediting bodies. Indeed, the "policymaking" for public programs often involves administrative decisions about what private standards of care should be used to form the basis or constitute coverage policy for public health plans.

The Medicare program has been the "flagship" health plan sponsor in terms of developing coverage policy.[11] With respect to the Medicaid program, states have the authority to make coverage policy for their own

Medicaid programs within the confines of federal law.[12] Regarding the State Child Health Insurance Program (SCHIP), health plans must have comparable benefits to the so-called benchmark plan within the state—that is, the standard Blue Cross and Blue Shield plan for federal employees, the health plan for state employees, or the commercial health maintenance organization (HMO) having the largest enrollment in the state.[13] Nevertheless, state Medicaid and SCHIP programs rely extensively on applicable Medicare coverage policy.[14] Further, sponsors of health plans for federal employees rely extensively on the Medicare coverage process.

Medicare covers three different types of benefits: (1) the amount and duration of conventional services; (2) medical devices and durable medical equipment; and (3) medical technologies and procedures. The Centers for Medicare and Medicaid Services (CMS)—formerly the Health Care Financing Administration (HCFA)—publishes national coverage policy in program manuals.[15] National coverage policy applies across the country and often drives coverage policy on similar issues for state Medicaid programs and private health plans. Medicare contractors continue to make coverage policy at the local level. Medicare contractors can also publish their own "local coverage determinations" for the Medicare program in their jurisdiction. In making coverage policy, Medicare contractors often follow a corporate policymaking model with little public involvement or subsequent publication.[16]

The Medicare national coverage policymaking process is the most prominent and important example of the administrative law model for coverage policymaking by a public health plan sponsor. In late 2000, Congress changed the national coverage decisionmaking process to provide more accessibility to interested parties (e.g., Medicare beneficiaries and medical device manufacturers) and imposed deadlines and other formal hearing requirements to make the CMS more accountable for its decisions.[17] These changes were to be implemented in October 2001, but have been postponed. Specifically, in making a national coverage determination, the CMS must ensure that the public has notice and opportunity to comment and that determinations are made on the record.[18] Further, in making the determination, the CMS must consider applicable information (including clinical experience and medical, technical, and scientific evidence) and provide a clear statement of the basis for the determination (including responses to comments received from the public) as well as the assumptions underlying that basis.[19] The CMS must make data used in the decisionmaking process available to the public. Further, in addition to requests for reconsideration available to all interested parties, Medicare beneficiaries have an opportunity to appeal national coverage decisions to the Departmental Appeals Board in the U.S. Department of Health and Human Services and to appeal local coverage decisions to an administrative law judge.[20] These and other extensive process requirements were designed to address long-standing concerns with the CMS's coverage decisionmaking process.

This legislation followed years of controversy between the Medicare program and manufacturers and suppliers of medical technologies over the Medicare national coverage policymaking process.[21] At the inception of the Medicare program in 1965, there was no formal process for making national coverage policy, and Medicare contractors made most coverage policy on a regional level. With advances in expensive new medical devices and technology and inconsistent coverage policy throughout the country, the Medicare program was faced with greater pressure to make definitive coverage decisions at the national level. For example, in the early 1980s, heart transplants were covered in California but not in other parts of the country.

A major source of pressure for national coverage policymaking has been the medical device manufacturers, which, as of 1976, had to get approval from the Food and Drug Administration (FDA) before marketing new medical devices to assure "the reasonable safety and effectiveness of medical devices intended for human use."[22] Medical device manufacturers were confounded when FDA approval did not necessarily result in Medicare coverage and further review was required.

The HCFA responded to this pressure by establishing an increasingly formal coverage decisionmaking process at the national level. In the 1980s, many organizations, including the Administrative Conference of the United States, the American Bar Association, and the U.S. General Accounting Office, expressed serious concerns about the closed character of the HCFA's coverage decisionmaking process.[23] In 1987, as part of the settlement in *Jameson v. Bowen*,[24] which contested the application of a national coverage policy, the HCFA issued a notice explaining its procedures for making coverage decisions[25] and stating its intention to promulgate a rule for making national coverage determinations. In 1989, the HCFA published a notice of proposed rulemaking—never promulgated as a final rule—to establish a more public, accountable process for making national and local coverage policy for the Medicare program.[26] In 1999, responding to criticism that its national coverage decisionmaking process was secretive and inaccessible, the HCFA appointed a Medicare Coverage Advisory Committee composed of outside experts that conducted public meetings on coverage issues and permitted manufacturers and other interested parties to present their views on specific coverage issues.[27]

The HCFA continued to struggle with the design of a coverage policymaking process that responds to the concerns of beneficiaries, device manufacturers, and other critics while maintaining tight control over decisionmaking. In April 1999, in response to pressure from the Republican Congress,[28] the HCFA published a notice outlining the administrative process for making national coverage policy.[29] This process has suggested time frames for HCFA action on outside requests for coverage, specific procedures enabling outside requesters to participate in the coverage decisionmaking process, and a specific program for publication of the process and its products through the Internet and other means. In 2000, Congress enacted the statutory changes to the Medicare coverage policymaking process described above.

The new legislation imposes an administrative law model with mandated notice and comment as well as some trial type requirements such as on-the-record decisionmaking. Prior to this legislation, both Congress and the courts seemed to acknowledge that a health services research model was appropriate for making Medicare coverage policy. In 1986, when it established administrative and judicial review for Part B claims, Congress expressly exempted national coverage determinations from judicial challenges on the grounds that they were not promulgated as legislative rules under Section 553 of the Administrative Procedures Act (APA).[30] Congress's rationale for this special treatment of national coverage policy was the fact that the HCFA had an established process for the solicitation of input from private medical organizations and the public health service.[31]

Further, after several court decisions holding Medicare coverage and payment policies invalid for not following notice-and-comment rulemaking requirements,[32] Congress expressly limited such procedural challenges to Medicare coverage policy.[33] Since then, federal courts have uniformly upheld this amendment and the authority of the CMS to promulgate Medicare coverage policy as interpretative rules.[34] While an administrative law model, which implies notice to affected parties and an opportunity for input in a structured process, is certainly appropriate for a public health insurance program, promulgation of coverage policy as interpretative rather than legislative rules is also appropriate given the need for public programs to be responsive to rapid changes in the medical sciences.

Policymaking by Private Health Plan Sponsors—the Corporate Policymaking Model. Private corporations, be they MCOs, health insurance companies, or institutional providers, make institutional policy as a corporation. As discussed in chapter 4, there are few, if any, state or federal legal requirements that specify processes for making corporate policy, and corporations vary greatly in the way in which they make and publicize different types of policies.

The process by which most private health plan sponsors make coverage policy for a given health plan is the proverbial black box. Health plan sponsors make decisions about coverage policy in the context of designing specific health plans. Generally, health plan sponsors make policy pertaining to quality, coverage, and price through corporate policymaking procedures. In making policy on quality and coverage, they rely heavily on medical standards of care set by private medical organizations and private accrediting bodies. If they are accredited, they must adopt some policies of private accrediting bodies.

In terms of medical standards of care, health plan sponsors generally make only medical review criteria used in utilization review and implementation of plan coverage policy. Medical review criteria are generally developed in a much less formal process by the health plan with little input from affected consumers or providers.[35] Medical review criteria are often the result of business decisions about the management of the utilization of health-care services in a health plan. Yet medical review criteria are extremely important to consumers because they are used to adjudicate decisions about coverage in individual cases and are often the basis of a plan's decision to deny coverage rather than a more general, published coverage provision. In general, but not necessarily, health plan sponsors establish medical review criteria on the basis of medical practice guidelines and standards of quality developed by private medical organizations.

Private health plan sponsors such as employers may leave the definition of coverage policy primarily to the insurance company or MCO that is offering or administering the plan. If a health plan sponsor elects to offer coverage through an MCO, the MCO will play a major role in defining coverage as an integral part of designing and pricing the health plan. Currently, with so much concern about quality, MCOs are increasingly seeking accreditation and thus adopting quality improvement systems as a condition of accreditation.[36]

Private policymaking by health plan sponsors at its best is usually informed by the standards of care that private medical organizations and private accrediting bodies develop. Specifically, to offer a high quality product and be competitive, responsible health plan sponsors generally base coverage policy on medical practice guidelines and standards of quality developed by private medical organizations. However, there is an inevitable tension between compliance with medical standards, particularly when they call for more intensive treatment, and the need to design a package of benefits that can be priced competitively. This tension is particularly pronounced with health plans that finance care on a capitated basis and that are often offered to employers and other private as well as public group health plan purchasers in a competitive environment.

Policymaking in Contracts with Health Plan Sponsors—the Contract Model. With the advent of managed care and the practice of public health plan sponsors contracting with MCOs to provide health plans for beneficiaries of government programs, coverage and other policies for health plans are being made in the contracts establishing the health plans. Most public health plan sponsors at both the federal and the state level contract with MCOs, HMOs, and traditional health insurers to offer and administer health plans for their beneficiaries. The Medicare+Choice program operates in this manner, as do the Medicaid program and SCHIP. Further, most government sponsors of health plans for public employees function in this manner as well.

The use of contract as a vehicle for making coverage and other policies for publicly sponsored health plans has not been studied extensively.[37] Frankly, this use of contract involves seemingly ad hoc processes about which little is known. Generally, the health plan sponsor publishes specifications for bids on health plans and invites MCOs, HMOs, and health insurers to bid competitively for the plan. Public health plan sponsors generally have to follow government contracting procedures in these bidding processes.[38] These process do not necessarily assure compliance with statutory specifications as to benefits and coverage for a government-sponsored health insurance program. However, there is some evidence with respect to the Medicaid program in the 1990s that state contracts with private health plans sharply curtailed Medicaid coverage in ways that were inconsistent with statutory and regulatory provisions.[39]

There is reason to be concerned about the processes for making policy in these contractual arrangements. One concern is the fact that policy that was once made by government agencies in public, accountable processes is now made in the course of negotiating and drafting contract terms. More important, the Supreme Court's decision in *American Manufacturers Mutual Insurance Company v. Sullivan*,[40] discussed in chapter 4, effectively insulates coverage decisions of private contractors such as MCOs from due process challenges by program beneficiaries. This decision thus constitutes a significant reduction of procedural due process protection in the benefits of government health insurance programs as often decisions about the amount, duration, and scope of benefits are made as coverage decisions.

Policymaking Processes Regarding Access within Providers

Institutional providers make important policies regarding access to their facilities for the uninsured. In doing so, these providers generally follow a corporate policymaking model (described above). Thus, there are few opportunities for potential or actual patients to participate in the policymaking activities of providers. Other than governance requirements such as board composition, there are generally no specific mandates on not-for-profit corporations regarding processes for making corporate policies. Consequently, there is considerable variation in the processes that providers use to make policies regarding the care of the uninsured and poor. It appears that, even where such processes for making such policies exist, they are not open to the public, nor are they publicized in a formal manner. Further, many of these policies are made in the course of business practice with little sensitivity to the process for making the policies.

POLICYMAKING REGARDING THE COST OF HEALTH-CARE SERVICES

There is great variation in the processes by which policy setting the price of health-care services is made. Providers are free to set the price of their services in general, although they are greatly constrained with respect to insured patients owing to provider payment policies of both public and private health plans. Public health plan sponsors may have statutory requirements for setting prices for providers' services or may regulate provider rates generally. Health insurers, MCOs, and HMOs have detailed payment formulas by which they pay physicians, hospitals, and other providers of health care.

These payment policies have a major effect on individual patients and consumers in need of health care. For example, the physician payment policies of capitated health plans—especially financial incentives that encourage physicians to curtail services to health plan members—have been very controversial in the patient protection debate of recent years because they arguably compromise physician commitment to patients. Provider payment policies also affect individuals as they influence the price that uninsured or underinsured individuals must pay for their health care. Yet there are few public processes used in setting the prices that individuals are charged for their health care. As a practical matter, consumers and patients have virtually no say in the pricing of health plans or provider services.

Payment Policy for Public and Private Health Plans

At the state level, there is insurance regulation, which regulates the price of coverage in health plans of health insurers and MCOs. State insurance regulators have traditionally regulated rates through a variety of mechanisms, including (1) state prescription of rates; (2) prior approval of rates; (3) the so-called file-and-use approach; and (4) open competition with effectively no regulation.[41] Under the third option, file and use, the insurer files rates with state regulators and proceeds to use these rates unless challenged by a regulator. An important variation of this approach, as well as of prior approval, is flex rating, in which regulators accord insurers a range in which to set rates. Generally, state insurance ratemaking procedures used for setting rates for health insurance and HMOs are fairly flexible, for most states use the file-and-use method of rate regulation for health insurance.[42] To the extent that Employee Retirement Income Security Act–regulated health plans purchase health-care coverage for employees through commercial insurance plans and HMOs, these latter entities are subject to state rate regulation.

Congress has established a special process for determining payment rates for MCOs providing Medicare+Choice plans for Medicare beneficiaries. For MCOs with compliant Medicare+Choice plan requirements,[43] Medicare will pay a capitated rate for Medicare beneficiaries in the area adjusted for such risk factors as age, disability status, gender, and institutional status.[44] While the setting of payment rates for Medicare+Choice plans is established in contracts between the CMS and the MCOs, the process is overseen by the congressional Medicare Payment Advisory Commission.[45]

Payment Policy of Institutional and Professional Providers

In general, when physicians, hospitals, and other providers deliver services to the uninsured or individuals receiving care independently of a health plan, they are free to set the prices of their services without regulation. As in other industries, pricing is generally an economic decision made independently in response to market conditions. Pricing becomes a political decision only when important constituencies are affected and call for government intervention in the pricing process through regulation. In theory, rate regulation makes aspects of pricing decisions political matters to be decided in a public forum and presumably with regard to the public interest.

Some states regulate the prices of some providers in various ways. In the past, some states had hospital rate-setting programs that regulated hospital charges, costs, prices, and/or revenues.[46] Regarding physician payment policies, Massachusetts has successfully precluded the practice of so-called balance billing as a consumer protection measure.[47] This prohibition prevents physicians and other providers from charging consumers a significant amount over insurance reimbursement for the same service.

In the 1990s, with the rise of managed care, health plan sponsors and MCOs contracted directly with physicians, hospitals, and other providers to serve their beneficiaries. In these contracts, the providers' prices and other terms were negotiated as part of the contract.[48] Further, physicians, hospitals, and other providers have joined together in networks to negotiate more effectively with health plan sponsors.[49] Regardless of arrangements, providers are often paid capitated rates negotiated in contracts.[50] It thus appears that states have less interest in regulating providers' rates directly and, as described in chapter 2, have turned their attention to the regulation of provider contracting practices.

The major federal regulation of the prices that providers charge consumers is through the Medicare program. The Medicare program strictly regulates payment rates charged by all the different types of providers with which the program contracts to provide care for its beneficiaries. Specifically, the Medicare statute limits the amounts that institutional providers can charge patients to deductibles and coinsurance and prohibits recouping charges in excess of Medicare payment levels.[51] The Medicare statute also contains elaborate measures to prevent physicians and other outpatient providers from charging and recouping additional funds for services over and above Medicare payment.[52] The Medicare program has, over the years, become much more formal about processes for setting prices given the great interest of the provider community in this issue.

With respect to Medicare, Congress specifically insulated all Medicare payment policies made before 1981 from judicial challenge for failing to comply with notice-and-comment rulemaking requirements under the federal APA.[53] Congress was responding to the Supreme Court decision *Bowen v. Michigan Academy of Family Physicians,*[54] which permitted direct challenges to methods of calculating Medicare payment policies. In a recent decision, *Shalala v. Illinois Council on Long Term Care,*[55] the Supreme Court sharply limited the scope of the *Michigan Academy* decision as authority for permitting direct challenges to Medicare payment and other policies. Further, with respect to hospital and physician payment rates, Congress has expressly precluded judicial review of the elements of established rates.[56]

The Medicare program has used an interesting model for setting rates for hospital and physician services, a model that marshals independent expertise in a public process. Congress created independent congressional commissions to analyze hospital and physician payment rates and make recommendations to the CMS about those rates.[57] In setting hospital and physician payment rates, the CMS must respond publicly to the recommendations of these commissions. The genesis of these commissions, in addition to seeking outside expertise, was concern that the HCFA was promoting cost containment above other priorities in setting payment rates. Now, the congressional Medicare Payment Advisory Commission oversees the establishment of all Medicare provider payment rates.[58]

POLICYMAKING AND DISSEMINATION: THE EXAMPLE OF DIABETES

To exemplify the processes of making and implementing policy and the interplay of all relevant actors in these processes, it is useful to look at policymaking for diabetes, a chronic disease affecting 7.6 million Americans.[59] What emerges is a pattern of interchange between the medical profession and its organizations, private accrediting bodies, and government agencies in making quality policy as well as between these entities and both public and private payers in making coverage policy.

There have been marked advances in the treatment of diabetes in recent years as well as controversy as to whether prepaid managed care plans were providing proper treatment for the care of patients with diabetes. Most important among this research is the National Institutes of Health (NIH)–funded ten-year trial in the 1980s and early 1990s, the Diabetes Control and Complications Trial (DCCT), which showed that strict control of blood sugar had a dramatic impact in preventing the complications of diabetes and profoundly changed professional opinion about the proper care of the disease.[60] The results of this trial have precipitated the development of new standards of care for diabetes.[61]

Further, with the cooperation of the American Diabetes Association (ADA) and other medical specialty societies and voluntary health organizations involved with diabetes, the NIH and the Centers for Disease Control have launched the massive National Diabetes Education Program to disseminate the findings of this ten-year trial to primary care practitioners, health plans, and the public.[62]

Also during this period, the FDA approved a generation of new drugs for the treatment of Type II diabetes, which generally afflicts older adults. These new drugs greatly enhanced the ability of practicing physicians to manage patient care and facilitate compliance with the recommendations of medical standards of care predicated on the findings of the DCCT and other research.

Medical organizations and the major voluntary health organization for diabetes, the ADA, played the major role in the development of standardized medical care for diabetes.[63] The ADA is a voluntary organization with both professional and nonprofessional members. With its large professional section of over thirteen thousand members, it has been the leading medical organization engaged in standard setting for diabetes over the last thirty years.[64] Working with other professional organizations and government agencies, the ADA sets medical standards of care through its system of professional councils on specific areas of diabetes research and care.[65] The standards of care developed in these processes are disseminated widely in the ADA's professional journal for clinical research, *Diabetes Care*.[66] Other medical organizations, such as the American College of Physicians (ACP), have also developed medical practice guidelines and standards of care for diabetes. The development of standards of care by the ADA, the ACP, and other organizations has been informed by the results of federally funded research.

Private accrediting bodies have picked up the revised medical quality standards based on these critical research findings and have revised quality performance measures accordingly. For example, the NCQA is a "collaborating research partner" in the Diabetes Quality Improvement Project along with the CMS, the ADA, and the Foundation for Accountability. The purpose of this project is to develop a common core set of diabetes performance measures that allows for fair comparisons and/or stimulates quality improvement among health plans and providers.

In the 1990s, there was great concern in the diabetes community that prepaid managed care plans, including those for Medicare and other public programs, did not have coverage policies that reflect the professional consensus and associated quality standards of care based on the DCCT findings that intensive treatment of diabetes would prevent future complications and thus should be available to all patients.[67] Indeed, some evidence suggests that MCOs use coverage policies designed to promote profits while minimizing the risk of medical liability and bad publicity.[68] Much of this effort responds to a prevailing criticism in recent years that prepaid managed care plans do not provide high quality care for people with chronic illnesses such as diabetes.[69] However, more recently, some MCOs have sought to incorporate medical standards of care into their treatment protocols for diabetes to provide better care for enrollees.[70]

Thus, the diabetes community successfully lobbied state legislatures and even Congress to mandate expanded coverage for diabetes care in managed care plans. These developments led Congress to enact special provisions regarding the care of people with diabetes in the Balanced Budget Act of 1997.[71] In 1997, fourteen states enacted legislation to improve healthcare coverage for diabetes in state-regulated health insurance plans, with the result that nearly half the states have such legislation.[72]

This experience with diabetes is exemplary of similar activity with respect to other diseases. The federal government funds research to expand the knowledge base about a disease. The pharmaceutical industry develops new treatments with the approval of the FDA. New knowledge is translated into clinical practice through the standard setting activity of private medical organizations. In turn, private accrediting bodies take the findings of research as well as the medical practice guidelines and medical quality standards that private medical organizations adopt and translate those standards into quality performance measures imposed on health plans and providers through private accreditation. Finally, health plan sponsors use these medical standards of care in making coverage and quality policy for their health plans and, in particular, in establishing the medical review criteria and other standards of care used in the day-to-day implementation of coverage and quality policy. To the extent that health plan sponsors are reluctant to adopt coverage policy reflecting professional quality norms and patient preferences, patients and providers may invoke the political process and obtain statutory mandates.

8 : Regimes for Tapping and Resolving Consumer

Concerns about Health Care

Because Americans obtain coverage in a wide variety of public and private health plans that are administered and regulated in different ways, different systems exist for identifying and resolving consumer concerns about their care.[1] For the most part, these systems operate independently of one another. Currently, there are two main ways in which consumers can raise their concerns about their health-care services and obtain some type of legal relief. First is internal review within health plans. Second is external review by an administrative agency or some other entity. These legal processes are available only for specific types of concerns and issues. The avenues for raising and resolving particular types of consumer disputes are presented in table 2 of chapter 5.

Clearly, there are many types of individual concerns about health care. The identification and resolution of these concerns is crucial. A central mission of this book is to assist individuals, providers, payers, and policymakers to sort out how to identify and resolve patient concerns about health care more effectively.

The terminology for describing different ways in which consumers present their concerns to responsible parties is important. When a consumer makes a concern known to a responsible party, particularly a legal institution, for adjudication and resolution, the consumer can be said to make a *complaint* or a *grievance*. However, the terminology describing consumer concerns about health care in existing systems for adjudicating concerns is, unfortunately, muddled. One prominent set of definitions is the Health Carrier Grievance Procedure Model Act of the National Association of Insurance Commissioners (NAIC).[2] This NAIC model act defines a *grievance* as a "written complaint" regarding the "availability, delivery or quality of health care services," "claims payment, handling or reimbursement for health care services," or "matters pertaining to the contractual relationship between a covered person and a health carrier."[3] However, the Centers for Medicare and Medicaid Services (CMS) has departed from this definition because the Medicare program has historically used the term *grievance* to refer to a nonappealable complaint.[4] Thus, the CMS uses the term *appeal* to refer to such an appealable complaint.[5] The National Committee for Quality Assurance (NCQA) defines an *appeal* as "a request from a member to change a previous decision made by the managed care organization."[6] The following definitions—based on a recent study of conflict resolution procedures in health maintenance organizations (HMOs) by the American Bar Association[7]—are offered for the key concepts *complaint, appeal,* and *grievance:*

> —*Complaint.* An oral or written expression of dissatisfaction by a plan member or some other health-care consumer.
> —*Appeal.* A request by a plan member or some other health-care consumer for review of a previous plan or provider decision about services or payment.
> —*Grievance.* A complaint or dispute other than one involving a plan or provider decision denying or limiting a service or a payment.

In sum, there is no consensus on the definitions of the major terms used to describe different types of complaints by which consumers express concerns in various adjudication systems. In the light of this lack of consensus, statutory definitions of terms are definitive particularly when delineating appeal rights in specific legal regimes for adjudicating concerns.

EXTRALEGAL INSTITUTIONS FOR TAPPING AND RESOLVING CONSUMER CONCERNS

Consideration of institutions for tapping and resolving consumer concerns about health care should begin with the informal mechanisms that most institutional providers and health plans have implemented. For many consumer complaints about health care are resolved informally without recourse to legal action or more formal appeals.

Customer Relations and Ombudsman Programs

Most health-care providers and health plans maintain some kind of customer-relations program to resolve identified consumer concerns about their health care.[8] These efforts are predicated on the theory that the best way to resolve disputes of any kind is direct, informal consultation between the parties and before a decisionmaker with power to accord relief for the complaint. Of note, an empirical study by the American Bar Association reports that the customer-relations departments in studied health plans handled from forty to over one hundred calls per day, resolving 80–90 percent of complaints.[9]

Customer-relations programs are especially helpful in resolving consumer concerns involving breaches of interpersonal competency that have offended the sensibilities of consumers but have not caused medical injury. In general, customer-relations programs employ very informal methods, such as conversations and correspondence, to resolve consumer concerns. However, some programs have used alternative dispute resolution (ADR) techniques such as mediation to resolve health-care disputes, including malpractice.[10] Most hospitals have now instituted such programs. Having a grievance program about which patients are notified on admission is now a condition for participating in the Medicare program.[11]

Internal review customarily involves a complaint-resolution procedure that the plan or provider maintains. The process includes so-called grievance procedures maintained by many HMOs and other health plans, often as a result of state and/or federal mandate.[12] Enrollees with a complaint or grievance must generally exhaust mandated internal review procedures before proceeding to administrative review, if available, or to judicial review. As discussed above, many providers have informal grievance procedures as part of their risk management programs, but these are not generally mandated by state or federal law.

Another effective strategy for early dispute resolution at the plan or provider level is ombudsman programs. Ombudsmen have been used successfully in other contexts to resolve disputes at early stages.[13] Ombudsmen are generally dispute resolution practitioners who serve as neutral facilitators in working confidentially and informally to resolve conflicts expeditiously.[14] Corporations and government agencies often have ombudsman offices to which individuals can bring concerns that they have with that corporation or agency for resolution. Now many federal agencies have adopted ombudsman programs.[15] Interestingly, the ombudsmen employed by state agencies on aging to act on behalf of the elderly in nursing homes, as mandated under the Older Americans Act,[16] tend to be advocates for their clients. The utilization of ombudsmen is just now gaining recognition as a dispute resolution technique for health-care disputes with managed care plans.[17] Ombudsmen have also been used in hospitals. One report indicates that nearly four thousand hospitals have ombudsman offices to handle patients' complaints.[18]

There have been numerous and disparate efforts on the part of providers and plans to require consumers to use contractual internal review.[19] Often, contractual review is a condition of obtaining treatment or enrolling in a health-care plan. The major types of disputes included in these contractual arrangements are medical malpractice claims and disputes over coverage. Contractual review has been used especially in the adjudication of medical malpractice claims.[20]

For the most part, contractual review involves the use of ADR methods.[21] Arbitration seems to be the predominant ADR method for the resolution of health-care disputes in contractual review processes.[22] In arbitration, parties ostensibly agree at some point to retain an individual arbitrator or a panel of arbitrators to render the decision instead of a court. Binding arbitration occurs when the parties agree that the arbitration will conclusively resolve the dispute, with limited appeal rights.

Arbitration has been promoted for the adjudication of malpractice claims on the grounds that it is more efficient, less costly, and less trying to the parties involved than conventional litigation is and that it marshals expertise more efficiently.[23] Others have found mandated arbitration or other ADR programs to be unfair to consumers who unknowingly surrender rights to common law tort remedies on enrolling in health plans or entering a treatment relationship with a provider.[24] Courts have invalidated binding arbitration agreements between providers and consumers on the grounds that the agreements were obtained under less-than-fair circumstances.[25] The contractual review arrangements—even binding arbitration—have fared better in judicial challenges.[26]

Empirical evidence on arbitration suggests that it has been effective in resolving malpractice disputes at lower costs.[27] A recent empirical study of the RAND Institute for Civil Justice found that binding arbitration is actually not used frequently to adjudicate health-care disputes, particularly malpractice claims.[28] Nevertheless, over two-thirds of studied HMO plans asked new enrollees to sign agreements to arbitrate contract disputes, including coverage disputes.[29] These findings are consistent with those of an earlier U.S. General Accounting Office (GAO) study showing that alternatives to litigation were not widely used for adjudicating malpractice claims.[30]

External review customarily involves a review process outside the plan or provider but exclusive of judicial review by a court. The most common type of external review is administrative review in procedures sponsored by administrative agencies for public health insurance programs described above.

Administrative review is available only for beneficiaries of public health insurance programs such as Medicare and Medicaid. It consists of adjudicative proceedings within administrative agencies, often with subsequent judicial review to ascertain if the administrative decision meets statutory standards. Administrative review proceedings for public programs must comport with constitutional principles of procedural due process.[31]

External review also includes other types of review by entities outside the health plan. For example, as discussed below, the CMS contracts with an outside organization to conduct external reconsiderations of decisions by Medicare+Choice plans for the Medicare program. In general, external review enjoys widespread confidence among patients and physicians as a fair review process.[32]

Indeed, external review of health plan decisions involving coverage denials and other primarily medical issues has emerged as an important strategy for protecting health-care consumers. Many states require such external review even for HMOs that contract with ERISA-regulated health plans.[33] As explained in chapter 2, the issue of whether states can mandate external review in this context is before the U.S. Supreme Court. Further, as also discussed in chapter 2, external review has been a consistent feature of most patient protection bills before Congress, although there has been some variation on its availability and cost to the consumer in the different bills.

State-Regulated Private Health Plans

States, as described in chapter 4, regulate insurance. While state insurance regulation chiefly addresses insurer solvency and market conduct, it also includes requirements for appeal procedures and other mechanisms by which consumers can raise complaints and have them adjudicated.

Two of the five model acts that constitute the NAIC's "Consolidated Licensure for Entities Assuming Risk" initiative, described in chapter 3, are aimed directly at the protection of consumers in health plans: the Utilization Review Model Act[34] and the Health Carrier Grievance Procedure

Model Act.[35] These two acts address the need for expedited review of certain insurer coverage denials. The Health Carrier Grievance Procedures Model Act calls for an initial review by health plans, with a written decision explaining the basis of the decision, further rights to appeal to the state's insurance commissioner, and also a subsequent oral appeal. These model acts have been adopted by a majority of states as they reform grievance-and-appeal procedures for state-regulated health insurers.[36] In addition, with recent legislation, at least eighteen states have mandated external review.[37]

State Requirements for HMOs. State insurance codes generally require HMOs to have grievance procedures as a condition of licensure.[38] Many states require HMOs to describe their grievance process as a condition of licensure, and some states authorize revocation of licenses for noncompliance with this requirement.[39]

The NAIC's Model HMO Act is the basis of most state HMO statutes.[40] Under the Model HMO Act, HMOs must establish and maintain approved procedures for the resolution of grievances initiated by enrollees.[41] The HMO must also maintain records regarding grievances. The NAIC Model HMO Act regulations also require contracts between providers and HMOs to explicitly address grievance procedures as well.[42] This regulation specifically requires the contract to provide for arbitration of patient grievances.[43] Most states have included this requirement in their HMO statutes.[44] The Model HMO Act does not explicitly provide for judicial review of HMO decisions in grievance proceedings.

There are other mandates on HMOs regarding internal review procedures. The Federal Health Maintenance Organization Act of 1973,[45] which formerly regulated federally qualified HMOs for the purpose of receiving federal grants, loans, and other benefits, required federally qualified HMOs to have "meaningful procedures for hearing and resolving grievances."[46] Interestingly, major HMO accrediting bodies (e.g., the NCQA) do not require grievance procedures, although they do require accredited plans to specify patient rights and responsibilities.[47] According to a GAO study, HMOs varied greatly in the degree to which they have effective grievance-and-appeal procedures in place.[48]

Other State-Regulated Private Health Plans. If a private health plan is not a prepaid health plan regulated as an HMO under state law or an employer-sponsored plan regulated by the Employee Retirement Income Security Act (ERISA), requirements for internal review are those that states otherwise impose.[49] Further, the NAIC Utilization Review Model Act[50] and the NAIC Health Carrier Grievance Procedure Model Act[51] apply to all state-regulated health insurance plans.

State insurance regulators regulate the claims settlement practices of all insurance companies and can sanction insurers that fail to comply with regulatory requirements.[52] Most states regulate insurer claim settlement practices under two NAIC model acts that either together or independently have been adopted in nearly all states.[53] The NAIC Unfair Claims Settlement Practices Model Act[54] designates specific forms of insurer misconduct as unfair claim practices, including failing to acknowledge with reasonable promptness pertinent communications regarding claims and failing to provide a prompt, reasonable, and accurate explanation of the basis for a claim denial or settlement offer. In addition, the NAIC's Unfair Trade Practices Model Act specifies that failure to maintain complaint-handling procedures and provide claims history are unfair trade practices.

Furthermore, like those holding other types of insurance, members of state-regulated plans have access to complaint procedures in the state's department of insurance or attorney general's office.[55] These procedures are quite varied and range from those comparable to HMOs' to more informal procedures.[56] Mostly, these complaint procedures do not involve an adjudicative proceeding that accords specific remedies to consumers who have filed a complaint. However, they may result in a favorable resolution of the complaint through informal negotiation with the intervention of state insurance regulators.

Finally, state regulators customarily perform "market conduct reviews" of the way in which insurers (regulated insurance companies and HMOs) treat consumers, focusing specifically on underwriting, advertising, rate-setting, and claims settlement practices.[57] State insurance regulators will consider consumer complaints in these reviews, and sanctions may be imposed against companies against which numerous complaints have been filed.[58] Empirical information is not readily available on the extent and nature of the complaints within state insurance departments.[59]

ERISA-Regulated Health Plans

The Employee Retirement Income Security Act of 1974 establishes requirements for health insurance plans and other employee benefit plans that are eligible for favorable federal tax treatment. ERISA Section 503 establishes extensive complaint review procedures for qualified employee benefit plans.[60] It requires plans to comply with Department of Labor (DOL) regulations giving notice to any participant or beneficiary whose claim for benefits has been denied and affording a reasonable opportunity for review of the claim denial decision.[61] Pursuant to DOL regulations under Section 503,[62] employee benefit plans must give notice to any participant or beneficiary whose claim for benefits has been denied and afford a reasonable opportunity for review of the decision denying the claim pursuant to specified deadlines. Every plan is required to establish a procedure to review decisions made in the grievance proceeding.[63] Further, for ERISA plans purchasing coverage through federally qualified HMOs, the claims review procedures of federally qualified HMOs are deemed to comply with the regulations under ERISA pertaining to claims procedures.[64]

In recent years, there has been much criticism of ERISA grievance procedure requirements, in particular the lack of external review.[65] Although historically reluctant to regulate in this area under past presidential administrations, the DOL decided to reform its complaint review procedures in part because of its recognition that beneficiaries were not adequately protected in prepaid managed care plans in the 1990s.[66] Reform of the ERISA grievance procedures was the major focus of the recent patient protection bills in Congress discussed in chapter 2.

In November 2000, the DOL promulgated a final rule reforming the ERISA grievance-and-appeal procedures that incorporated the expedited review procedures recently adopted by the Medicare program for Medicare prepaid health plans.[67] The rule clarified required disclosures to plan participants and beneficiaries, shortened time limits for making health benefit claim decisions, particularly for emergency care, and required plans to provide better information about appeal rights and coverage denials. The new rule also required employee benefit plans to provide claimants with extensive information, including records and other materials on the basis of decisions, in cases involving adverse determination of benefits.[68] Despite concerns of health plans, the DOL maintained that such availability of information was important to empower beneficiaries to appeal effectively. Also of interest, the DOL limited the use of mandatory contractual ADR in adjudicating appeals under ERISA. The limits imposed ensure that beneficiaries can appeal arbitrators' decisions and do not have to bear the cost of proceedings, among other measures.[69] This rule sought to comply with

President Clinton's executive order requiring federal agencies to implement the recommendations of the Presidential Commission on Consumer Protection and Quality in the Health Care Industry.[70]

Programs for Government Employees

States and the federal government often contract with managed care organizations (MCOs) and insurance companies to provide health plans for their employees. Thus, as a practical matter, except for government oversight, these health plans resemble private health plans more than government programs. Nevertheless, the sponsoring government may impose statutory or regulatory requirements on private health plans for their employees. For example, federal programs for government employees as well as military personnel and their dependents also have consumer protection requirements, some of which are described below. Further, as of 1999, these programs must implement President Clinton's executive order mandating adoption of the protections in the presidential commission's consumer bill of rights.[71]

Federal Employee Health Benefit Plan. Under the Federal Employee Health Benefit Plan (FEHBP), internal review of a carrier denial of a claim or denial of enrollment is available in the federal Office of Personnel Management.[72] HMOs serving federal employees under the FEHBP must meet specific consumer protection requirements.[73] Further, Department of Defense regulations establish administrative hearing and appeal procedures for the TRICARE program for military personnel.[74]

State Employee Health Plans. State statutes generally address administrative appeal procedures for health plans for state employees. Customarily, plans for state employees are underwritten and administered by commercial health insurers and regulated under state insurance codes. To the extent that states purchase health insurance on the private market, administrative appeal procedures are specified under state insurance codes. (Such publically sponsored health plans do not qualify as employee benefit plans under ERISA.)[75] However, because a state sponsors a plan, enrollees would be entitled to procedural due process notice and hearing requirements under both federal and state constitutional law.

Medicare beneficiaries have two options for obtaining their benefits—the traditional fee-for-service program and the Medicare+Choice program, which replaces the old Medicare HMO program. As a result, there are different methods by which Medicare beneficiaries can raise concerns with the Medicare program and its contractors.

Requirements for the Fee-for-Service Medicare Program. For fee-for-service Medicare, there is internal review of some disputes over denied claims, denied services, and bills before Medicare contractors.[76] In the Medicare, Medicaid, and State Child Health Insurance Program Benefits Improvement and Protection Act of 2000,[77] Congress changed the beneficiary appeal process for Part B of the Medicare program with respect to appeals involving Medicare coverage decisions.

There are still separate administrative appeal systems for beneficiaries dissatisfied with determinations under Parts A and B of the Medicare program.[78] Under Part A, beneficiaries can appeal a denial of hospital services to a peer review organization[79] and can appeal claims involving other providers to the fiscal intermediary.[80] For Part B appeals, beneficiaries could have a fair hearing for claims before the carrier that administers them.[81]

The new Medicare appeals requirements under the Medicare, Medicaid, and SCHIP Benefits Improvement and Protection Act (BIPA) established additional steps in the appeals process involving challenges to Medicare coverage decisions.[82] Included reforms are direct administrative review of national and local coverage determinations, an expedited review process, and strict time frames for decisionmaking at all levels of review.

Also, there is a new level of independent review by a qualified independent contractor. This contractor provides review at the reconsideration of the Medicare contractor's initial determination. If the issue raised is whether services were reasonable or necessary, the independent contractor must provide a panel of physicians or other health-care professionals in support of its decision. In this review, national coverage determinations are binding, but local coverage policies are not.

Requirements for Prepaid Health Plans under Medicare+Choice. The Balanced Budget Act established grievance-and-appeal procedures for Medicare+Choice plans.[83] In addition to having meaningful grievance procedures for so-called organizational determinations made by health plans and external review for reconsiderations, plans must also have a procedure for determining an individual's entitlement to a health service and any financial liability for the service. The plan must give detailed notice of coverage denials in writing and procedures for reconsideration of coverage denials. The time frame for reconsiderations shall be no later than sixty days from the date of receiving the request or within an earlier time period set by the CMS.

Further, Medicare+Choice plans must also maintain procedures for expediting organizational determinations and reconsiderations when, at the request of either an enrollee or a health-care professional, the plan determines that the application of the normal time frame for making a determination (or a reconsideration involving a determination) could seriously jeopardize the life or health of the enrollee or the enrollee's ability to regain maximum functioning.[84] In such cases, the plan shall notify the enrollee (and the physician involved, as appropriate) of the determination or reconsideration under time limits established by the secretary of DHHS, but not later than seventy-two hours from the time of receipt of the request for the determination or reconsideration (or receipt of the information necessary to make the determination or reconsideration) or some longer period, which the CMS may grant in specified cases. Further, the CMS shall contract with an independent, outside entity to review and resolve in a timely manner reconsiderations that affirm denial of coverage.[85]

The prior Medicare HMO program, which the Medicare+Choice program replaced, had a comprehensible and publicized grievance-and-appeal process.[86] Several important judicial decisions imposed requirements on this program that would likely pertain to the Medicare+Choice program. In *Levy v. Sullivan*,[87] the HCFA entered a settlement agreement to improve timeliness and notice in reconsiderations. As a result of *Levy*, the HCFA arranged for an outside contractor to conduct reconsiderations.[88] This outside contractor, the Center for Health Dispute Resolution, continues to handle reconsiderations for the Medicare+Choice program.[89]

Clearly, the most important decision regarding Medicare HMO procedures is the Ninth Circuit's in *Grijalva v. Shalala*,[90] which ruled that extant Medicare HMO reconsideration procedures failed to secure minimum due process for Medicare beneficiaries and that the CMS's notice and hearing procedures were deficient. The deficiencies pertained chiefly to the fact that beneficiaries did not have access to immediate reconsiderations for denials of acute services needed immediately.

The Ninth Circuit Court of Appeals also confirmed that HMO service denials did constitute federal action for purposes of the procedural due process clause. On appeal, the U.S. Supreme Court remanded the case to the Ninth Circuit for reconsideration in view of its March 1999 decision *American Manufacturers Mutual Insurance Company v. Sullivan*[91] and the Balanced Budget Act of 1997 and the regulations thereunder establishing the Medicare+Choice program.[92] (In *American Manufacturers,* the Supreme Court held that a private insurer's decision to withhold payment for disputed medical treatment in a state-mandated workers' compensation program was not state action under the procedural due process doctrine and that claimants had no property interest in payment for a medical treatment before the insurer's determination that it was reasonable and necessary.)[93] Nevertheless, the CMS has proposed improvements in the Medicare+Choice grievance-and-appeal procedures in the light of *Grijalva.*[94]

Administrative Review. The Medicare statute also makes express provision for administrative and judicial review of all beneficiary disputes. For fee-for-service Medicare, the Benefits Improvement and Protection Act retains administrative review for all Part A and Part B beneficiary appeals of $100 or more to an administrative law judge (ALJ), with an appeal to the Departmental Review Board in the U.S. Department of Health and Human Services.[95] The new Medicare+Choice program retains the same system for administrative hearings before an ALJ with an appeal to the Departmental Appeals Board.[96] Of note, in *Gray Panthers v. Schweiker,*[97] the District of Columbia Circuit ruled that the CMS must provide an oral hearing for Medicare claims under $100 but can use a toll free telephone system for such hearings.

The Medicaid Program

Medicaid beneficiaries generally receive care through prepaid managed care plans or on a traditional fee-for-service basis. Only recipients in managed care plans have access to internal grievance-and-appeal procedures within a health plan.

Internal Review for Medicaid Managed Care Plans. Regarding internal review, Medicaid regulations have always required prepaid health plans to maintain an internal grievance procedure that is approved by the state Medicaid agency.[98] The advocacy community has often expressed concern about grievance-and-appeal procedures in Medicaid managed care plans.[99]

The Balanced Budget Act of 1997 established protections for beneficiaries of Medicaid MCOs and those receiving benefits through a primary care case manager.[100] Medicaid managed care plans must also establish grievance procedures, although no specific requirements for expedited review in emergency situations are mandated. The HCFA's proposed rule on Medicaid managed care requirements specifies features of the required grievanceand-appeal procedure.[101] Specifically, the proposed rule requires that MCOs make plan enrollees aware of the grievance system and how to use it and imposes recordkeeping and monitoring requirements. The proposed rule also prescribes procedures for expedited appeals in emergency situations. In addition, according to President Clinton's executive order, state Medicaid grievance-and-appeal procedures should comport with the procedural protections recommended by the President's Commission on Consumer Protection and Quality in the Health Care Industry (see chap. 2).

Administrative Review. State Medicaid programs are to provide an opportunity for a fair hearing before the state agency for any Medicaid beneficiaries whose claims are either denied or not acted on with reasonable promptness or in those situations where the agency otherwise acted erroneously.[102] Under the new Medicaid managed care rules, a Medicaid beneficiary who is dissatisfied with the decision in an HMO grievance proceeding can obtain a fair administrative hearing before the state Medicaid agency.[103] There must be evidentiary hearings at the local level before state Medicaid agencies will grant an appeal to a state agency.[104]

The Veterans Medical System

The appeal system for the Department of Veterans Affairs (VA) is managed by the Board of Veterans' Appeals (BVA).[105] Veterans can appeal to the BVA any decision, such as a denial of eligibility for medical treatment, made by the VA regional office or a VA medical center.[106] However, decisions concerning the need for medical care or the type of medical treatment needed are not within the jurisdiction of the BVA.[107] Appeals are made first to the VA local office, then to the BVA.[108] Independent expert evaluation is also available from physicians who are not members of the VA system.[109]

JUDICIAL REVIEW

For many consumer concerns, legal recourse is also available in state and/ or federal courts. If the concern was adjudicated in an administrative proceeding, judicial review may be available. In general, a concern raised directly in court must fit within available common law or statutory causes of action. Not all consumer concerns fit neatly into available causes of action, with the result that many concerns cannot be maintained successfully in court. Historically, judicial review has played an important role in protecting the interests of health-care consumers, particularly the most vulnerable—the uninsured poor.[110]

De Novo Judicial Review under ERISA for Employer-Sponsored Plans

As described above, ERISA Section 502(a) accords ERISA plan members de novo judicial review of plan determinations under Section 503 as well as enforcement of ERISA plan requirements in federal district court.[111] Specifically, plan participants or beneficiaries may sue to enforce their rights under the terms of the plan and to clarify rights to future benefits under the terms of the plan if they have exhausted administrative remedies under Section 503.[112] Also, plan requirements that parties submit to arbitration are generally enforceable.[113] Of note, the DOL regulations regarding ERISA claims procedures prohibit the practice of requiring arbitration.[114]

Plan participants and beneficiaries as well as fiduciaries can also sue for equitable relief for violations of ERISA requirements.[115] ERISA remedies for challenges to plan requirements and benefits are exclusive and completely preempt available state remedies.[116] Of note, the 10th Circuit recently ruled that a court could not review the medical review criteria used by a third-party administrator for an ERISA-regulated plan to make a coverage determination in an individual case.[117]

ERISA also preempts substantive state laws that relate to employee benefit plans.[118] However, ERISA explicitly excludes state insurance codes from preemption but then provides that employee benefit plans will not be deemed insurers for purposes of state insurance regulation.[119] Consequently, a self-insured employee health plan clearly will be subject only to ERISA. If the employer purchases a health insurance plan from an MCO, an HMO, or a commercial insurance company, aspects of the health plan that relate to the business of insurance may be regulated by state insurance laws.[120] Thus, as described in chapter 4, many employers have self-insured their employee health insurance plans to avoid state regulation[121] and, in particular, to avoid compliance with state mandates for inclusion of benefits in plans.[122] Also, as discussed in chapter 2, there has been much litigation over this preemption provision, with some indication that the Supreme Court and lower courts are moving toward a more restrictive vision of the scope of the preemption.

Health Insurance Programs for Government Employees

Judicial review is also available for individuals enrolled in federal employee health insurance programs. Specifically, for the FEHBP, judicial review is available in any district court of the United States.[123] The action must be brought against the Office of Personnel Management, which administers the FEHBP, not against the private insurance carrier, and recovery is limited to the amount of benefits in dispute. For the Civilian Health and Medical Program of the Uniformed Services (CHAMPUS), judicial review is available in federal district court with original jurisdiction.[124] Judicial review of health insurance programs for state employees is generally available under common law principles for judicial review so long as the enabling legislation for such programs does not preclude review.[125]

Public Health Coverage Programs

Judicial review is customarily available for adjudicative decisions of administrative agencies that manage public health insurance programs. Generally, the enabling legislation expressly permits judicial review and specifies the conditions under which it is available.[126] If the enabling legislation is silent, judicial review is available at common law if the consumer has standing, the agency action is ripe for review, and review is sought in the proper form of action and at the appropriate time. Judicial review may also be applicable for review of federal agency actions under the federal Administrative Procedure Act (APA)[127] or of state agency actions under state administrative adjudication acts.[128] Under the APA, decisions can be overturned if they are found to be arbitrary, capricious, and an abuse of discretion or otherwise not in accord with the law or not supported by substantial evidence, among other grounds.[129] State administrative procedure acts have similar standards for judicial review.[130]

The Medicare Program. Following administrative review, beneficiaries under all parts of the Medicare program can obtain judicial review of claims and disputes over a certain monetary threshold.[131] However, the

Social Security Act proscribes federal question jurisdiction[132] of all issues except for administratively adjudicated claims under the Social Security Act.[133] Thus, judicial review of Medicare disputes is sharply constrained by the authority and terms of Medicare statutory provisions regarding judicial review.

In the 1986 decision *Bowen v. Michigan Academy of Family Physicians*,[134] the U.S. Supreme Court permitted a provider organization to challenge directly a Medicare physician payment policy. The Court ruled that Section 205(h) did not bar federal question jurisdiction on an issue for which the Medicare statute contained no express provision for judicial review. Reiterating the fundamental administrative law principle favoring judicial review in the absence of express statutory preclusion, the Court concluded that the relevant provision of the Medicare Act "simply does not speak to challenges mounted against the *method* by which such amounts are to be determined rather than the *determinations* themselves."[135] This decision opened up an avenue for judicial review of Medicare policies that Congress quickly sought to limit with new provisions regarding judicial review of Medicare coverage and payment policies.[136]

More recently, in *Shalala v. Illinois Council on Long Term Care*,[137] the Supreme Court sharply limited *Michigan Academy*, concluding that, now, unlike when *Michigan Academy* was decided, judicial review of all Medicare claims is available. Further, the court reasoned, the jurisdictional bar in Section 205(h) requires the "channeling" of virtually all legal attacks through the agency.[138] *Illinois Council on Long Term Care* thus significantly restricts, if it does not vitiate, the authority of *Michigan Academy* to permit prospective challenges of Medicare program rules and policies.

Further, the Medicare statute does limit judicial review of Medicare's national coverage policy.[139] Specifically, the Medicare statute precludes procedural challenges of policy for failing to comply with rulemaking and publication procedures in Chapter 5 of the federal APA[140] and requires that a court remand a challenged policy back to the CMS for amplification before invalidating it on any grounds.[141] A line of cases since the 1980s has strictly construed requirements for exhaustion of administrative remedies and limited nonstatutory judicial review under the Social Security Act.[142] Courts have also given great deference to administrative determinations on judicial review.[143]

The Medicaid Program. The federal Medicaid statute is silent on the availability of judicial review for decisions of state agencies in administrative appeals. Thus, federal courts do not have jurisdiction to hear disputes over Medicaid claims as the Medicaid statute is Title XIX of the Social Security Act. Section 205(h) of the Social Security Act explicitly bars federal question jurisdiction[144] for all actions "to recover on any claim" arising under the Social Security Act.[145]

Judicial review of state Medicaid agency decisions may be reviewable under the Civil Rights Act of 1871, commonly referred to as Section 1983,[146] which creates a private cause of action against any person who, under color of state law, abridges rights created by the Constitution and laws of the United States. In *Maine v. Thiboutot*,[147] the Supreme Court ruled that Section 1983 also offered protection for state violations of federal statutory obligations. And, in *Wilder v. Virginia Hospital Association*,[148] the Court ruled that a provision of the Medicaid statute establishing payment standards for institutional providers created a federal cause of action under Section 1983 to challenge state compliance with federal statutory criteria for provider payment.[149]

The Veterans Health Program. Judicial review of decisions of the BVA is available to to the U.S. Court of Appeals for Veterans Claims, a special Article I court under the federal Constitution.[150] However, in the case of a finding of material fact made in reaching a decision in a case before the department with respect to veterans' benefits, the standard for review of a finding is clearly erroneous. The U.S. Court of Appeals for the Federal Circuit may review Veterans Court decisions on issues of law.[151]

TORT CAUSES OF ACTION

The law of torts offers several theories for advancing consumer complaints. Tort remedies are pursued through state courts, unless there is a state statute imposing an alternative method for handling the tort claim. Many states have modified the common law tort system for the adjudication of medical malpractice claims,[152] but have not changed other tort causes of action relevant to consumer quality concerns. While many have criticized the common tort system as being inefficient and irrational,[153] recent empirical studies suggest that such critiques of the tort system are not accurate and that the tort system does perform relatively well.[154]

An important concern about tort reform is measures that reduce provider and health plan exposure to malpractice claims but also compromise access to the tort system for the uninsured poor. A noteworthy example of such a tort reform is 1995 legislation making federally funded community health centers, which expressly serve the poor and uninsured federal employees for purposes of malpractice claims.[155] Thus, clients of community health centers, who are by definition poor, must pursue their medical liability claims under the Federal Tort Claims Act[156] rather than the more familiar state court system.[157] While such tort reform is beneficial to providers, it places extensive burdens on the most vulnerable health-care consumers in pressing legitimate disputes about their health care. Such ramifications are unfortunate and should be considered when contemplating any legislative change to the common law tort system.

The Tort of Medical Malpractice to Address Quality Concerns

Medical malpractice ostensibly addresses a very different type of issue—situations in which the quality of medical care does not meet generally accepted professional standards and that inadequate care causes injury. Medical malpractice is the tort of negligence committed by physicians and other health-care professionals. Processes for bringing medical malpractice lawsuits vary among states, for medical malpractice litigation has been the subject of tort reform efforts since the 1970s. Some states have external review of medical malpractice claims independent of courts.[158] Basically, these are medical review panels, which are convened by the state department of insurance or some other state agency.[159] The model for many state programs is the medical review panel system in Indiana, which has been in place since 1975 without a successful judicial challenge.[160] At least two states, Virginia and Florida, have enacted no-fault administrative systems to adjudicate malpractice claims involving catastrophic obstetric injuries.[161]

Of all consumer health-care disputes, probably most is known empirically about medical malpractice claims. As suggested by Felstiner and his colleagues (see chap. 5),[162] all people with actionable claims regarding medical injury do not bring malpractice suits. Research indicates that there is no consistent correspondence in patient injury and the filing of a malpractice claim and that many malpractice suits do not involve medical injury.[163] Further, pressing a medical malpractice claim is an expensive proposition, and many claimants' attorneys are reluctant to bring small claims.[164]

The Tort of Bad Faith Breach to Challenge Coverage Denials

The tort of bad faith breach allows for recovery in disputes between an insured and an HMO or some other insurer over bad faith coverage denials and other forms of misconduct.[165] This theory provides tort along with contract remedies for the insured when the insurance company acts in bad faith in rejecting a claim. The cause of action in some states has developed as essentially a contract action with contract damages and also as a tort action with damages for emotional injury and other noncontract injuries. Most states recognize a tort cause of action for insurer conduct that goes beyond lack of good faith or negligence but demonstrates that the insurer had no reasonable basis, whether actual or perceived, for its conduct.[166]

Tort Actions to Challenge Denials of Care

Uninsured poor people have often sought to enhance access to needed health-care services through a variety of tort theories.[167] Although neither the law of torts nor that of contracts requires physicians and institutional providers to serve the uninsured, several state courts have imposed liability in tort for a hospital's failure to provide emergency services, particularly when it operates emergency rooms for the public or has a type of corporate control that otherwise requires care for the indigent.[168] Departing from the tort theory that liability attaches for negligent conduct once an individual has begun to rescue another to whom no duty was owed initially,[169] courts have imposed liability on providers that have initiated treatment for an uninsured individual who lacks the funds to pay for care.[170] These later cases have often been based on a strained malpractice theory that the physician's termination of care constituted malpractice.[171]

Nevertheless, these tort causes of action are highly inefficient vehicles for handling the health-care concerns of the uninsured. Yet often they are the only means available for an uninsured consumer to access a legal institution to seek legal redress because grievance procedures and administrative review are often available only to insured consumers in health plans. Further, while the uninsured do have access to provider complaint-and-grievance procedures, they may feel constrained from pressing complaints against a provider that offers them uncompensated care and may be their only source of care in the future.

Federal Preemption of State Tort Causes of Action and Remedies

For most plans regulated under federal law, there is the question of whether a common law tort cause of action under state law is preempted by federal law. Affected plans include ERISA, the FEHBP, CHAMPUS, and the Medicare program.

The most controversial federal preemption is the provision in ERISA that preempts all state laws that relate to ERISA-regulated employee benefit plans.[172] The statutory provisions for this preemption scheme are described earlier in this chapter and in chapter 4. In brief, in *Pilot Life Insurance Co. v. Dedeaux*,[173] the Supreme Court ruled that ERISA provided exclusive remedies for employer violation of plan requirements and preempted state causes of action in tort for bad faith breach against employee welfare benefit plans and the commercial insurers that funded these plans. The Court concluded that a plan participant or beneficiary may recover benefits under the civil enforcement provisions of Section 502(a).[174]

A controversial issue in recent years is the degree to which these enforcement provisions as well as the ERISA preemption clause generally supplant other state common law tort causes of action besides bad faith breach. Courts have exhibited considerable confusion about whether ERISA preemption principles preclude relief under state tort causes of action.[175] Courts have permitted tort claims based on vicarious liability and direct negligence theories. Further, they permit challenges based on the quality of plan service or the design of plan policies and procedures. However, they have precluded challenges to plan decisionmaking about benefits and claims.

The ERISA preemption poses a significant barrier to individuals who have had a dispute with the plan over coverage of benefits or the quality of benefits accorded by plan providers and have sought to obtain damages and other relief through tort causes of action. Many states are concerned about ERISA's preemption of state law remedies for managed care plans, and some states have enacted legislation making it easier to sue health plans in spite of the ERISA preemption.[176] At least one federal court has ruled that ERISA preempts these state reform laws to the extent that they impose obligations on employee welfare benefit plans.[177] Further, as discussed in chapter 2, plan liability for decisions of plan physicians has been a most contentious issue in the debate over patient protection legislation and a major reason for its demise.

The issue of federal preemption of tort remedies has arisen in other contexts. With respect to the FEHBP, the federal government asserts that state law tort causes of action are preempted by federal law. However, courts are split as to whether there is federal preemption of any description.[178] Interestingly, some courts have recognized that Medicare beneficiaries may bring state tort claims against Medicare HMOs.[179]

CONTRACT CAUSES OF ACTION

Another important source of common law judicial remedies for a subset of consumer concerns about health care is the law of contract. Specifically, if the consumer has a contract with a plan or provider that has generated the concern and that concern constitutes a violation of the contract, then breach of the contract may have occurred and contract remedies may be available. Despite the major role of the law of contract in organizing the relationships for consumers in the American health-care sector (see chap. 4), consumers do not often resort to suits in contract to protect their health-care interests.

There are several reasons for this limited role of contract remedies in addressing consumer concerns about health care. Other than billing disputes, most concerns that consumers have with providers concern the quality of the rendered health-care services. The effective remedies for these concerns, such as damages for personal injury, are generally available in tort. Consumers that have private health insurance have contractual remedies against health plans and health plan sponsors. However, as discussed above, members of ERISA-regulated plans have only those remedies available under ERISA due to ERISA's preemption of state common law. Furthermore, as discussed above, consumer actions for bad faith breach are tort rather than contract actions in most states.

STATUTORY CAUSES OF ACTIONS

There are many statutory causes of action under both state and federal law. These statutory causes of action are generally based on statutory mandates to provide emergency and other services to the uninsured poor who are unable to pay for care. Consequently, these statutory causes of action are extremely important, albeit incomplete, sources of remedies for the uninsured poor who seek needed health-care services.

There are several federal statutory causes of action designed to facilitate access to health-care facilities and services. Some arise out of statutory obligations for hospitals and other health-care facilities to provide emergency services to the indigent without health insurance coverage. A second group is statutes that prohibit discrimination on the basis of disability or other specified characteristics.

The Hill-Burton Community Service Assurance. The Hill-Burton community service assurance requires hospitals that receive Hill-Burton grants, loans, or loan guarantees for the construction or expansion of their facilities not to discriminate on the basis of race, creed, color, national origin, or ability to pay.[180] This antidiscrimination provision requires that Hill-Burton hospitals be open to all in the relevant geographic area and not discriminate against individuals in need of emergency services who are unable to pay for care.[181] In *Cook v. Ochsner Foundation Hospital,*[182] a federal district court recognized an implied private right of action for consumers to challenge the Hill-Burton obligations.[183] In the National Health Planning and Resources Development Act of 1974,[184] Congress restated the obligation and further authorized a private right of action if the Department of Health and Human Services does not take action on the complaint.

The Emergency Medical Treatment and Active Labor Act. The Emergency Medical Treatment and Active Labor Act (EMTALA) requires, as a condition of receiving Medicare funding, that hospitals screen and stabilize all patients presenting for emergency treatment.[185] In addition to administrative imposition of civil penalties,[186] the EMTALA authorizes a private cause of action in tort for damage and equitable relief for aggrieved parties.[187]

There has been much controversy over the scope of the EMTALA as consumers have sought to use the statute to enhance access to health-care services. Courts have generally refused to impose additional duties on hospitals beyond stabilization and have not considered health insurance status as a justification for further access.[188] Courts have also resisted expanding the private cause of action under the EMTALA to include conventional medical malpractice claims.[189]

The Americans with Disabilities Act and Other Federal Civil Rights Laws. Federal civil rights laws prohibit discrimination on the basis of race, religion, national origin, age, and gender.[190] The Americans with Disabilities Act of 1990 (ADA) prohibits discrimination on the basis of disability.[191] The ADA tracks the language of Section 504 of the Rehabilitation Act of 1973, which prohibits discrimination on the basis of disability in federally funded programs or services.[192] Discrimination on the basis of disability with respect to health care is difficult to determine because decisions about services are predicated on clinical decisions about disability and disease. Thus, it is often difficult to distinguish between a clinical decision not to treat on medical grounds and an act of discrimination on disability grounds.

Many disability discrimination cases have involved patients with AIDS whom providers have refused to serve[193] and also situations in which providers have refused health-care services on grounds that they would be futile.[194] The ADA has a potentially crucial effect with respect to discrimination by employer-sponsored health plans against people with specific types of disabilities that generate heavy medical expenses.[195] Recently, in *John Doe and Richard Smith v. Mutual of Omaha Insurance Company*,[196] the Supreme Court ruled that caps in insurance policies for the care of AIDS or AIDS-related complex did not violate the ADA provision prohibiting discrimination in public accommodations, and interpretation of the ADA to prohibit such caps was barred by the McCarran-Ferguson Act.[197] This decision limits the usefulness of the ADA in challenges to the benefit and coverage policies of health plans that exclude or limit coverage for specific, potentially costly diseases.

State Statutory Causes of Action to Challenge Denials of Care

Many states have imposed obligations by statute on public and private not-for-profit hospitals to provide emergency services. Specifically, several states have statutes that set an emergency standard of care and define guidelines for hospital transfers.[198] Other states require hospitals to offer emergency services to all persons regardless of ability to pay as a condition of licensure.[199] At least one state, Virginia, requires licensed hospitals that provide obstetric services to establish protocol for the admission or transfer of all pregnant woman in labor.[200] In addition, most states have civil rights laws that prohibit discrimination on the basis of race, religion, national origin, and gender.[201]

9 : Principles of Sound Procedural Protections

This chapter presents principles of sound procedural protections for all patients and consumers of health care in the United States, including the uninsured.[1] Presented first are principles for making health-care policies that affect the content, quality, and price of and access to health care. Presented second are principles for sound procedures for adjudicating the concerns of consumers about their health care. These principles should serve as criteria for evaluating the fairness and justice of procedures for making health-care policies and adjudicating concerns about health care. Policies made utilizing these procedures should have validity, credibility, and democratic legitimacy. Disputes adjudicated in procedures conforming to these principles should be settled fairly and justly.

These proposed principles are offered with the recognition that, in truth, little is known about the nature and extent of consumers' concerns about their health care, their knowledge of and participation in health-care policymaking, or their use of existing legal processes to adjudicate concerns. This lack of empirical information greatly inhibits efforts to design effective reforms. Thus, this chapter closes with a plea for more empirical research on these issues.

PRINCIPLES OF SOUND POLICYMAKING PROCEDURES

All health-care policy and the standards of care that inform such policy should exhibit three core values: (1) validity; (2) credibility; and (3) democratic legitimacy. The values of validity and credibility address the reasonableness and scientific accuracy of a policy. The value of democratic legitimacy addresses the process by which policy is made.

If policies were made with these three core values in mind, physicians would view them as scientifically based and consistent with clinical experience and would therefore not feel constrained in recommending courses of care in line with them even when that care is more conservative and less costly than other treatment options. Patients would have confidence in their physicians' recommendations, particularly if those recommendations were demonstrably consistent with sound medical standards of care developed by prestigious and credible medical organizations and accrediting bodies. Decisions about care made in these circumstances would hopefully be less likely to lead to patient concerns about poor quality care, coverage denials, or other matters affected by health-care policies.

Presented below are four principles for fair and accurate policymaking procedures that directly govern the content, quality, and cost of health-care services as well as access to these services for all consumers of health care. These principles should assist consumers, providers, payers, and policymakers in evaluating policies pertaining to health care as well as the standards of care that inform such policies. Policymaking procedures conforming to these four criteria should exemplify the core values of validity, credibility, and democratic legitimacy. These principles are the following:

—A designated process must exist for adopting any policy that significantly affects the interests of consumers in health care or any standard of care used in the formulation of such policy.

—Procedures should assure that relevant scientific and clinical information is marshaled, made available, and expertly considered by the decisionmakers formulating policies.

—Procedures should exist that provide consumers with an opportunity to influence the content of policies should they desire to do so even after organizations have adopted the policies.

—All policies must be publicized and easily accessible to consumers as well as physicians and other health-care providers.

Designated Process for the Adoption of Policies

The first principle, a designated process for policy adoption, is essential for making all policies and standards of care that significantly affect the interests of health-care consumers. The concept embodied in this first principle is the identification of decisions that are, as a practical matter, policies that will define the content, coverage, quality, and price of health-care services. This concept goes to the democratic legitimacy of the policy.

Two issues are important with respect to this criterion. First is a consciousness that the organization is indeed making policy that will substantially affect the interests of health-care consumers. Second, the organization must consider how that policy is made and publicized and design procedures to follow in making the policy.

This first issue is significant. It is likely that many organizations, especially private corporations, are often not conscious of the fact that their policies significantly affect the interests of health-care consumers. For example, in the early years of the Medicare program, Medicare carriers and fiscal intermediaries seemed unaware of how their coverage policies affected program beneficiaries. In later years, they become more careful and formal about coverage policymaking only after pressure from patient advocates and the medical device industry.[2]

The second issue pertains to the processes employed in making policy of interest to consumers and their health-care providers. In public agencies, statutes and published agency procedural rules generally outline the internal procedures for making policy and, in some cases, impose comparable structural characteristics on policymaking processes. However, public agencies do not always use explicit policymaking processes for making health-care policy. Specifically, when they contract with managed care organizations (MCOs) and other private health plan sponsors to purchase a health plan for their beneficiaries, the contract often contains relevant policy not made in established agency processes.

In a private organization, processes for making policies are generally not subject to legal mandates. Thus, the design and implementation of policymaking procedures are determined by the organization, and a wide range of choices exist as to the processes for making policies. Specifically, will policies be made by a single individual and simply recorded in corporate files to be used by staff as needed? Or will they be made in a more formal process by designated individuals or bodies with a publicized agenda, formal adoption procedures, and, perhaps, opportunity for outside input? Obviously, a policy position that is made by a few individuals with an established point of view is markedly different than one adopted in a designated process, such as a committee process with scientific and clinical input or a formal adoption process in a constituent assembly.

As indicated, the internal structural characteristics of an organization involved in policymaking are useful in assuring a sound policymaking process. Especially important in this regard are a representative governing board, published bylaws, the public election of board members and officers, a constituent assembly, a federated structure, and a nonexclusive membership policy. The presence of these structural characteristics and their use in a policymaking process are good indicators that the policymaking process is sound and that resulting policies have credibility and democratic legitimacy.

Private medical organizations, voluntary health organizations, and private accrediting bodies are more likely to have the structural characteristics that accord credibility and democratic legitimacy to their standards of care. Specifically, private medical associations and voluntary health organizations may have processes through which their membership, for example, in constituent assemblies, formally adopts the policies that the organizations endorse. With respect to medical practice guidelines and standards of quality made by private medical organizations and quality performance measures made by private accrediting bodies, formal committees may make such standards of care, which are then recognized as organization policy. In some cases, the organization's board of directors or constituent assembly may give its imprimatur to the policy. Such procedures accord credibility, democratic legitimacy, and, presumably, even scientific validity to the policy.

Regarding coverage and pricing policies of public and private health plans, the situation is quite varied. The Medicare program has the most institutionalized process for making both coverage policy. State insurance regulation sets forth criteria for coverage and payment policy and, in most states, requires state-regulated health insurers to file health insurance contracts with the state insurance commissioner to ensure compliance with regulatory requirements. Also, the states that regulate hospital payment rates have criteria for reviewing those rates. Otherwise, public and private health plan sponsors make coverage and payment policy virtually in private.

The selective contracting processes that public and private health plan sponsors use to contract with health plans and providers for their beneficiaries are, frankly, problematic. Selecting contracting processes are not generally public. While the specifications for coverage and pricing in requests for proposals may be available publicly, they are not published in readily accessible formats. Further, the contracts with health maintenance organizations (HMOs), provider networks, and other providers establishing the plans are not generally published, nor are they readily available to consumers in an accessible format. The contracts are generally so technical and long that they are inaccessible to all but the most knowledgeable consumers. While these characteristics of the contracting process are probably unavoidable, more thought and theory are necessary to accord validity, credibility, and democratic legitimacy to the contracting process and the health-care policies embedded in these contracts.

Serious problems also exist with respect to policymaking procedures for medical review criteria used by health plans. In many cases, health plans are insensitive to the fact that these medical review criteria affect the interests of health-care consumers. The procedures for making medical review criteria are less formal, if they exist at all. Their publication and availability to consumers have been a major reform proposed in patient protection legislation before recent congresses. While it is unlikely that most medical review criteria (e.g., screens that identify problem claims) would be determined in an open policymaking process, health plans should be conscious of the importance of these policies and specify internally the processes by which they are made, maintained, and publicized. Further, medical review criteria should be informed by the credible medical practice guidelines and medical quality standards of medical professional associations and private accrediting bodies. Medical review criteria that are based on business assessments of legal liability risks and financial considerations—such as those that have been used by some managed care companies in the treatment of diabetes—are completely inappropriate.[3]

Similarly, institutional providers do not generally utilize formal processes when making policies regarding the terms of access to and the pricing of their services. Nor are these policies usually publicized or otherwise made available to consumers. In many cases, they are corporate decisions that may or may not be formulated and recorded as corporate policies. Consequently, these policies are extremely difficult for consumers to access. Here again, a consciousness that the organization is making policy that significantly affects the health-care interests of consumers is warranted. Institutional providers should designate a process for making, and maintaining, and even publicizing policies that set prices or govern access to health care.

It is not meant to suggest that all policies of health-care plans and providers that affect health care must be made in formal processes with consumer participation and subsequent publication. Such an eventuality would be neither possible, practical, nor desirable. However, health plans, health-care providers, and their policymakers should be conscious of the fact that they are constantly making policies that affect the interests of health-care consumers. They must therefore be sensitive to when such policy should be made in a designated process and when the making of that policy warrants outside input and subsequent publication.

Procedures to Enhance and Assure Scientific Accuracy

The second principle for fair and accurate policymaking procedures addresses the scientific and clinical integrity of policies with medical content—hence their validity and credibility. This principle is extremely important to all policies relating to the quality and coverage and also the cost of health-care services and the standards of care developed by private organizations and public agencies. The Centers for Medicare and Medicaid Services (CMS)—formerly the Health Care Financing Administration (HCFA)—and many private medical organizations have policymaking processes designed to marshal expertise, formulate professional consensus, and achieve formal adoption by appropriately designated bodies such as elected officers or even constituent assemblies. These procedures enhance the credibility and democratic legitimacy of the policies.

The key question is the degree to which procedures are designed to assure the accuracy of the policy. Health researchers have given much attention to this issue and have developed policymaking theory that goes beyond the notice-and-comment model of prevailing administrative law theory. In addition to process, they have given much attention to the nature of the medical evidence needed to justify the policy and confirm its scientific accuracy. The demand for high quality medical evidence to support medical practice guidelines and other medical standards of care has done much to provide guidance to providers and payers alike in the financing and delivery of high quality care in the United States.

Opportunity for Consumer Input

The third principle for fair and accurate policymaking procedures is that a process should exist that provides consumers with an opportunity to influence the content of relevant policies should they desire to do so—even after an organization has adopted those policies. Consumer involvement in policymaking is an intractably difficult issue. Two major, virtually insurmountable barriers exist in achieving genuine consumer involvement in policymaking.

First, individual consumers generally do not have sufficient medical knowledge to make informed decisions about the accuracy of a medical standard of care. Even organizations that represent consumers do not have this information unless they retain their own medical experts. Second, given that there are many complicated policies affecting the health care of particular consumers, it is difficult for any consumer to be sufficiently familiar with all all of them. Further, consumers have little motivation to be involved. Unless they have a choice among health plans, they are unlikely to conduct a careful study of the policies delineating the content, quality, and cost of health care. In reality, most consumers are actively concerned about a policy only when they have been negatively affected by that policy, that is, when they or their family members are sick. Often, in this situation, they are looking at short term concerns rather than taking a long term view of future needs.

Frankly, however, it is difficult to envision strategies that will adequately address these two barriers. For example, it is not sufficient simply to publish a notice that a policy is being made and then wait for affected consumers to provide input. Nor is it sufficient to conclude that organizations that historically represent consumer interests will do so adequately in health-care policymaking processes. Other strategies must be devised to involve health-care consumers or representatives truly acting on their behalf. Many scholars have struggled with this problem and suggested ideas for enhancing consumer protection, such as putting consumer representatives on MCO boards and requiring MCOs to take account of consumer views about their policies and procedures.[4]

One problem in harnessing consumer representation in policymaking processes is the limitations of organizations advocating for consumers. There are numerous consumer advocacy programs—such as the National Health Law Program, the National Senior Citizens Law Center, the Medicare Advocacy Center, the Children's Defense Fund, the American Association of Retired Persons, and Families USA—that served as powerful and distinct voices on behalf of consumers and their health care, especially with respect to state and federal legislation. However, these organizations generally do not have the requisite medical expertise to become effectively involved in processes for establishing medical standards of care. In this regard, voluntary health organizations—with their combined professional and nonprofessional membership—have been far more effective advocates for consumers in making health-care policies for specific diseases.

One helpful strategy would be to permit consumers to challenge the validity or appropriateness of a policy when it is invoked against them in a coverage or quality dispute. To do so, consumers would clearly need to present their own expert testimony, which would be costly. While this sounds radical and is also a potential nightmare for insurers, which want and need certainty when determining risk, this approach enables consumers to have real input into the content of policy at a time when they have the greatest incentive to do so. If responsible parties permit flexibility in the application of a policy, then consumers have the opportunity to make a persuasive case that a policy is inappropriate and, at least, should not be applied in their case. To the extent that disputed coverage denials reach the courts, judges and juries decide the appropriateness of the application of a medical standard of care. Such flexibility could be accorded in grievance-and-appeal procedures, thus permitting consumers to challenge policies that might not have been applied appropriately.

Another approach is to appreciate the potential role of voluntary health organizations in serving consumer interests in the formation of health-care policies regarding quality and coverage. Voluntary health organizations are unique in that they have consumer members who are vitally concerned about progress in the treatment and cure of a particular disease and therefore have a direct and current interest in health-care policy, albeit with a narrow focus. Physicians and other health-care professionals are also involved with voluntary health organizations. They bring specialized knowledge and expertise to bear when the voluntary health organization is making health-care policy or is involved in the policymaking processes of other organizations or government. This combination of consumers and experts is potentially a great resource to be mobilized on behalf of the protection of the interests of individuals in their health care.

Publication

The fourth principle for fair and accurate policymaking procedures—publication—is essential for a policy's democratic legitimacy. Publication also serves to improve the validity and ultimately the credibility of a policy. Further, publication is important for medical standards of care and policies based on these standards to ensure greater scientific validity as policymakers would presumably be more careful knowing that policy would be accessible to the public and their peers. In sum, publication is essential for ensuring the accountability of policymakers.

Publication of all policy is also necessary if consumers are to make informed choices about the health care that they need and the providers and health plans that can provide such care. For example, with respect to health plans, it is just as important to publish the medical review criteria used in the implementation of coverage policy as it is to publish the coverage policy itself. Use of unpublished and essentially secret medical review criteria, in the form of computer "screens" and algorithms, has been problematic. Indeed, most federal patient protection legislative proposals discussed in chapter 2 have called for the express publication of such policy. This example clearly exemplifies the problem if relevant health-care policy is not publicized and made available to consumers.

PRINCIPLES FOR BETTER WAYS TO TAP AND RESOLVE CONSUMER CONCERNS ABOUT HEALTH CARE

The principles of a theory of procedure should appropriately proceed from the proposition that the goal of any procedure is to be fair. As discussed in chapter 1, the concept of fairness in Western legal thought is generally aligned with equal treatment in a given procedural context. In other words, as long as adversaries in a given proceeding are treated equally by the manager of the process, the process is deemed to be fair. Assuring the fairness of a process also accommodates differences in status and power among parties associated with socioeconomic and other cultural factors, with a view toward mitigating these power differences in the proceeding. It is not enough simply to treat parties equally; accommodating differences in power is essential.

For the purposes of this discussion, an adjudicative procedure is probably fair when all disputants believe that, at the inception of the process, the requisite procedural characteristics are present to assure that the process will enable the development and consideration of all relevant evidence and arguments by all parties and, at the end of the process, disputants will remain satisfied with the process regardless of its outcome. A fair procedure should have the effect of leaving all participants with the legitimate perception that—regardless of outcome—their concerns have been taken seriously, that the ultimate decision has been based on appropriate facts and policies, and that they have had adequate opportunity to present their case.

Seven principles clearly influence the fairness of procedures for tapping and resolving consumer concerns about health care. These principles are as follows:

—Voice and Resolve Consumer Concerns Early in a Nonconfrontational Forum. There should be a process prior to the invocation of more formal legal procedures enabling consumers to voice their concerns about health care and have these concerns rectified in a satisfactory manner. Efforts should be made to link these processes with quality assurance mechanisms that identify problems with health-care services that might remain unidentified.

—Address Power Disparities between Consumers and Plans and/or Providers. Consumers should have adequate status and power in any dispute resolution process, including contractual and judicially supervised alternative dispute resolution (ADR) procedures, vis-à-vis providers and plans to assure that they are likely to prevail if the merits of their case warrant it.

—Simplify and Consolidate Dispute Resolution Processes. The grievance-and-appeal procedures of providers and health plans should be as simple and comprehensible as possible, coordinated with one another whenever possible, and expansive enough to address as many of the different types of consumer concerns about health care as possible.

—Ensure Access to Adjudicative Procedures for the Uninsured. Uninsured consumers have limited access to more informal, less costly dispute resolution procedures, which are customarily available only to members of health plans. They need forums to raise and resolve concerns as at present they can, as a practical matter, resort only to court proceedings or providers' customer relations programs.

—Design Nonjudicial Adjudicative Procedures That Empower Consumers and Achieve Fairness. Adjudicative procedures for resolving consumer concerns should ensure accurate and complete consideration of the consumer's concern and accord the greatest opportunity for an accurate and fair decision by an unbiased decisionmaker.

—Ensure Access to Relevant Policy and Expert Opinion. Consumers should have timely and complete access to the relevant policies governing the subject matter of their concern or dispute. More important, when necessary, they should have access to independent expert medical opinion to evaluate the application to their situation of policies with medical content.

—Ensure the Legal Accountability of Public and Private Health Plans and Providers. This effort involves documentation of the demise of constitutional and common law tort doctrines that have historically enforced the accountability of sponsors of public and private health plans. It also calls for the development of legal doctrines and requirements that assure that providers and especially health plans and their sponsors are required to provide pro-

cedures for tapping and resolving consumer concerns about health care and otherwise protect the interests of the consumer.

Voice and Resolve Consumer Concerns Early in a Nonconfrontational Forum

Provider organizations and health plans should establish a concrete process in an established location to enable consumers to identify and voice their concerns about health care and have these concerns rectified in a satisfactory manner in a nonconfrontational forum prior to the invocation of more formal legal procedures. This process should be closely linked to the institution's quality assurance and risk management programs. Most health plans and providers have informal processes for consumers to present concerns about health care. These processes often take the form of a complaint department or even an ombudsman office.

Characteristics of the Process. These processes must have goals beyond just ameliorating patient concerns in order to discourage lawsuits or complying with legal mandates. They must seek genuine resolution, including even appropriate compensation, of legitimate consumer complaints about their health care. Specifically, such processes should have the following characteristics to function effectively for the genuine protection of consumers. First, they should be located in identifiable offices that are known and easily accessible to consumers at the time they seek and obtain health care—not just after an incident arises. Second, the process should provide a means through which a consumer can voice a concern and be assured that the responsible parties within the provider or plan have at least heard and considered the concern. The managers of the process should have the authority to apologize on behalf of the organization as well as provide compensation if necessary. Consumers often proceed to litigation more to attract the attention of the wrongdoer than to obtain legal redress.

If underlying facts are in dispute and/or some remedy other than an apology is called for, the process should have established procedures in place for resolving factual issues and making decisions. One crucial element of this early dispute resolution process is the right to "discovery," which enables consumers to get more information about the underlying facts giving rise to a concern without having to resort to a more formal legal process. For example, such a process would get all relevant medical records and any plan or provider policies regarding coverage and quality. Such information would be helpful in the early resolution of disputes over breaches of technical competence or coverage disputes—both of which generally involve technical medical facts. In addition, discovery opportunities designed to get at explanations of situations giving rise to breaches of interpersonal competence could be very useful in defusing tensions and resolving concerns.

Perhaps most important, discovery should permit a consumer to determine whether the injury sustained is serious enough to warrant tort damages. In that event, the process should accommodate the consumer's retention of legal counsel and the involvement of the relevant insurance carriers in determining damages and arranging for compensation. In no event should the early dispute resolution process endeavor to "buy off" a consumer with a serious claim, withhold information about the seriousness of a claim, or deny damages to which a consumer is entitled under law.

Regarding redress and remedies, the complaint department or ombudsman office should have the discretion and flexibility to craft mutually satisfactory settlements, including the payment of monetary compensation. In the final disposition of the matter, the office should send the consumer a letter explaining the disposition of the concern and the perspective of the provider or plan regarding its disposition, a letter written in nonbureaucratic, respectful, and humane language. Furnishing an aggrieved consumer with a written explanation of the decision, including an apology if appropriate and even monetary relief, can do much to ameliorate the situation. Besides avoiding future litigation, it is the right thing to do. However, it is difficult and sometimes even unfair to require a plan or provider to provide a written apology, especially if future litigation is a real possibility.

Relations with Quality Assurance and Risk Management. Another important characteristic of early identification and resolution is actually identifying most, if not all, consumer concerns in a systematic process. Specifically, tapping patient satisfaction through a quality assessment process that utilizes surveys has enormous potential for generating information about issues that concern consumers. A sound consumer satisfaction survey and data collection process can provide crucial information about the incidence, prevalence, and scope of consumer issues as well as what factors may influence their development. These data can inform appropriate reforms and reduce consumer concerns in the future.

A consumer satisfaction survey may identify consumer concerns that warrant redress but that might not otherwise surface. Such use of consumer satisfaction data is unlikely except when an exceptionally serious injury has occurred. It cannot realistically be expected that either providers or plans will take affirmative action to redress concerns unless the consumer steps forward and complains. Not all consumers will complain, for the complaint process is time consuming and involved. Nevertheless, in a perfect world, the early dispute resolution process would endeavor to resolve concerns identified in the quality assurance and risk management programs even when consumers do not step forward.

Address Power Disparities between Consumers and Plans and/or Providers

Consumers should have adequate status and power in any dispute resolution process vis-à-vis providers and plans to assure that their concerns are fairly adjudicated. Perhaps the greatest problem in current systems is the power imbalance between consumers and their health-care provider or plan, an imbalance manifested in two major ways.

First, there is an imbalance in knowledge, particularly medical knowledge, of the matters at issue in the dispute. Consumers with little medical knowledge are inevitably and inherently disadvantaged in several respects. Often, they cannot recognize that they even have cause for concern, especially when breaches of technical competence and denials of care that occur in a clinical context are involved. Consumers also often have difficulty accurately conceptualizing their concerns in a way that will command a remedy. This disadvantage is enhanced when they are poor, uneducated, and sick.

Second, there is an imbalance of power when providers and plans control the dispute resolution process. Extralegal processes, such as grievance-and-appeal and ADR procedures, are usually administered and often "owned" by the plan or provider against which a complaint is raised. In such cases, the plan and/or provider has control over access to the medical facts underlying the dispute and may not necessarily make this information available to the consumer. Consumers, particularly those of lower socioeconomic backgrounds, are especially powerless in this situation because they have fewer monetary and other resources enabling them to obtain the legal and medical expertise needed to press concerns effectively. Uninsured consumers are, for obvious reasons, even more powerless.

The power imbalance between consumers and health plans and providers in health-care disputes is especially problematic in contractual arrangements for dispute resolution. Clearly, contract enables opportunities for the development of innovative dispute resolution arrangement in lieu of the common law tort system—provided that the parties involved have adequate bargaining power to influence the terms of the contract. Nevertheless, the use of contractual internal review procedures is problematic in the health-care context, especially when plans or providers require consumers to sign contracts to use binding ADR as a condition of enrollment or treatment. As a practical matter, consumers have no say in the imposition of these ADR arrangements in health plan contracts, which are usually made between employers or other sponsors of health plans and MCOs. Thus, it is inappropriate to defend contractual ADR on the grounds of consumer choice. Rather, the process must be defended on the grounds that it saves costs, promotes justice, or achieves other policy goals.

It is significant that the American Arbitration Association/American Medical Association/American Bar Association task force recommended that binding ADR be used only where both parties agree to it after the dispute arises.[5] This should be the norm. It is hard to believe that health-care consumers ever have the requisite information or appreciation of the consequences to make truly informed decisions prior to a dispute. Yet, at the time a dispute arises, consumers may well find that an ADR process that offers faster relief than the civil judicial process might be very attractive and should be available.

Finally, the imbalance of power between consumers and their health plans and providers is greatly exacerbated by the inadequacy of current legal doctrines to ensure accountability of public and private health plans (discussed below). Specifically, these doctrines result in diminished procedural due process protections for consumers in managed care plans and limited access to the tort system for enrollees in plans subject to preemptions of state common law.

Simplify Dispute Resolution Processes

All consumers should have access to simple and comprehensible processes to raise all their concerns about their health care. Simplicity and comprehensiveness require reforms on several fronts. First is coordination of health plan grievance-and-appeal procedures for the insured. Internal review (e.g., grievance-and-appeal procedures, most external review, and administrative review) is available only to consumers in health plans. Second is access to comprehensive dispute resolution processes for the un-insured—an issue addressed in the next section.

For the insured, procedures differ markedly depending on the type of health plan in which the consumer is enrolled, the sponsor of the health plan, and the subject matter of the consumer concern. Now, the physical location and management of the review process vary among health plans and are not always evident to consumers. For plans regulated by the Employee Retirement Income Security Act (ERISA), the grievance-and-appeal process may be housed in the employer's personnel department or the offices of a third party administrator. If the employer-sponsored plan has contracted with an HMO, the consumer may proceed through the HMO's grievance-and-appeal procedures. A Medicaid recipient in the same HMO would proceed through the HMO's grievance-and-appeal procedures for Medicaid recipients with an opportunity for administrative review before the state agency. A Medicare recipient in the same HMO would proceed through the HMO's grievance-and-appeal procedure for Medicare bene-ficiaries and then onto external review for reconsideration and further administrative review. An individual who joined the HMO independently would have access to the HMO's grievance-and-appeal process and possibly further external review, depending on the state. These differences in pro-cedural arrangements makes little intuitive sense to consumers, who are largely unfamiliar with the administrative arrangements and the sponsor-ship of their health plan.

Then there are the grievance procedures of institutional providers and the ADR procedures established pursuant to contracts between providers and consumers at the inception of care. These procedures generally ad-judicate a different set of issues. It should be noted that the uninsured, if treated by the provider, have access to these procedures. However, they may well be reluctant to use them given fears about future access to free or lower cost care from that provider.

The selection of the grievance-and-appeal system often depends on the subject of the concern in question. It is often not apparent to consumers that different concerns are adjudicated in different venues. (The array of consumer concerns about access, quality, and cost are displayed in table 2 (see chap. 5).) Nor is it always clear to consumers which venue provides the best forum. Consumers may in fact have to litigate the same set of facts in several venues—first the health plan's internal processes, next the pro-vider's contractual ADR procedures, and finally state court.

The case of coverage disputes and medical malpractice claims is especially exemplary of this phenomenon. Specifically, malpractice claims are generally brought in state court if not resolved informally through early insurance settlements, having been identified in provider or plan risk management programs. If plan coverage policy or utilization review influenced medical treatment, a claim for bad faith breach against the plan as well as a malpractice claim against the provider may arise out of the same circumstances. If the health plan sponsor is an employer or the federal government, or if the consumer is bound to use binding contractual ADR with either the plan or the provider, state tort remedies may not be available.

Finally, in designing fair procedures for health-care consumers, one must look beyond specific procedures for specific plans or a specific subject matter and consider the possibilities of a more integrated, more inclusive system. Consolidation of dispute resolution procedures for all health plans and providers into a single process within a single organization for a specific geographic region would do much to simplify the maze. President Clinton's executive order implementing the Patient Bill of Rights will do much to integrate and rationalize internal appeal processes for consumers in federally sponsored health insurance and health-care services programs. But more consolidation and inclusion of all processes is needed.

Ensure Access to Adjudicative Procedures for the Uninsured

Uninsured consumers have limited access to more informal, less costly dispute resolution procedures, which are customarily available only to members of health plans. Most mandated grievance procedures and all administrative appeal procedures are available only to members of health plans, who, by definition, are insured. The uninsured basically have three options: (1) internal grievance-and-appeal procedures of providers; (2) common law tort remedies; and (3) state and federal statutory remedies for denials of emergency care in state or federal court. As discussed above, in utilizing providers' internal grievance-and-appeal procedures, the poor justifiably fear compromising future access to care with that provider. Judicial remedies are cumbersome, expensive, and often difficult to access unless the consumer has suffered significant damage and has counsel.

The problems faced by the uninsured in pressing their concerns about health care are serious and have been largely unaddressed in the current patient protection debate at both the state and the federal levels. In part, this deficiency is due to the fact that the problem of lack of insurance has been conceived and addressed in a separate context from the problem of procedural protections for patients in health plans. Consequently, the uninsured are virtually ignored in the patient protection debate and in existing procedures for identifying and resolving consumer concerns. A most important benefit of an independent, integrated dispute resolution institution would be its availability to uninsured consumers with disputes with providers from whom they obtained care and also from whom they sought but were denied care.

Further, when the federal government and the states do establish public programs to expand coverage for the uninsured, they tend to design them in ways that curtail the rights of beneficiaries to challenge the denial of benefits specified by statute. Specifically, in recent legislation establishing the new welfare reform programs—Temporary Assistance for Needy Families and the State Child Health Insurance Program—Congress stated that program benefits were not entitlements, thus eliminating open-ended obligations to actual and potential program clients.[6] Further, courts have supported this arrangement. For example, in *Colson v. Sillman,*[7] the Second Circuit ruled that a program client had no constitutionally protected entitlement interest in program benefits because the enabling legislation accorded discretion to the state in determining need for benefits and limited benefits to those funded from fiscal appropriations. This combination of statutory denial of entitlement and thus property status with subsequent judicial approval and justification spells potential doom for the protection of vulnerable beneficiaries in existing and new public health insurance programs.

Design Nonjudicial Adjudicative Procedures That Empower Consumers and Achieve Fairness

All procedures used to adjudicate and resolve consumer concerns should contain the requisite elements of process to ensure accurate and complete consideration of the consumer's concern and its underlying facts and accord the greatest opportunity for an accurate and fair decision before an unbiased decisionmaker. The design of an adjudicative process determines its ability to achieve the ideals contemplated in this principle.

Much has been written about how to design a fair hearing procedure, particularly for the resolution of health-care disputes. There are several sources of relevant theory regarding what procedural elements assure a fair adjudicative process, including procedural due process jurisprudence, scholarship from the ADR movement, and empirical research from social psychology in addition to a more recent analysis of health-care dispute resolution. Such theory and scholarship endeavor to identify characteristics of fair process through empirical experiments with simulated or actual adjudicative models in which research subjects offer perceptions of the fairness of models with different process elements.[8]

Several important observations can be gleaned from this theoretical work. One major lesson is that no single design or ideal list of process elements guarantees fairness to consumers. However, there are some design approaches that do seem to promote the overall fairness of an adjudicative procedure for health-care disputes. These key elements and the supportive empirical research findings are described below.

Proper Development of Medical Facts. Procedures for the adjudication of medical issues call for special care since health-care disputes often involve medical facts or policies beyond the knowledge of most consumers. Often, ADR processes have limited discovery to save time and money. In such cases, the party with control over the information has a distinct advantage in the proceeding. Discovery rules in ADR proceedings adjudicating health-care disputes must assure that such an unfair advantage does not accrue to providers and health plan sponsors. This element of process is so important that it is the basis of a separate principle described below.

Independence and Authority of the Decisionmaker. The decisionmaker must be knowledgeable and unbiased. This becomes a problem when the plan or provider "owns" the adjudicative process. In *Schweicker v. McClure,*[9] the U.S. Supreme Court clearly rejected the idea that carrier employees serving as decisionmakers in the appeals of Medicare beneficiaries constitutes unconstitutional bias. Nevertheless, the issue of the "ownership" of the decision remains problematic. It is especially so in the context of contractual ADR procedures within health plans. Unlike Medicare hearings before Medicare contractors, there is no public agency or judicial oversight to ensure the accountability of the decisionmaker. Some attention to the process by which decisionmakers are selected may do much to assure their independence. For example, for a three-member panel, each side could appoint one decisionmaker each, and these two could then appoint the third.

In addition, the decisionmaker should have the requisite discretion and authority to decide the matter at hand and to provide relief. The decision-maker should also, like a judge, have the authority to resolve a matter without necessarily adjudicating liability. Such authority would greatly enhance the decisionmaker's ability to resolve disputes in a manner that is satisfactory to all parties. Further, the decisionmaker must be required to adjudicate the matter expeditiously.

Rights to Reconsideration and Judicial Review. Consumers should have the right to reconsideration and judicial review of an adverse decision in any adjudicative proceeding "owned" by the provider or plan. An important issue is the scope of judicial review. Specifically, are courts conducting a complete de novo review of all matters previously adjudicated, or is judicial review limited to whether the initial decision met legal standards, such as lack of bias, no manifest disregard for the law, or was supported by substantial evidence?

According to empirical evidence,[10] the availability of further review greatly enhances litigants' perceptions of the process. It is more likely that consumers will be satisfied with the decision in an internal process if they know that it can be appealed. The availability of review also mitigates the effect of procedures that a participant would otherwise find unfair.[11] Of note, empirical research has found that permitting disputants an opportunity to present their positions and to appeal an unfair decision dramatically improved the perceived fairness of an inquisitorial type process.[12]

Empowerment of Consumers. Methods for empowering consumers should be present in the process. A process should be informal and comprehensive enough so that appeals can be negotiated by consumers themselves (at their option). However, consumers should also have available to them representation by counsel or another advocate of their choice and facilitated access to free legal counsel. Thibaut and Walker, exploring the role of "control" over process and decisions between disputants and the decisionmaker in empirical research, found that disputants with greater power over the presentation of their cases, as in adversary court proceedings, were more likely to perceive that the process was fair.[13]

Numerous organizations exist that have historically been effective in representing consumer interests in adjudicative proceedings. Specifically, the Legal Services Corporation and such organizations as the Medicare Advocacy Center provide an important source of legal counsel for consumers and have often litigated landmark cases that have changed the policies and practices of public and private health plans as well as providers. Voluntary health organizations are, to a lesser extent, also active in judicial advocacy, but they generally press issues of concern to people with a particular disease. The contribution of these organizations to the effective advocacy of consumer interests should be recognized and facilitated.

Interaction of Process Elements. Finally, it is crucial to appreciate the critical influence that the combination and interaction of various elements of an adjudicative proceeding can have on its ultimate fairness. The interaction of different process elements is especially important in empowering consumers in a procedure. Of note, important empirical research found that the interaction of the elements of processes affected perceptions of fairness more than the presence or absence of specific elements.[14]

Furthermore, the elements of process that assure fairness are often very subtle. Seemingly minor features of a process that may be entirely defensible from a policy or even a moral perspective can have a critical impact on the fairness of a process. This important phenomenon is well exemplified by a debate over the elements of the grievance-and-appeal procedures for Medicaid MCOs mandated in the Balanced Budget Act of 1997.[15] In September 1998, the HCFA (now CMS) proposed grievance-and-appeal procedures for MCOs.[16] In the proposed rule, the HCFA decided not to require MCOs to provide complainants with information about legal and patient advocacy services in the area and invited comment on this decision.[17] Yet perhaps no other procedural step could empower poor Medicaid recipients in an appeal against a corporate MCO better than facilitating access to free, knowledgeable legal counsel to assist in the preparation and execution of an appeal. One might suspect that MCOs appreciated this fact and pressed the HCFA on this procedural point.

Ensure Access to Relevant Policy and Expert Opinion

A lack of medical knowledge puts virtually all consumers—irrespective of socioeconomic status—at an inevitable disadvantage vis-à-vis providers and plans. Thus, consumers should have full rights of discovery and credible expert assistance in the development of a case when medical facts are at issue. Specifically, there should be adequate mechanisms for timely and complete access to and discovery of all the medical facts on which a decision is based, including any applicable medical practice guideline or other standard of care used by the plan or provider to govern a prior relevant judgment. Fairness is compromised when the sponsor of the plan also has control over the medical facts and testimony needed to resolve a consumer's dispute.

Further, if medical facts are definitive, consumers should have access to independent expert medical opinion during the process to evaluate the application of policies with medical content to their situation. At the very least, the decisionmaker should have access to neutral expert testimony to evaluate the relevant medical facts in the adjudicative proceeding and in any appeal process. Common law rules of evidence have long relegated the determination of medical issues to expert testimony.[18]

The issue of whether and how to structure fair processes for independent medical review has been critical in the patient protection debate of the late 1990s. Specifically, external review is a central component of the reform proposals of the President's Commission on Consumer Protection and Quality.[19] Many of the patient protection bills before Congress in recent years included provisions for external review of varying designs.[20]

There are various options for the design of independent medical review. Four important design issues are involved: how independent medical reviewers are selected, how the review process is designed, what issues are subject to independent review, and who pays for the review. Ideas for designing independent medical reviews are presented in chapter 10.

In designing independent review systems, some empirical research by Poythress and his colleagues is particularly relevant.[21] In one hybrid model, the judge selected the expert, and, in the other, the judge arranged for an empirical survey of physicians in the relevant field and the geographic area to determine breach of the standard of care. Both hybrid models were perceived to be more just and fair than the purely adversarial model, in which the disputants arranged for their own expert testimony. These findings suggest that designers have considerable flexibility in crafting a fair process for independent review and that the credibility and independence of the expert probably plays the greatest role in assuring fairness from the perspective of consumers.

Ensure the Legal Accountability of Public and Private Health Plans and Providers

Ensuring the legal accountability of public and private health plans and providers has been a most important and problematic issue in recent years. Legal doctrines should be sufficient to ensure the genuine accountability of providers and/or plans, thereby addressing the legitimate concerns of consumers about their health care. But such doctrines are in retreat. There has been a demise of constitutional and common law tort doctrines that have historically enforced the accountability of sponsors of public and private health plans, and there have also been efforts to limit the tort liability of health-care providers through tort reform and contractual ADR.

Receding Constitutional Protections. Procedural due process protections for beneficiaries of public health insurance programs have diminished significantly. The U.S. Supreme Court has issued several decisions recently that bode ill for the promise of due process jurisprudence ensuring the accountability of public health plan sponsors.

If, as suggested in *American Manufacturers Mutual Insurance Company v. Sullivan,*[22] due process protections do not even attach until after a private insurer, which has a contractual relationship with the public agency health plan sponsor, has made a decision on coverage, then beneficiaries have no rights to be heard on coverage denials. Now, health plans can make coverage decisions with impunity, especially with the Court's conclusion that benefits under the public health insurance program do not constitute a protected property interest until the coverage decision is made. This decision effectively removes coverage decisions from judicial oversight and also overrules the Ninth Circuit in *Grijalva v. Shalala,*[23] which reached a contrary decision with respect to Medicare HMOs. The Supreme Court remanded *Grijalva* for further consideration in the light of *American Manufacturers* as well as the grievance-and-appeal procedures in the Balanced Budget Act of 1997 for HMOs in the Medicare+Choice program and the regulations thereunder.[24]

The *American Manufacturers* decision represents a sharp cutback in constitutional procedural protections, which have historically been a great source of empowerment and protection for beneficiaries of public benefit programs. Without this constitutional oversight, sponsors of public health-care programs, and, especially, the private health plan sponsors with whom they contract, have greater latitude to trim benefits inappropriately in meeting cost containment and other goals.

Compromised Access to the Tort System. In recent years, there has been a movement to limit health-care consumers' access to the common law tort system. Consumers do retain limited access to the tort system, which allows them to press certain types of concerns against health plans. But there is confusion as to whether common law tort remedies are available to members of ERISA-regulated and government-sponsored health plans. At common law, insurance companies in most states are subject to the tort of bad faith breach of contract for egregious conduct toward insureds in such matters as coverage decisionmaking. However, this cause of action is not available to all members of all health plans. Specifically, because of the ERISA preemption, members of employer-sponsored plans—even those enrolled in state-regulated HMOs—cannot sue plans in tort for bad faith breach in coverage decisions. Similarly, many courts have ruled that members of health plans sponsored by the Federal Employees Health Benefit Plan and the Civilian Health and Medical Program of the Uniformed Services also do not have access to these state tort remedies.

The fact that limiting consumer access to the common law tort system to sue HMOs has been a very contentious issue in the patient protection debate in the 105th and 106th Congresses may reflect on the effectiveness of tort remedies in protecting health-care consumers and redressing their concerns. For example, in the 105th Congress, the managed care industry reportedly spent $60 million to defeat patient protection legislation in Congress in the first half of 1998—four times more than the $14 million spent by medical organizations, trial lawyers, unions, and consumer groups to promote passage.[25]

Categorically, it is unfair to treat similarly situated consumers differently with respect to available legal remedies for similar conduct. If the tort of bad faith breach and other common law torts are important sources of remedies for legitimate consumer concerns, they should be available to all. If they are not, then it is appropriate to limit or eliminate them, but on an equitable basis.

Regarding the tort liability of providers, there has been a concerted press for moving medical malpractice litigation out of the common law tort system and into ADR or limiting claims altogether. While many of these proposed reforms are warranted (the common law tort system is by no means perfect), it does seem that many others focus on limiting the frequency and severity of malpractice claims, not on streamlining the process for claimants.[26] Also, HMOs and other health plans as well as provider organizations have contractual ADR mechanisms that consumers must agree to use should medical malpractice claims arise as a condition of joining the plan or receiving care from the provider. As indicated above, these arrangements are often "owned" by the provider or plan and are operated in ways that compromise the fairness of the adjudication process from the perspective of consumers.

Blocking access to the common law tort system is a serious step. The common law tort system greatly empowers all people who have been injured through the tortious conduct of others, including consumers with concerns over health care. With access to the system, consumers can initiate tort actions themselves and need not rely on regulatory authorities to take action on their behalf. Further, courts are independent of health plans and providers, and consumers stand on an equal footing with plans and providers in a proceeding that is supervised by a judge. This circumstance alone greatly empowers health-care consumers in pressing their concerns against providers or plans. Also, tort law enables consumers to achieve accountability from plans and/or providers for injuries sustained through compensatory and even punitive damages. Finally, the fact that juries have awarded multimillion dollar verdicts to consumers in tort suits against HMOs cannot be ignored as an indicator of serious misconduct on the part of some HMOs.

A CALL FOR BETTER EMPIRICAL INFORMATION ABOUT CONSUMER CONCERNS

Little empirical information is available on the incidence of different types of consumer concerns about health care generally or even those that surface in various dispute resolution processes for disposition. Data could easily be collected for some categories of disputes, such as consumer concerns raised in the grievance-and-appeal process in health plans. Besides malpractice, data are systematically collected only on reconsiderations of Medicare HMO decisions and on analyses of reported appellate opinions on coverage disputes, although these data are reported in widely available databases such as Lexis-Nexis and Westlaw. Further, and perhaps most important, consumer satisfaction data from HEDIS (see chap. 5) and other instruments is more readily available to indicate the epidemiology of consumer concerns about health care.

As a general matter, public and private health plans and their sponsors should collect data on plan members' concerns about health care and the disposition of all plan members' complaints systematically and in a uniform fashion. They also need to make data on their experience with disputes available to researchers. It is encouraging that the stewards of the Medicare and Medicaid programs as well as many state insurance regulators are becoming more sensitive to the need for data and are requiring the MCOs and HMOs over which they have authority to collect and make available such data.

The experience of research on medical malpractice is instructive. In the mid-1980s, scholars initiated much theoretical and empirical research on medical malpractice. The Robert Wood Johnson Foundation has funded two initiatives to support empirical research on medical malpractice. Several federal agencies have committed resources to research on malpractice and its relation to quality. As a result, much more is known about the nature of medical malpractice claims. The information thus collected has been important in designing and evaluating reforms of the tort system. More important, information on the nature of malpractice claims has been utilized in the processes by which many standards of care are set, which in turn has had a beneficial effect on health-care quality.

The whole problem of identifying, adjudicating, and resolving the disputes of health-care consumers could well benefit from a comprehensive, highly visible program of sponsored research such as occurred with malpractice. Empirical work should also focus on the barriers to legal processes for consumers with concerns about health care. Specific issues to be addressed include what types of concerns consumers have, to what extent they have or are planning to take action, and what relief is sought or obtained. Empirical work should also focus on the concerns of all consumers, not just those in health plans. For all the empirical work in recent years on lack of access to high quality health-care services for the uninsured, there has been virtually no discussion of how such disempowered consumers can seek relief for violations of the few extant rights they do have with respect to health care.

In sum, a better empirical understanding of consumer concerns about health care is necessary to craft genuine reform of procedures to protect consumers' interests in access to affordable and high quality health care. Thus, the list of principles presented in this chapter is preliminary. Further, the vision of reform offered in the final chapter of this book is, at best, preliminary as well.

10 : A Vision of Reform

After a book of theory and criticism—the bread and butter of academic endeavor—it is time to envision what reformed procedural protections might look like. This chapter offers a vision of ideal procedural protections for individuals as they seek and use health-care services. However, real protection of consumers comes with adequate health-care coverage for all. As discussed in chapter 1, procedural justice has its limits. Only distributive justice as implemented through policy approaches that assure access to high quality, affordable health care for all can accomplish genuine protection of the interests of all individuals in their health care. Further, in terms of genuine protection of individuals' interest in their health care, there is no substitute for the relevant actors—providers and payers—taking competent action in good faith in the first instance.

As described in this book, the current systems for identifying, tapping, and resolving consumer concerns are uncoordinated, inaccessible, inequitable, and noninclusive. Even when individuals recognize that they have legitimate concerns about their health care, obtaining remedies is difficult, and relief is not always available. Furthermore, even if complaints are raised before responsible authorities, the dispute resolution process is governed by policies determining the quality, coverage, cost, and other aspects of health care. These policies have been made previously in processes of which consumers have had little notice, to which they are not likely to have had access, and in which they have only recently become personally interested. In what follows are offered ideas for concrete reforms based on the principles enunciated in chapter 9.

MORE DEFINITE ALLOCATION OF REGULATORY RESPONSIBILITY

A vision of reform begins with clarification of regulatory responsibility for procedural protections for individuals as they need and seek health care. Historically, as discussed above, regulatory authority over procedural protections has been split between the states and the federal government—to the extent that it exists at all. Administrative and contractual processes for adjudication of consumer disputes have been regulated by the authorities that regulate health plans, and neither the states nor the federal government mandates processes to which uninsured individuals have access.

Further, the states and the federal government do not regulate—nor should they—the processes by which private organizations establish medical standards of care. Nevertheless, reforms of the processes by which policy is made and used to define the content, quality, and price of as well as access to health care are in order. First, there is a need for greater awareness within the health-care sector generally of the extent to which health-care policies govern the generation and resolution of individual concerns about health care. Second, there needs to be a better understanding of the dominant role that private organizations play in making these policies. This private role is manifested in two contexts: that in which private medical organizations, voluntary health organizations, and private accrediting bodies establish medical standards of care and that in which public and private health plan sponsors contractually establish health plans for their beneficiaries. Third, there must be strategies in place that assure that affected individuals know about relevant policies and that these policies do not compromise rights to which those individuals are otherwise entitled under state or federal law.

Clarification of Federal Responsibilities

The role of the federal government in the regulation of procedural protections for individuals with an interest in health care must be clarified and reformed. Specifically, the current situation in which plans regulated under the Employee Retirement Income Security Act (ERISA) are exempt from state regulation and state tort liability, with no comparable federal regulation or compensation rules, results in lack of protections for many consumers and unequal treatment of similarly situated consumers. At least, Congress should enact legislation similar to the patient protection legislation considered by recent Congresses to assure adequate procedural protections for enrollees in ERISA.[1]

Congress should also recognize state tort liability for bad faith breach on the part of health plans or expand the remedies under ERISA allowing the adequate compensation of consumers for damages resulting from comparable conduct on the part of ERISA-regulated health plans. As discussed below, such liability has great potential for the protection of consumers from the wrongful application of medical standards of care and, more particularly, medical review criteria and contract provisions that threaten the legitimate interests of individuals in their health care.

An Expanded Role for States

States are ideally positioned to organize and implement procedural protections for consumers and, specifically, to develop institutions within state government for this purpose. States already regulate health insurers and managed care organizations (MCOs) as well as institutional health-care providers and professionals. They administer the Medicaid program and the State Child Health Insurance Program. Thus, they have administrative expertise and experience in the management of health insurance programs, particularly programs serving vulnerable groups. They also have the primary responsibility for public health and have state health departments to execute this function. In addition, the common law of torts and contracts is state law. Thus, state courts have the responsibility for adjudicating common law tort and contract matters. Further, entities of state government are bound by constitutional guarantees of procedural due process under the federal constitution as well as by state constitutional guarantees. State officers are also subject to Section 1983 of Civil Rights Act of 1871 and liable for violations of federal constitutional guarantees.[2]

It should be noted, however, that, in taking on an expanded regulatory role, the states would be disadvantaged by the fact that most insured Americans—an estimated 85 million—are covered under employer-sponsored health plans or federal programs that are regulated or administered under federal law.[3] As such, employer-sponsored plans need essentially relate to state authorities only voluntarily or, if required to do so, by federal statute. Federal programs could be authorized or even required to contract with the state institutions designed to provide procedural protections for individuals residing within the state. How such relationships might be accomplished is also described below.

POLICYMAKING REFORMS

A vision of true reform calls for reforms in the ways in which the policies that govern the content, quality, and price of health-care services are made, publicized, and used in the health-care sector. As most relevant policy is made by various private organizations, the only available strategy that can affect policies and the processes in which they are made, publicized, or used is state and/or federal regulation. However, given the many different types of organizations involved in making private policies and the vast array of policies made, it is unlikely that regulatory mandates can be crafted that are sensitive or effective enough to assure real consumer input or the scientific integrity of policy, or achieve other objectives. Regulation can promote fairly straightforward goals, such as mandating publication of policy to interested parties and requiring procedural minimums (including providing notice that policymaking will occur and giving interested parties the opportunity to offer input). However, even these minimal procedural mandates are problematic, given the wide variety and purposes of policies that private organizations make.

Opportunity for Procedural Challenge

A far more effective strategy to promote sound policymaking, and one that complies with the cardinal characteristics of sound policy (validity, credibility, and democratic legitimacy), is to have rules for the construction and management of policies used in mandated adjudicative procedures. Such rules could address whether the policy to be applied against an individual was made in a process that comports with the principles of sound policymaking enunciated in chapter 8. The review criteria would be the following four principles: (1) a designated process was used to make the policy; (2) procedures were used to assure the marshaling and consideration of relevant scientific and clinical information; (3) procedures were used to assure consumers an opportunity to influence the content of policy; and (4) the policy was publicized properly. Ideally, policies made in processes that did not comport with these criteria would be subject to substantive review and possible invalidation in adjudicative proceedings. In that event, the complainant would then have an opportunity to present other evidence, including expert opinion, to convince the decisionmaker to adjudicate the concern in a manner contrary to that required by the the policy. If there were mandates for such review under state and/or federal law, policymaking organizations would have greater incentives to make policy in open and accessible forums and in conformity with democratic procedures. Such an approach also accommodates the myriad ways in which policies are made, including contracting processes, without imposing detailed regulation designed to meet individual situations.

Maintenance of Tort Liability

To ensure the integrity of policy and its application from an individual patient's perspective, tort liability with damages to compensate for resulting injuries is valuable, if not essential. In a situation such as widespread private policymaking and implementation of private policy in a variety of contexts, tort offers an effective enforcement mechanism that can deal with varied circumstances. Regulatory schemes can rarely be designed to deal as effectively with the same array of varying circumstances. Thus, current arrangements, such as the preemption of state tort liability for bad faith breach under ERISA and other laws governing federally sponsored health plans, are undesirable unless they provide for comparable remedies, including damages for tortious injury, under federal law.

Government Leadership in the Policymaking Process

The states and the federal government can play an important role in ensuring that the policies defining the content and quality of health-care services are appropriate and sound. The federal government has moved away from direct policymaking regarding medical standards of care and toward fostering this effort in the private sector. Not all states have been active in the process by which medical standards of care are determined, and, given the limited resources of most state health departments, most are probably unable to sustain such an effort. Nevertheless, both the federal government and the states, especially in their roles as stewards of public health insurance programs, should be mindful of the processes in which private organizations determine the medical standards of care and how these standards of care are used in public health insurance programs. The states and the federal government should be especially careful that significant policies regarding the content and quality of care are not made inadvertently in their own contracting processes with MCOs to provide health plans for their beneficiaries.

One important function of government is to stimulate the development of medical standards of care, especially those pertaining to quality. Unlike private organizations, government has the authority to convene advisory panels and marshal experts to assist plans and providers in developing medical policy. This role is markedly different from actually determining medical standards of care. Rather, it is more of a facilitator role—mobilizing private organizations, setting an agenda, and, especially, funding the research providing the data that inform the content and ensure the scientific validity of medical standards of care developed by private organizations.

Given the fact that medical standards of care are universal in application and in scope, the federal government should retain an important role in the standard setting process. For one thing, it has greater resources at its disposal as well as access to a wider range of expertise on which to base medical standards of care than do state governments, whose resources are much more limited. However, despite the desirability of government involvement, mechanisms should exist to ensure pluralism and debate in the process of developing medical standards of care by different medical specialty societies, medical professional organizations, and private accrediting bodies.

Nevertheless, the states have an important role to play as well. States, especially given their responsibility through licensure for the quality of health care, gather and publish information on quality, including the best practices, the results of research, and other relevant information. They can also provide a forum in which providers, concerned about the quality of medical policies in specific health plans in the state, can raise complaints and initiate debate or the investigation of policies that might be undesirable or even illegal. States are also well positioned to disseminate information about extant health-care policies and their implications to consumers in ways that could possibly prevent future consumer concerns over health care that develop into legal disputes with providers and/or health plans.

REFORMS FOR TAPPING AND RESOLVING CONSUMER CONCERNS ABOUT HEALTH CARE

Reformers of systems for adjudicating consumer disputes, particularly those with programmatic and regulatory responsibilities, understandably think mainly in terms of working within the boundaries of their system's authority. They generally do not look beyond these jurisdictional constraints to imagine different and arguably more effective reforms. However, greater coordination with movement toward a unified consumer dispute resolution process is possible and would constitute a much needed and useful reform. In what follows are presented some ideas of what a more coordinated system might look like.

Better Coordination of Existing Systems

The most pressing need in the reform of the dispute resolution process for consumer complaints is the simplification and coordination of existing processes for adjudicating disputes that result from the current balkanized system of financing and delivering health-care services in the United States. Absent the adoption of a national single payer system that includes the uninsured, creating a single national set of procedural protections is currently not practical. Nevertheless, despite current realities, movement for simplification and even consolidation of processes for adjudicating consumer concerns is possible. However, there are ways to coordinate existing procedural protections and thereby minimize consumer confusion and enhance access to process and remedies. Just small steps toward coordination can do much to improve procedural protections for individuals with concerns about health care. In that regard, President Clinton's executive order calling for administrative implementation of the Consumer Bill of Rights of the Presidential Advisory Commission on Consumer Protection and Quality in the Health Care Industry has done much to move federal agencies to coordinate and reform their grievance-and-appeal procedures and take other measures to enhance the protection of consumers' interest in their health care.[4]

The typology of consumer concerns about quality, cost, and access presented in chapter 5 reveals opportunities for coordination of grievance procedures in different insurance programs and plans. One major opportunity is that all concerns, except for concerns over costs and denials of care, present themselves in the same manner through consumer complaints, consumer satisfaction surveys, incident reports, and litigation. The fact that many consumer concerns are handled initially in similar informal processes suggests that the consolidation of informal procedures for adjudicating claims through a centralized dispute resolution institution is feasible. These patterns suggest that much can be done by providers and plans internally to identify and resolve disputes at a very early stage before they "mature" into legal claims.

But, if disputes and concerns are not resolved informally and must proceed to a grievance-and-appeal process for more formal adjudication, there is no reason that they could not be resolved in a centralized dispute resolution institution of the type described below. The fact that the law locates in different types of consumer concerns different causes of action for judicial review should not be a problem. The institution could help individual complainants locate the appropriate paths of subsequent external administrative and judicial review.

Uniform regulatory requirements for grievance-and-appeal procedures would create opportunities for the evolution of common dispute resolution institutions for the adjudication and resolution of disputes that individuals have with health plans and providers. Such reforms should facilitate use of common processes for tapping independent medical expertise either at the provider or at the plan level. Common requirements would enable providers and plans to contract with organizations to manage their grievance-and-appeal procedures and thereby tap the expertise and resources garnered from those organizations' contacts with multiple health plans and their sponsors. Such contractors, given economies of scale, could offer a wide variety of dispute resolution techniques for the resolution of consumer concerns.

The coordination of regulatory mandates would also paradoxically permit the decentralization of dispute resolution processes and thereby greatly enhance the accessibility of these processes to consumers. To move toward "seamless" grievance-and-appeal procedures, requirements for federally sponsored or regulated as well as state-regulated health plans should be coordinated. To facilitate coordination of state-regulated health plans, the National Association of Insurance Commissioners should consider adopting reform measures, implemented in federally sponsored and/or regulated health insurance programs, recommended in the Patient Bill of Rights.[5]

Models for Dispute Resolution Institutions

There are many possible models for the design of such dispute resolution institutions, including the following: (1) an agency of a state health department; (2) an agency of the state court or even a state subject matter court; and (3) a private organization that operates on a multistate or national basis. The models are not mutually exclusive. The advantages and disadvantages of these design options are presented below.

A State Administrative Agency. A dispute resolution institution could be established as an administrative agency within state government. Models exist for such state agencies in the state workers' compensation agencies. As state agencies, their adjudicative procedures would be subject to well-developed principles of administrative law (described in chap. 4). One chief advantage of a state agency would be its ability to address the needs of the uninsured, who have limited or no access to most nonjudicial review processes. Arguably, state health departments would be especially sensitive to the needs of the uninsured because they have a public health mission that serves the uninsured in other contexts. At the very least, they might provide an ombudsman to enable the uninsured to press their concerns about health care outside the common law tort system and independent of provider grievance procedures.

One possible and important disadvantage is the fact that private health plan sponsors and providers are unlikely to use the services of government agencies to handle their grievance-and-appeal system. To invoke the services of a government agency when not required to do so by regulation is contrary to the business culture of most private health plan sponsors and providers. Further, most state contracting procedures may be too bureaucratic to facilitate the private use of dispute resolution procedures within a state agency.

The State Court System. The dispute resolution institution could be lodged in the state court system. The state court system could operate grievance-and-appeal procedures for providers and health plans. It could also manage existing and new systems for adjudicating medical malpractice and other tort claims. Arguably, state courts could attract better judges than state agencies as state court judges are customarily better compensated than state administrative law judges.[6]

There are multiple reasons to tap the expertise of state courts in ensuring procedural protections for individuals with concerns about their health care. Patient disputes involving medical injury and, for claimants in some health plans, disputes over bad faith coverage decisions and other adverse conduct are already adjudicated in state courts. Thus, locating the adjudication of other disputes in state courts would allow for consolidation. Further, as tort litigation is a major portion of civil trial work,[7] state court judges have experience adjudicating medical issues as well as many of the tort actions through which health-care consumers raise concerns.

State courts have also been actively involved with the administration of many tort reforms for medical malpractice, such as medical review panels as well as mandated alternative dispute resolution (ADR). Many state courts have adopted ADR mechanisms, including mediation, for all their civil case-loads.[8] These ADR processes would be available to claimants with disputes over health care. ADR under state court supervision alleviates many of the problems with ADR used in the health plan context. Specifically, judicial oversight in a truly independent process would do much to address the inequities inherent in the undue power that plans and providers wield in contractual ADR processes. Unfortunately, under current law, ERISA-regulated plans would not be subject to the jurisdiction of these health courts.

States could, pursuant to statute, also establish a separate subject matter court to adjudicate health-care cases. Subject matter courts at both the state and the federal levels are not unprecedented.[9] At the state level, probate and juvenile courts are long-standing examples of state subject matter courts. A subject matter state court for health would adjudicate all consumer health-care disputes under state law. Its jurisdiction could include appeals under the Medicaid program, state-regulated health plans, as well as state common law and statutory actions ranging from medical malpractice and insurer bad faith breach to implied causes of action under state laws requiring hospitals to provide emergency services. Ideally, a state health court would have the public status and authority to invest it with the neutrality that is not currently present in contractual ADR processes operated by plans and their sponsors. At the very least, however, it should have the sponsorship of state government, which would institute public accountability through political and legal processes. Unfortunately, under current law, ERISA-regulated plans would not be subject to the jurisdiction of these health courts.

A Private Dispute Resolution Entity. The dispute resolution institution could also be a private entity with which public and private health plan sponsors and also providers contract to administer their grievance-and-appeal systems. This idea is not without precedent. The Centers for Medicare and Medicaid Services already contracts with the Health Care Dispute Resolution Center to adjudicate reconsiderations of determinations in health maintenance organization (HMO) grievance procedures and also contracts with private peer review organizations and insurance companies to hear a wide variety of other claimant disputes with the traditional Medicare fee-for-service program within states.

One great advantage of a private entity is the flexibility that it has under corporate law to perform a variety of functions in innovative ways. Because of this characteristic, a private entity is likely to be more attractive to private health plans and providers as a source of dispute resolution services than either a public administrative agency or a court. Also, a private entity that operated in many states might be particularly attractive to employer sponsors of health plans or MCOs that operate nationally.

One disadvantage of private organizations is that their relationships with health plan sponsors and providers would be made through contract. For the law governing contracts for the privatization of public functions is not well developed, especially from the perspective of protecting the interests of affected individuals.[10] In this regard, regulation of these private entities or at least the plan sponsors or providers that contract with them is probably imperative to set minimal requirements for grievance-and-appeal procedures and to ensure that their operations comply with these requirements.

Required Functions of Dispute Resolution Institutions

Regardless of design, the dispute resolution institutions should be required to perform three functions. First, they should provide processes through which the uninsured can raise complaints and grievances against providers and other parties with whom they have a concern about their health care. Second, they should provide access to affordable external review by qualified experts to resolve complaints at any stage involving medical issues. Third, they should offer a full complement of dispute resolution procedures to accommodate the preferences and needs of all individuals raising concerns.

Meeting the Needs of the Uninsured. Meeting the needs of the uninsured is one of the most difficult challenges for the dispute resolution institution. Specifically, the uninsured are often poor and otherwise disadvantaged. They may have difficulty recognizing and presenting complaints easily. Thus, special outreach and publication strategies may be needed to make the uninsured aware of this service. Second, the uninsured poor, in particular, have difficulty raising complaints. To address this problem, the dispute resolution institution may want to establish an ombudsman type office that works with complainants to resolve concerns with providers, especially about their care. There is precedent for an ombudsman-like function in state agencies to protect residents of nursing homes under the Older Americans' Act of 1965.[11] As discussed above, a public administrative agency—lodged in the state health department, for example—would probably be the most effective way of implementing and operating a grievance-and-appeal system for those uninsured with disputes with providers over their health care.

The dispute resolution institution may also want to contract with legal services organizations to represent clients in more complex and advanced proceedings. These organizations have extensive experience in advocating for the health-care interests of the poor. Also, funding a program for the uninsured will require external funding as the institution cannot rely on contract revenues, as it can with programs for health plan beneficiaries. In sum, either the states or the federal government is going to have to fund this important function to ensure that it is consistently and adequately funded.

Enhancing Independent External Review. One ideal feature of a centralized dispute resolution institution would be external review. The majority of states now require external review for state-regulated health plans.[12] Specifically, the institution could retain an independent panel of physicians and other health-care professionals to provide expert testimony in the adjudication of medical issues. A precedent already exists for such review in the system of mandated medical review panels for adjudicating malpractice claims in some states.[13] An independent panel of experts would ideally be composed of acknowledged experts, giving its decisions additional credibility. Many health plans are already using independent panels of experts in dispute resolution to achieve just such credibility.[14] A centralized dispute resolution institution with a panel of independent experts would provide for real independence in the decisionmaking process, particularly with respect to crucial medical issues. External review would mitigate many of the concerns about power imbalances between consumers and plans that arise when the health plan sponsor also operates the dispute resolution procedure.

Particularly important research findings are those of Poythress and his colleagues[15] that tight judicial control over expert testimony is perceived as more fair than the development of expert testimony by the parties involved in the action. If consumers are comfortable relinquishing control over medical expert testimony to decisionmakers, then there is greater flexibility to design processes that can marshal neutral expert testimony more efficiently and inexpensively. For example, a plan could contract with leading physicians in the community to conduct external expert review that would be persuasive both to consumers and to health plans and providers involved in the dispute.

Facilitating Diversity in Dispute Resolution Mechanisms. The state institution for the procedural protection of health-care consumers could offer a wide variety of methods ranging from a traditional jury trial to administrative review and conventional ADR methodologies such as arbitration and mediation. Further, a centralized dispute resolution institution could also use ADR methods such as mediation and arbitration more easily than could contractual dispute resolution processes operated by plans or providers. A truly independent process, especially coupled with review by a truly independent medical expert, would greatly mitigate the problem that plagues the use of contractual ADR methods in many contexts today—the power imbalance between the consumer and the plan or provider. The sponsor of the process would not be the consumer's adversary. Nor would it have exclusive possession and/or control of the requisite expert knowledge of the relevant medical facts. In such a context, ADR methods might well work as originally envisioned.

Further, the dispute resolution institution, regardless of model, should permit judicial supervision of all ADR processes. As discussed in chapter 9, much of the criticism of ADR in the health-care field—particularly when medical malpractice is involved—is the disparity of power between the provider/plan, with its hold on medical expertise, and the consumer. Judicial supervision can mitigate the adverse consequences of this disparity and assure consumer protection. In general, such proposed judicial supervision of ADR will mitigate one of the major critiques of ADR generally—that private dispute resolution leads to undesirable limitations on public oversight on the development of law, to the detriment of consumers' interests.[16]

Legal Constraints on the Design of Reforms

In envisioning reforms that involve government, it is noteworthy that the law accords considerable flexibility in the design and architecture of agencies and programs. In the twentieth century, legislatures have become quite inventive when designing administrative agencies and special courts to address problems requiring a special response by the government. States too have demonstrated such flexibility. Early on, they recognized that many private rights adjudicated in the common law tort system were really public matters requiring public law solutions. At the beginning of the twentieth century, states established statutory workers' compensation programs to handle the adjudication of claims for injury formerly handled in the common law tort system.[17] In the 1960s and 1970s, many states adopted statutory compensation schemes when the common law tort system proved incapable of efficiently handling tort claims for automobile injury.[18] In the 1970s and 1980s, some states adopted statutory schemes for the adjudication and compensation of medical malpractice claims, for similar reasons.[19] State supreme courts, to varying degrees, have not always supported these innovations, although, in recent years, they seem to have become more accepting of structural innovations in state agencies and courts to meet important problems.[20]

Congress has established comparable innovations, beginning with the independent commission beyond the control of the executive branch.[21] Since 1980, Congress has established unique government bodies to address particular social, economic, and political problems that traditional structures seem incapable of handling efficiently.[22] Further, Congress has the authority to assign the adjudication of a wide variety of disputes arising under regulatory programs to administrative agencies, including ancillary common law claims.[23] Congress also has the authority to identify or create an administrative tribunal or subject matter court (such as the U.S. Tax Court),[24] which will adjudicate disputes more expeditiously and with greater expertise than Article III courts with general subject matter jurisdiction. Finally, Congress has the authority to use private regulators, such as private accrediting organizations, to perform some regulatory functions.[25]

The creation of these unique structures and arrangements and their validation by courts in lawsuits challenging their constitutionality on the grounds of violation of the separation of powers doctrine confirm the great flexibility of legislatures in crafting government bodies capable of solving particular problems. Clearly, states have the requisite authority to visualize institutions that will establish procedural protections for all health-care consumers, even the uninsured.

Whatever institutional design and authority is selected, the profile of the institution should be quite high in the state so that consumers are aware of its existence. The institution should be designed in such a way as to marshal the best expertise in the state, in terms of both staff and advisory boards, to assist in its work. The institution should capitalize on existing resources with strong reputations.

THE LIMITS OF PROCEDURAL JUSTICE
WITHOUT DISTRIBUTIVE JUSTICE

In the short run, for insured individuals, the greatest hope for procedural reform lies in improved processes for making coverage, quality, and other policy that defines the content and amount of health-care services offered through health plans. If concerns arise, straightforward, accessible processes should be in place giving individual enrollees the power and information to press and resolve their concerns effectively. Also, efforts should be made on the part of responsible parties to survey patients and engage in other activities that reduce consumer concerns about their health care in the first instance. For the uninsured, the greatest hope lies in access to health-care services through existing public programs or through providers that are programmatically capable of and committed to providing comprehensive health-care services.

In the long run, the most effective protection for the interests of all Americans—especially the uninsured—in their health care is comprehensive, adequately funded health-care coverage that is based on sound, scientific policies that define the quality of covered benefits. In other words, the book closes where it opened—with the observation that it is distributive justice that ultimately protects the interests of individuals in their health care and prevents or alleviates many of their concerns about health care.

It is fair to say that the United States has not yet faced seriously problems of distributive justice in health care. Since the 1980s, the confident liberalism of the 1960s, with its rhetoric of expanded opportunity for the poor, has been on the defensive. The prevalent conservative paradigm extolled individual liberty, market economics, and the reduction of government. This conservative paradigm precluded theoretical and practical consideration of how government could and should address major deficiencies in distributive justice. Yet the persistent inability of private health insurers to reach all in need is evidence of failure in the private health insurance market. In that event, government might act—either directly, through public programs or regulation, or indirectly, through subsidies and taxation—to expand needed health-care coverage. Indeed, both the states and the federal government have, through direct programs and substantial tax subsidies, done much to expand coverage. Nevertheless, the dominant conservative paradigm of recent years rejects this idea.

To conclude, in the current American political and cultural environment, the requisite rhetorical consensus does not exist to establish universal health-care coverage today. This fact poses a significant barrier to the protection of the many Americans who need some subsidy if they are to have access to adequate health-care services. To the extent that their health-care concerns stem from their inability to pay or otherwise secure financing for health care, the types of protections discussed in this book, which are procedural in nature, will be of little help.

Notes

1 Introduction

1 See, e.g., Clark C. Havighurst, "The Backlash against Managed Health Care: Hard Politics Make Bad Policy," 34 *Ind. L. Rev.* 395 (2001); Alain C. Enthoven et al., "Consumer Choice and the Managed Care Backlash," 27 *Am. J. L. and Med.* 1 (2001); Robert J. Blendon et al., "Understanding the Managed Care Backlash," *Health Aff.,* July–Aug. 1998, at 80; Atul Gawande et al., "Does Dissatisfaction with Health Plans Stem from Having No Choice?" *Health Aff.,* Sept.–Oct. 1998, at 184; and Thomas Bodenheimer, "The HMO Backlash— Righteous or Reactionary?" 335 *New Eng. J. Med.* 1601 (1996).

2 See Henry J. Kaiser Family Foundation, "Kaiser/Harvard Recent Findings on Public Attitudes toward Patients' Rights and Managed Care: Chart Pack" (June 2000). See generally Robert J. Blendon and John M. Benson, "Fifty Years of Consumers' Views on Health," *Health Aff.,* Mar.–Apr. 2001, at 33.

3 See Eleanor D. Kinney, "Tapping and Resolving American Concerns about Health Care," 25 *Am. J. L. and Med.* 335 and n. 2 (2000).

4 See, e.g., Moran v. Rush Prudential HMO, Incorporated, 230 F.3d 959 (7th Cir. 2000), rev'd 1999 WL 417384 (N.D. Ill. 1999), cert. granted, 121 S.Ct. 2589 (Jun. 29, 2001); Bauman v. U.S. Healthcare, Inc., 1 F. Supp., 193 F.3d 151 (3d Cir. 1999), cert. denied, 530 U.S. 1242 (2000); Pegram v. Herdrich, 120 S.Ct. 2143 (2000); Shea v. Esensten, 107 F.3d 625 (8th Cir. 1997), cert. denied, 522 U.S. 914 (1997); Goodrich v. Aetna US Healthcare of CA, Inc., 1999 WL 181418 (Cal. Super. Mar. 29, 1999) (discussed in Julie Margquis, "Widow's Lawsuit against HMO Ends with $120 Million Verdict," *L.A. Times,* Jan. 21, 1999, at E7); and Fox v. Healthnet, No. 219/692 (Riverside Cty. Sup. Ct. Ca. Dec. 28, 1993) (discussed in Jody C. Collins, "Comment: Experimental Medical Treatments: Who Should Decide Coverage?" 20 *Seattle U. L. Rev.* 451, 451 (1997)).

5 Cara S. Lesser and Paul B. Ginsburg, "Update on the Nation's Health Care System, 1997–1999," *Health Aff.,* Nov.–Dec. 2000, at 206.

6 For general theories, see, e.g., John Rawls, *A Theory of Justice* (1971); and Hans Kelson, *What Is Justice?* (1957).

7 See Mark A. Hall, *Making Medical Spending Decisions: The Law, Ethics, and Economics of Rationing Mechanisms* (1997); Paul T. Menzel, *Strong Medicine: The Ethical Rationing of Health Care* (1990); Daniel Callahan, *Setting Limits: Medical Goals in an Aging Society* (1987); Larry R. Churchill, *Rationing Health Care in America* (1987); Victor R. Fuchs, *Who Shall Live? Health, Economics, and Social Choice* (1974); Mark A. Hall, "Rationing Health Care at the Bedside," 69

N.Y.U. L. Rev. 693, 778 (1994); Einer Elhauge, "Allocating Health Care Morally," 82 *Cal. L. Rev.* 1449 (1994); Richard D. Lamm, "Rationing of Health Care: Inevitable and Desirable," 140 *U. Pa. L. Rev.* 1511 (1992); Henry Aaron and William B. Schwartz, "Rationing Health Care: The Choice before Us," 247 *Science* 418 (1990); David Orentlicher, "Practice Guidelines: A Limited Role in Resolving Rationing Decisions," 46 *J. Am. Geriatrics Soc'y* 369 (1998); and David Eddy, "Health System Reform: Will Controlling Costs Require Rationing Services?" 272 *JAMA* 324 (1994).

8   See President's Commission for the Study of Ethical Problems in Medicine and Biomedical and Behavioral Research, *Security Access to Health Care* (1983). See also, e.g., James Blumstein, "Rationing Medical Resources: A Constitutional, Legal, and Policy Analysis," 59 *Tex. L. Rev.* 1345 (1982); and Rand Rosenblatt, "Rationing 'Normal' Health Care: The Hidden Legal Issues," 59 *Tex. L. Rev.* 1401 (1982).

9   See, e.g., Norman Daniels et al., *Benchmarks of Fairness for Health Care Reform* (1996); Tom L. Beauchamp and James F. Childress, *Principles of Biomedical Ethics* (4th ed. 1994); Larry Palmer, *Law, Medicine, and Social Justice* (1989); Norman Daniels, *Just Health Care* (1985); *Justice and Health Care* (Earl E. Shelp ed., 1981); and American Medical Association, Council on Ethical and Judicial Affairs, "Ethical Issues in Health Systems Reform: The Provision of Adequate Health Care," 272 *JAMA* 1056 (1994).

10 Beauchamp and Childress, supra note 9, at 328–31.

11 Rawls, supra note 6.

12 Daniels, *Just Health Care,* supra note 9, at 39.

13 See Uwe Reinhardt, "Uncompensated Hospital Care," in *Uncompensated Hospital Care: Rights and Responsibilities* (Frank A. Sloan, James F. Blumstein, and James M. Perrin eds., 1986).

14 U.S. Census Bureau, *Health Insurance Coverage: 1999* 1 (fig. 1) (Current Population Reports 2000).

15 Wendy K. Mariner, "Going Hollywood with Patient Rights in Managed Care," 281 *JAMA* 861, 861 (1999). See also George J. Annas, "A National Bill of Patients' Rights," 338 *New Eng. J. Med.* 695 (1998); and Wendy K. Mariner, "Standards of Care and Standard Form Contracts: Distinguishing Patient Rights and Consumer Rights in Managed Care," 15 *J. Contemp. Health L. and Pol'y* 1 (1998).

2 The Patient Protection Debate

1   "President Clinton's Health Care Reform Proposal and Health Security Act as Presented to Congress on October 27, 1993" (1993), in *Medicare and Medicaid Guide* (CCH) (Rep. No. 773, Nov. 1, 1993).

2   H.R. 3600, Health Security Act, 103d Cong., 2d Sess. §§5201–43 (1994). See, e.g., Eleanor D. Kinney, "Rule and Policy Making under Health Reform," 47 *Admin. L. Rev.* 403 (1995); Timothy S. Jost, "Administrative Adjudication under Health Care Reform," 47 *Admin. L. Rev.* 425 (1995); Eleanor D. Kinney, "Protecting Consumers and Providers under Health Reform," 5 *Health Matrix* 83 (1995); Mark R. Fondacaro, "Toward a Synthesis of Law and Social Science: Due Process and Procedural Justice in the Context of National Health Care Reform," 72 *Denv. U. L. Rev.* 303 (1995); Louise G. Trubeck and Elizabeth A. Hoffman, "Searching for a Balance in Universal Health Care Reform: Protection for the Disenfranchised Consumer," 43 *DePaul L. Rev.* 1081 (1994); and Coalition for Consumer Protection and Quality in Health Care Reform, "White Paper on Consumer Due Process Protections in Health Care Reform," 28 *Clearinghouse Rev.* 506 (1994).

3   This useful conceptual framework was developed in Jill A. Marsteller and Randall R. Bovbjerg, *Federalism and Patient Protection: Changing Roles for State and Federal Government* (1999).

4   See, e.g., Program on Negotiation and Conflict Resolution and the Medication Group, Inc., *Dispute Resolution in Managed Care: A Modular Self Assessment Protocol* (2001); American Bar Association, Commission on Legal Problems of the Elderly, *Resolution of Consumer Disputes in Managed Care: Insights from an Interdisciplinary Roundtable* (1997); "Symposium: Conflict Resolution and Managed Health Care: The Challenge of Achieving both Equity and Efficiency," 34 *Forum* 1 (1997).

5   See Marc A. Rodwin, *Promoting Accountable Managed Health Care: The Potential Role for Consumer Voice* (2000).

6   See, e.g., Peter V. Lee and Debra L. Roth, *Improving Quality: Opportunities for Intervention by Consumer Groups* (Center for Health Care Rights 2000); Public Welfare Foundations, *Community Catalyst 2000, Health Care Justice: Linking Grassroots Leadership and Legal Advocacy* (2000); Consumer Coalition for Quality Health Care, *Health Plan Complaint Procedure and Administrative and Judicial Review Requirements* (1997); Center for Health Care Rights, *Managed Care Ombudsman Programs: New Approaches to Assist Consumers and Improve the Health Care System* (1996); and Center for Health Care Rights, *Consumer Protection in State HMO Laws* (1995).

7   See Karen Ignagni and Kathryn Wilber, "Encouraging Innovation in Resolving Disputes between Health Plans and Their Members," 34 *Forum* 1 (1997); and David Richardson, "Dispute Resolution Systems: Fitting the Pieces Together," 34 *Forum* 16 (1997).

8   See, e.g., State Issues Forum, *Designing Consumer Protection Standards* (American Hospital Association 1996); and National Society for Patient Representation and Consumer Affairs, *In the Name of the Patient: Consumer Advocacy in Health Care* (American Hospital Association 1994).

9   American Arbitration Association et al., *Health Care Due Process Protocol: A Due Process Protocol for Mediation and Arbitration of Health Care Disputes* (1998).

10   See Families USA, *Hit or Miss: State Managed Care Laws* (1998); Geraldine Dallek, Carol Jimenez, and Marlene Schwartz, *Consumer Protections in State HMO Laws* (1995); and National Conference of State Legislatures, Health Policy Tracking Service, "Internal and External Grievance Procedures: A Fifty State Overview" (1998), in *Health Care Quality: Grievance Procedures: Hearings before the Senate Committee on Labor and Human Resources,* 105th Cong., 2d Sess. 46 (1998). See also Michael E. Ginsberg, "Recent Legislation: HMO Grievance Processes," 37 *Harv. J. on Legis.* 237 (2000); and Tracy E. Miller, "Managed Care Regulation: In the Laboratory of the States," 278 *JAMA* 1102 (1997).

11   Marsteller and Bovbjerg, supra note 3, at 3–7.

12   See Karen Pollitz et al., *External Review of Health Plan Decisions: An Overview of Key Program Features in the States and Medicare* (1998); Geraldine Dallek and Karen Pollitz, *External Review of Health Plan Decisions: An Update* (2000); National Association of Insurance Commissioners, *Issues Involving External Grievance Review Procedures* (2000).

13   Texas Health Care Liability Act, Tex. Civ. Prac. and Rem. Code Ann. §§88.001– 88.003 (Vernon Supp. 1999). See Shannon Turner, "Note: ERISA Preemption of Direct Liability Claims: Texas Throws Down the Gauntlet," 78 *Tex. L. Rev.* 211 (1999); and Ron Paterson et al., *Implementation of Managed Care Consumer Protections in Missouri, New Jersey, Texas, and Vermont: Full Report* (Kaiser Family Foundation 1999).

14   See President's Advisory Commission on Consumer Protection and Quality in the Health Care Industry, *Quality First: Better Health Care for All Americans* (1998); and President's Advisory Commission on Consumer Protection and Quality in the Health Care Industry, *Consumer Bill of Rights and Responsibilities: Report to the President of the United States* (1997).

15   H.R. 2967, S. 1499, Health Insurance Consumer's Bill of Rights, 105th Cong., 2d Sess. (1998); H.R. 358, S. 6, Patients' Bill of Rights Act of 1999, 106th Cong., 1st Sess. (1999).

16   See Memorandum on Federal Agency Compliance with the Patient Bill of Rights, 1 Pub. Papers 260 (Feb. 20, 1998).

17   Pub. L. No. 93-406, 88 Stat. 832 (codified as amended at 29 U.S.C. §§1001– 1191c).

18   Marsteller and Bovbjerg, supra note 3, at 7.

19   See U.S. Congress, Congressional Research Service, *CRS Issue Brief: Managed Health Care: Major Issues in the 105th Congress* (1998). See also Amy Goldstein and Helan Dewar, "Senate Kills Patients' Bill of Rights," *Wash. Post,* Oct. 10, 1998, at A1.

20   See U.S. Congress, Congressional Research Service, *CRS Issue Brief for Con-*

gress: Patient Protection and Managed Care: Legislation in the 106th Congress (1999).

21 S. 1052, Bipartisan Patient Protection Act, 107th Cong., 1st Sess. (2001); H.R. 2563, Bipartisan Patient Protection Act, 107th Cong., 1st Sess. (2001). See U.S. Congress, Congressional Research Service, *Patient Protection and Managed Care: Legislation in the 107th Congress* (2001).

22 H.R. 2723, Bipartisan Consensus Managed Care Improvement Act of 1999, 106th Cong., 1st Sess. (1999); S. 1344, Patients' Bill of Rights Act of 1999, 106th Cong., 1st Sess. (1999).

23 S. 283, Bipartisan Patient Protection Act of 2001, 107th Cong., 1st Sess. (2001).

24 S. 1052, Bipartisan Patient Protection Act, 107th Cong., 1st Sess. (2001); H.R. 2563, Bipartisan Patient Protection Act, 107th Cong., 1st Sess. (2001).

25 Robert Pear, "Deal Is Reached on a Bill to Set Patients' Rights," *N.Y. Times,* Aug. 1, 2001, at A1.

26 29 U.S.C. §1144 (1994 and Supp. V 1999).

27 De Buono v. NYSA-ILA Medical and Clinical Services Fund, 520 U.S. 806 (1997); California Division of Labor Standards Enforcement, N.A., Inc., 519 U.S. 316 (1997); Boggs v. Boggs, 520 U.S. 833 (1997). See also New York State Conference of Blue Cross Blue Shield Plans v. Travelers Ins., Inc., 514 U.S. 645 (1995) and Robert N. Covington, "Amending ERISA's Preemption Scheme," 8 *Kan. J. L. and Pub. Pol'y* 1 (1999).

28 See, e.g., Peter D. Jacobson and Scott D. Pomfret, "Form, Function, and Managed Care Torts: Achieving Fairness and Equity in ERISA Jurisprudence," 35 *Hous. L. Rev.* 985 (1998); Karen A. Jordan, "The Shifting Preemption Paradigm: Conceptual and Interpretive Issues," 51 *Vand. L. Rev.* 1149 (1998); Karen A. Jordan, "Tort Liability for Managed Care: The Weakening of ERISA's Protective Shield," 25 *J. L. Med. and Ethics* 160 (1997); Margaret G. Farrell, "ERISA Preemption and Regulation of Managed Health Care: The Case for Managed Federalism," 23 *Am. J. L. and Med.* 251 (1997); and Jack K. Kilcullen, "Grouping for the Reins: ERISA, HMO Malpractice, and Enterprise Liability," 22 *Am. J. L. and Med.* 7 (1996).

29 530 U.S. 211 (2000), rev'g, 54 F.3d 362 (7th Cir. 1998). See "Symposium: Introduction to *Pegram v. Herdrich,* 530 U.S. 211 (2000), and Responses," 1 *Yale J. Health Pol'y L. and Ethics* 159 (2001); Thomas R. McLean and Edward P. Richards, "Managed Care Liability for Breach of Fiduciary Duty after *Pegram v. Herdrich:* The End of the ERISA Preemption for State Law Liability for Medical Care Decision Making," 53 *Fla. L. Rev.* 1 (2001); and William M. Sage, "U R Here: The Supreme Court's Guide for Managed Care," *Health Aff.,* Sept.–Oct. 2000, at 219.

30 530 U.S. 211, 215 (2000) (citations omitted).

31 215 F.3d 526 (5th Cir. 2000), petition for cert. filed, 69 USLW 3317 (Oct. 24,

2000) (No. 00-665). See Christine Lockhart, "The Safest Care Is to Deny Care: Implications of *Corporate Health Insurance, Inc. v. Texas Department of Insurance* on HMO Liability in Texas," 41 *S. Tex. L. Rev.* 621 (2000).

32 230 F.3d 959 (7th Cir. 2000), rev'd 1999 WL 417384 (N.D. Ill. 1999), cert. granted, 121 S.Ct. 2589 (Jun. 29, 2001).

33 410 Ill. Comp. Stat. 50/3 (2000).

34 See Clark C. Havighurst, "Consumers versus Managed Care: The New Class Actions," *Health Aff.*, Jul.–Aug. 2001, at 8.

35 Racketeer-Influenced and Corrupt Organizations Act, §1962, 18 U.S.C. §1961 (1994 and Supp. V 1999).

36 29 U.S.C. §§1022(a)(1) and 1024(b)(1) (1994 and Supp. V 1999).

37 See Maio v. Aetna Inc., 221 F.3d 472 (3d Cir. 2000); Ehlmann v. Kaiser Foundation Health Plan of Texas, 198 F.3d 552 (5th Cir. 2000); Weiss v. CIGNA Healthcare, Inc., 972 F. Supp. 552 (S.D.N.Y. 1997).

38 See Shea v. Esensten, 107 F.3d 625 (8th Cir.), cert. denied, 522 U.S. 914 (1997); Drolet v. Healthsource, Inc., 968 F. Supp. 757 (D.N.H. 1997).

39 See Humana, Inc. Managed Care Litigation, S.D. Fl. MDL No. 1334.

40 See Marshall B. Kapp, "Health Care in the Marketplace: Implications for Decisionally Impaired Consumers and Their Surrogates and Advocates," 24 *S. Ill. U. L. J.* 1 (1999).

41 See, e.g., Russell Korobkin, "The Efficiency of Managed Care 'Patient Protection' Laws: Incomplete Contracts, Bounded Rationality, and Market Failure," 85 *Cornell L. Rev.* 1 (1999); David A. Hyman, "Regulating Managed Care: What's Wrong with a Patient's Bill of Rights?" 73 *Cal. L. Rev.* 221 (2000); and David A. Hyman, "Consumer Protection in a Managed Care World: Should Consumers Call 911?" 43 *Vill. L. Rev.* 409 (1998).

42 See George J. Annas, "Patient's Rights in Managed Care—Exit, Voice, and Choice," 337 *New Eng. J. Med.* 210 (1997); and Walter A. Zelman, "Consumer Protection in Managed Care: Finding the Balance," *Health Aff.*, Jan.–Feb. 1997, at 158.

43 See Rodwin, supra note 5; Marc A. Rodwin, "The Neglected Remedy: Strengthening Consumer Voice in Managed Care," *Am. Prospect*, Sept.–Oct. 1997, at 45; Marc A. Rodwin, "Consumer Protection and Managed Care: The Need for Organized Consumers," *Health Aff.*, May–June 1996, at 110; and Marc A. Rodwin, "Consumer Protection and Managed Care," 22 *Hous. L. Rev.* 1319 (1996).

44 See Andrew Ruskin, "Empowering Patients to Act Like Consumers: A Proposal Creating Price and Quality Choice within Health Care," 73 *St. John's L. Rev.* 651 (1999).

45 See Cathy Charles and Suzanne DeMaio, "Lay Participation in Health Care Decision Making: A Conceptual Framework," 18 *J. Health Pol. Pol'y and L.* 881 (1993).

46 See ICA Resource Center, *Health Insurance Counseling and Assistance Programs: Resource for Older Persons Caught in the Health Care Maze* (1996).

47 See Sylvia A. Law, "A Right to Health Care That Cannot Be Taken Away: The Lessons of Twenty-five Years of Health Care Advocacy," 61 *Tenn. L. Rev.* 771 (1994).

48 See Havighurst, supra note 34; and Kathy L. Cerminara, "The Class Action Suit as a Method of Patient Empowerment in Managed Care," 24 *Am. J. L. and Med.* 7 (1998).

49 See James E. Eggleston, "Patient Advocacy and Consumer Protection through Union Activism: Protecting Health Care Consumers, Patients, and Workers during an Unprecedented Restructuring of the Health Care Industry," 41 *St. Louis U. L. J.* 925, 928–29 (1997).

50 See Maxwell J. Mehlman, "Medical Advocates: A Call for a New Profession," 1 *Widener L. Symp. J.* 299 (1996).

51 See Karen Markus, "Comment: The Nurse as Patient Advocate: Is There a Conflict of Interest?" 29 *Santa Clara L. Rev.* 391 (1989).

52 See Susan L. Goldberg, "A Cure for What Ails? Why the Medical Advocate Is Not the Answer to Problems in the Doctor-Patient Relationship," 1 *Widener L. Symp. J.* 325 (1996).

53 See William M. Sage, "Physicians as Advocates," 35 *Hous. L. Rev.* 1529 (1999); Lawrence C. Kleinman, "Health Care in Crisis: A Proposed Role for the Individual Physician as Advocate," 265 *JAMA* 1991 (1991); and Robert Baker et al., "Crisis, Ethics, and the American Medical Association: 1847 and 1997," 278 *JAMA* 163, 164 (1998). See also Mark J. Hanson and Daniel Callahan, *The Goals of Medicine: The Forgotten Issue in Health Care Reform* (1999); E. Haavi Morreim, *Balancing Act: The New Medical Ethics of Medicine's New Economics* (1991); and David Mechanic, *From Advocacy to Allocation: The Evolving American Health Care System* (1986).

54 See David Mechanic and Mark Schlesinger, "The Impact of Managed Care on Patients' Trust in Medical Care and Their Physicians," 275 *JAMA* 1693 (1996); Linda L. Emanuel, "A Professional Response to Demands for Accountability: Practical Recommendations regarding Ethical Aspects of Patient Care," 124 *Annals of Internal Med.* 240 (1996); Ezekiel J. Emanuel and Linda L. Emanuel, "What Is Accountability in Health Care?" 124 *Annals of Internal Med.* 229 (1996); Council on Ethical and Judicial Affairs, American Medical Association, "Ethical Issues in Managed Care," 273 *JAMA* 330 (1995); Ezekiel J. Emanuel and Nancy N. Dubler, "Preserving the Physician-Patient Relationship in the Era of Managed Care," 273 *JAMA* 323 (1992); *Conflicts of Interest in Clinical Practice and Research* (Roy G. Spece et al. eds., 1996); and George Anders, *Health against Wealth: HMOs and the Breakdown of Medical Trust* (1996). For law review articles on the subject, see Mark Hurt, "Doctors as Double Agents— Conflicting Loyalties in the Contemporary Doctor-Patient Relationship," 2 *J. L.*

and Med. 25 (1997); David Orentlicher, "Health Care Reform and the Patient-Physician Relationship," 5 *Health Matrix* 141 (1995); Marc A. Rodwin, "Conflicts in Managed Care," 332 *New Eng. J. Med.* 604 (1995); and Marc A. Rodwin, "Strains in the Fiduciary Metaphor: Divided Physician Loyalties and Obligations in a Changing Health Care System," 21 *Am. J. L. and Med.* 241 (1995).

55 See, e.g., David Orentlicher, "Paying Physicians to Do Less: Financial Incentives to Limit Care," 30 *U. Rich. L. Rev.* 155 (1996); and Alan L. Hillman, Mark V. Pauly, and Joseph J. Kerstein, "How Do Financial Incentives Affect Physicians' Clinical Decisions and the Financial Performance of Health Maintenance Organizations?" 321 *New Eng. J. Med.* 86 (1989).

56 See, e.g., Tracy E. Miller and William M. Sage, "Disclosing Physician Financial Incentives," 281 *JAMA* 1424 (1999); Ezekiel J. Emanuel and Lee Goldman, "Protecting Patient Welfare in Managed Care: Six Safeguards," 23 *J. Health Pol. Pol'y and L.* 635 (1998); and Deven C. McGraw, "Financial Incentives to Limit Services: Should Physicians Be Required to Disclose These to Patients?" 83 *Geo. L. J.* 1821 (1995).

57 See, e.g., Barry R. Furrow, "The Ethics of Cost-Containment: Bureaucratic Medicine and the Doctor as Patient-Advocate," 3 *Notre Dame J. L. Ethics and Pub. Pol'y* 187 (1988); and Mark A. Hall and Robert A. Berenson, "Ethical Practice in Managed Care: A Dose of Realism," 128 *Annals of Internal Med.* 395 (1998). See also Allen Buchanan, "Rationing without Justice," 23 *J. Health Pol. Pol'y and L.* 617 (1998).

58 See, e.g., Kathy L. Cerminara, "Contextualizing ADR in Managed Care: A Proposal Aimed at Easing Tensions and Resolving Conflict," 33 *Loy. U. Chi. L.J.* (forthcoming 2002); Ann H. Nevers, "Consumer Managed Care Appeals: Are the Available Procedural Protections Fundamentally Fair?" 33 *J. Health L.* 287 (2000); Louise G. Trubek, "Informing, Claiming, Contracting: Enforcement in the Managed Care Era," 8 *Annals of Health L.* 133 (1999); Tracy E. Miller, "Center Stage on the Patient Protection Agenda: Grievance and Appeal Rights," 26 *J. L. Med. and Ethics* 89 (1998); Eleanor D. Kinney, "Procedural Protections for Patients in Capitated Health Plans," 22 *Am. J. L. and Med.* 301 (1996); Eleanor D. Kinney, "Resolving Consumer Grievance in a Managed Care Environment," 6 *Health Matrix* 147 (1996); Phyllis E. Bernard, "Social Security and Medicare Adjudication at HHS: Two Approaches to Administrative Justice in an Ever Expanding Bureaucracy," 3 *Health Matrix* 339 (1993); Margaret G. Farrell, "The Need for a Process Theory: Formulating Health Policy through Adjudication," 8 *J. L. and Health* 201 (1993); and Susan J. Stayn, "Securing Access to Care in Health Maintenance Organizations: Toward a Uniform Model of Grievance and Appeal Procedures," 94 *Colum. L. Rev.* 1674 (1994).

59 See Roderick B. Mathews, "ADR for Managed Care Disputes," 25 *Hum. Rts.* 21 (1998); and Marvin Lieberman, "The Consumer, Managed Health Care, and Dispute Resolution," 34 *Forum* 21 (1997).

60 American Arbitration Association et al., supra note 9.

61 See, e.g., Thomas B. Metzloff, "The Unrealized Potential of Malpractice Arbitration," 31 *Wake Forest L. Rev.* 203, 204 (1996); and Thomas B. Metzloff, "Alternative Dispute Resolution Strategies in Medical Malpractice," 9 *Alaska L. Rev.* 429 (1992).

62 See, e.g., Alice A. Noble and Troyen A. Brennan, "The Stages of Managed Care Regulation: Developing Better Rules," 24 *J. Health Pol. Pol'y and L.* 1275 (1999); Jon Gabel, "Ten Ways HMOs Have Changed during the 1990s," *Health Aff.*, May–June 1997, at 134; and Larry Katzenstein, "Beyond the Horror Stories, Good News about Managed Care," *N.Y. Times*, June 13, 1999, at §15-6.

63 Donald M. Berwick, "Payment by Capitation and the Quality of Care," 335 *New Eng. J. Med.* 1227 (1996); Fred J. Hellinger, "The Effect of Managed Care on Quality," 158 *Archives of Internal Med.* 833 (1998); Robert H. Miller and Harold S. Luft, "Does Managed Care Lead to Better or Worse Quality of Care?" *Health Aff.*, Sept.–Oct. 1997, at 17; Robert H. Miller and Harold S. Luft, "Managed Care Plan Performance since 1980: A Literature Analysis," 271 *JAMA* 1512 (1994); and Harold S. Luft, "HMOs and the Quality of Care," 25 *Inquiry* 147 (1988).

64 Noble and Brennan, supra note 62.

3 Health Insurance Coverage in the United States

1 U.S. Census Bureau, *Health Insurance Coverage: 1999* 1 (fig. 1) (Current Population Reports 2000).

2 See American Association of Health Plans, *The Regulation of Health Plans* (1999); U.S. Congress, Congressional Research Service, *Managed Health Care: Federal and State Regulation: CRS Report for Congress* (1997); and Eleanor D. Kinney, "Procedural Protections for Patients in Capitated Health Plans," 22 *Am. J. L. and Med.* 301 (1996).

3 See generally Paul Starr, *The Social Transformation of American Medicine* (1982).

4 Abraham Flexner, *Medical Education in the United States and Canada: A Report to the Carnegie Foundation for the Advancement of Teaching* (1910).

5 Randall R. Bovbjerg et al., "U.S. Health Care Coverage and Costs: Historical Development and Choices for the 1990s," 2 *J. L. Med. and Ethics* 140 (1993).

6 Id. at 142 (table 1).

7 Katharine Levit et al., "Health Spending in 1998: Signals of Change," *Health Aff.*, Jan.–Feb. 2000, at 124, 131 (exhibit 6).

8 Some material in this chapter has been presented in Eleanor D. Kinney, "Clearing the Way for an Effective Federal-State Partnership in Health Reform," 32 *U. Mich. J. L. Ref.* 899 (1999).

9 Employee Retirement Income Security Act of 1974, §503, Pub. L. No. 93-406, 88 Stat. 832 (codified as amended at 29 U.S.C. §§1001 et seq.).

10 See Herman M. Somers and Anne R. Somers, "Private Health Insurance, Part One: Changing Patterns of Medical Care Demand and Supply in Relation to Health Insurance," 46 *Cal. L. Rev.* 376 (1958); and Herman M. Somers and Anne R. Somers, "Private Health Insurance, Part Two: Problems, Pressures, and Prospects," 46 *Cal. L. Rev.* 508 (1958).

11 Social Security Amendments of 1965, Pub. L. No. 89-97, 79 Stat. 286 (codified as amended in 42 U.S.C. §1396).

12 Social Security Amendments of 1972, Pub. L. No. 92-603, §301, 86 Stat. 1471 (codified as amended at 42 U.S.C. §1382c).

13 Social Security Amendments of 1965, §102(a), Pub. L. No. 89-97, 79 Stat. 286 (codified as amended at 42 U.S.C. §1395 (Medicare)); id. at §121(a) (codified as amended at 42 U.S.C. §1396 (Medicaid)). For histories of Medicare, see, e.g., Judith M. Feder, *Medicare: The Politics of Federal Hospital Insurance* (1977); Sylvia Law, *Blue Cross—What Went Wrong?* (2d ed. 1976); Theodore Marmor, *The Politics of Medicare* (1973); Robert J. Myers, *Medicare* (1970); and Herman Miles Somers and Anne Ramsay Somers, *Medicare and the Hospitals: Issues and Prospects* (1967). For histories of Medicaid, see, e.g., Rosemary Stevens and Robert Stevens, *Welfare Medicine in America: A Case Study of Medicaid* (1974); and Karen Davis and Kathy Schoen, *Health and the War on Poverty* (1978).

14 42 U.S.C. §1395a (1994 and Supp. V 1999). See also id. at §1396a(a)(23) (for similar guarantees for the Medicaid program).

15 Wilber Cohen, "Reflections on the Enactment of Medicare and Medicaid," *Health Care Fin. Rev.*, 1985 Ann. Supp., at 3, 5. See generally William D. Fullerton, "Politics of Federal Health Policy, 1960–1975: A Perspective," *Health Care Fin. Rev.*, winter 1996, at 169.

16 See Staff of Senate Committee on Finance, 91st Cong., 1st Sess., *Medicare and Medicaid: Problems, Issues, and Alternatives* 53, 140–43 (Comm. Print 1970). See also Marian Gornick et al., "Twenty Years of Medicare and Medicaid: Covered Populations, Use of Benefits, and Program Expenditures," *Health Care Fin. Rev.*, 1985 Ann. Supp., at 13, 35–45.

17 Jana K. Strain and Eleanor D. Kinney, "The Road Paved with Good Intentions: Problems and Potential for Employer-Sponsored Health Insurance under ERISA," 31 *Loy. U. Chi. L. J.* 29, 30 (1999).

18 See Daniel M. Fox and Daniel C. Shaffer, "Health Policy and ERISA: Interest Groups and Semipreemption," 14 *J. Health Pol. Pol'y and L.* 239 (1989).

19 See Gail A. Jensen and Jon R. Gabel, "The Erosion of Purchased Health Insurance," 25 *Inquiry* 328 (1988).

20 See, e.g., Mary Ann Chirba-Martin and Troyen A. Brennan, "The Critical Role of ERISA in State Health Reform," *Health Aff.*, spring (II) 1994, at 142; Vicki Gottlich, "ERISA Preemption: A Stumbling Block to State Health Care Re-

form," 26 *Clearinghouse Rev.* 1469 (1993); Wendy K. Mariner, "Problems with Employer-Provider Health Insurance—the Employee Retirement Income Security Act and Health Care Reform," 327 *New Eng. J. Med.* 1682 (1992); and Deborah A. Stone, "Why the States Can't Solve the Healthcare Crisis," *Am. Prospect,* spring 1992, at 174.

21 Eleanor D. Kinney, "Rule and Policy Making under the Medicaid Program: A Challenge to Federalism," 51 *Ohio St. L. J.* 855, 866 (1990).

22 Balanced Budget Amendments of 1997, §4901a, Pub. L. No. 105-33, 111 Stat. 552 (codified at 42 U.S.C. §1397aa).

23 See House Subcommittee on Health of the Committee on Ways and Means, 94th Cong., *National Health Insurance Resource Book* (1976); and Karen Davis, *National Health Insurance: Benefits, Costs, and Consequences* (1975).

24 See Kenneth J. Arrow, "The Economics of Moral Hazard: Further Comments," 58 *Am. Econ. Rev.* 537 (1968). See also Paul Joskow, *Controlling Hospital Costs: The Role of Government Regulation* (1981); and *The Role of Health Insurance in the Health Services Sector* (Richard Rosett ed., 1976).

25 See, e.g., Department of Health, Education, and Welfare, *Medical Technology: The Culprit behind Health Care Costs?* (1977); Louise Russell, *Technology in Hospitals: Medical Advances and Their Diffusion* (1979); and U.S. Congress, Office of Technology Assessment, *Medical Technology under Proposals to Increase Competition in Health Care* (1982).

26 See Brian Biles, Carl J. Schramm, and J. Graham Atkinson, "Hospital Cost Inflation under State Rate Setting Programs," 303 *New Eng. J. Med.* 664 (1980); and Carl J. Schramm, "State Hospital Cost Containment: An Analysis of Legislative Initiatives," 19 *Ind. L. Rev.* 919 (1986).

27 See Bonnie Lefkowitz, *Health Planning: Lessons for the Future* 13 (1983); and James B. Simpson, "Full Circle: The Return of Certificate of Need Regulation and Health Facilities to State Control," 19 *Ind. L. Rev.* 1025 (1986).

28 Social Security Amendments of 1972, Pub. L. No. 92-603, 86 Stat. 1329 (codified as amended at scatter sections of 42 U.S.C.).

29 National Health Planning and Resource Development Act of 1974, Pub. L. No. 93-641, 88 Stat. 2251 (1975).

30 See Kenneth R. Wing and Andrew M. Silton, "Constitutional Authority for Extending Federal Control over the Delivery of Health Care," 57 *N.C. L. Rev.* 1423 (1979).

31 Executive Office of the President, Office of Management and Budget, *Budget of the United States Government: Fiscal Year 1983* 3–23 (1982).

32 Tax Equity and Fiscal Responsibility Act of 1982, Pub. L. No. 97-248, §§101 and 141–50, 96 Stat. 324 (codified as amended at 42 U.S.C. §§1395ww(a)–(c) and 1320c).

33 Social Security Amendments of 1983, Pub. L. No. 98-21, §601(c)(1), 97 Stat. 65 (codified as amended at 42 U.S.C. §1395ww).

34 See David M. Frankford, "The Complexity of Medicare's Hospital Reimbursement System: Paradoxes of Averaging," 78 *Iowa L. Rev.* 517 (1993); David M. Frankford, "The Medicare DRGs: Efficiency and Organizational Rationality," 10 *Yale J. on Reg.* 273 (1993); Wendy K. Mariner, "Prospective Payment for Hospital Services: Social Responsibility and the Limits of Legal Standards," 17 *Cumb. L. Rev.* 379 (1987); and Eleanor D. Kinney, "Making Hard Choices under the Medicare Prospective Payment System: One Administrative Model for Allocating Medical Resources under a Government Health Insurance Program," 19 *Ind. L. Rev.* 1151 (1986).

35 Levit et al., supra note 7.

36 Omnibus Budget Reconciliation Act of 1989, §6102, Pub. L. No. 101-239, 103 Stat. 2111, 2169 (codified as amended at 42 U.S.C. §1395w-4(a)). See "Physician Payment Symposium," *Health Aff.*, spring 1989, at 5; William Roper, "Perspectives on Physician Payment Reform," 319 *New Eng. J. Med.* 865 (1988); and Mark A. Hall, "Institutional Control of Physician Behavior: Legal Barriers to Health Care Cost Containment," 137 *U. Pa. L. Rev.* 431 (1988).

37 See Jon Gabel et al., "The Changing World of Group Health Insurance," *Health Aff.*, summer 1988, at 48.

38 See Bovbjerg et al., supra note 5, at 153–55; and Jon Gabel et al., "The Commercial Health Insurance Industry in Transition," *Health Aff.*, fall 1987, at 46.

39 See Jensen and Gabel, supra note 21; and Patricia McConnell et al., "Self-Insured Health Plans," *Health Care Fin. Rev.*, winter 1986, at 1.

40 See Sara Rosenbaum et al., "Who Should Determine When Health Care Is Medically Necessary?" 340 *New Eng. J. Med.* 229 (1999); William M. Sage, "Judicial Opinions Involving Health Insurance Coverage: Trompe l'Oeil or Window on the World?" 31 *Ind. L. Rev.* 49 (1998); Mark Hall et al., "Judicial Protection of Managed Care Consumers: An Empirical Study of Insurance Coverage Disputes," 26 *Seton Hall Legis. J.* 1055 (1996); Richard Saver, "Reimbursing New Technologies: Why Are the Courts Judging Experimental Medicine?" 44 *Stan. L. Rev.* 1095 (1992); and Mark A. Hall and Gerald F. Anderson, "Health Insurer's Assessment of Medical Necessity," 140 *U. Pa. L. Rev.* 1637 (1992).

41 Jacob S. Hacker and Theodore Marmor, "How Not to Think about 'Managed Care,'" 32 *U. Mich. J. L. Ref.* 661 (1999).

42 See Alain C. Enthoven, "The History and Principles of Managed Competition," *Health Aff.*, Supp. 1993, at 25.

43 Federal Health Maintenance Organizations Act of 1973, Pub. L. No. 93-222, 87 Stat. 914 (codified as amended at 42 U.S.C. §§300e(1–17)). See Michele M. Garvin, "Health Maintenance Organizations," in *Health Care Corporate Law: Managed Care* (Mark Hall and William Brewbaker III eds., 1996).

44 See Troyen A. Brennan and Donald M. Berwick, *New Rules: Regulation, Markets, and the Quality of American Health Care* 152 (1996).

45 See Alain Enthoven, *Health Plan: The Only Practical Solution to the Soaring Cost*

of Medical Care (1980); Alain Enthoven, "Consumer Choice Health Plan: A National Health Insurance Proposal Based on Regulated Competition in the Private Sector," 298 *New Eng. J. Med.* 650, 709 (1978); Clark C. Havighurst, *Deregulating the Health Care Industry* (1982); and *National Health Insurance: What Now, What Later, What Never* (Mark Pauly ed., 1980). See also "Symposium: Competition and Regulation in Health Care Markets," 59 *Milbank Mem. Fund Q.* 107 (1981); and "Special Symposium: Market Oriented Approaches to Achieving Health Policy Goals," 34 *Vand. L. Rev.* 849 (1981).

46 See Randall R. Bovbjerg and John Holahan, *Medicaid in the Reagan Era: Federal Policy and State Choices* (1982); and Kenneth Wing, "The Impact of Reagan-Era Politics on the Federal Medicaid Program," 33 *Cath. U. L. Rev.* 1 (1983).

47 See Eleanor D. Kinney, "Medicare Managed Care from the Beneficiary's Perspective," 26 *Seton Hall L. Rev.* 1163 (1996).

48 See Paul Starr, *The Logic of Health Care Reform: Transforming American Medicine for the Better* (1992); and Jackson Hole Group, "Managed Competition II: A Proposal," 46 *Wash. U. J. Urb. and Contemp. L.* 33 (1994).

49 H.R. 3600, Health Security Act of 1993, 103d Cong., 1st Sess. (1993).

50 See Robert Pear, "Health Industry Is Moving to Form Service Networks," *N.Y. Times,* Aug. 21, 1993, at A1.

51 See, e.g., *Strategic Choices for a Changing Health Care System* (Stuart H. Altman and Uwe E. Reinhardt eds., 1996); Walter A. Zelman, *The Changing Health Care Market Place: Private Ventures, Public Interests* (1996); Stephen M. Shortell et al., *Remaking Health Care in America: Building Organized Delivery Systems* (1986); and "Symposium: Integrated Delivery Networks," *Health Aff.,* summer 1996, at 7.

52 Jon Gabel et al., "Job-Based Health Insurance in 2000: Premiums Rise Sharply while Coverage Grows," *Health Aff.,* Sept.–Oct. 2000, at 144, 148.

53 Id. See also Gail A. Jensen et al., "The New Dominance of Managed Care: Insurance Trends in the 1990s," *Health Aff.,* Jan.–Feb. 1997, at 125.

54 See U.S. General Accounting Office, *Medicare Managed Care Plans: Many Factors Contribute to Recent Withdrawals; Plan Interest Continues* (1999).

55 Cara S. Lesser and Paul B. Ginsburg, "Update on the Nation's Health Care System, 1997–1999," *Health Aff.,* Nov.–Dec. 2000, at 206.

56 U.S. Census Bureau, supra note 1, at 1 (fig. 1).

57 5 U.S.C. §§8901–13 (1994 and Supp. V 1999). See also Office of Personnel Management, *The 2000 Guide to Federal Employees Health Benefit Plan* (2000).

58 I.R.C. §§162(a) (employer deduction) and 106 (tax treatment for individuals) (1994 and Supp. V 1999).

59 John Sheils and Paul Hogan, "Cost of Tax-Exempt Health Benefits in 1998," *Health Aff.,* Mar.–Apr. 1999, at 176.

60 See Paul B. Ginsburg et al., "Tracking Small-Firm Coverage, 1989-1996,"

Health Aff., Jan.–Feb. 1998, at 167; and Gail Jensen et al., "Cost-Sharing and the Changing Pattern of Employer-Sponsored Health Benefits," 65 *Milbank Mem. Fund Q.* 4 (1987). See also U.S. General Accounting Office, *Employment-Based Health Insurance: Costs Increase and Family Coverage Decreases* (1997).

61 Pamela Farley Short and Jessica Banthin, "New Estimates of the Underinsured Younger Than 65 Years," 274 *JAMA* 1302 (1995).

62 Pub. L. No. 79-15, 59 Stat. 33 (codified as amended at 15 U.S.C. §§1011–14). See Banks McDowell, *The Crisis in Insurance Regulation* 41–44 (1994).

63 See Kathleen Heald Ettlinger et al., *State Insurance Regulation* (1995).

64 *The NAIC: A Tradition of Consumer Protection,* http://www.naic.org/1misc/aboutnaic/about/about02.htm (visited Feb. 2, 1999).

65 See National Academy for State Health Policy, *Emerging Challenges in State Regulation of Managed Care: Report of a Survey of State Agency Regulation of Prepaid Managed Care Entities* (1996).

66 Model HMO Act, in National Association of Insurance Commissioners, *NAIC Model Laws, Regulations, and Guidelines* (1998).

67 See National Association of Insurance Commissioners, *Compendium of State Laws on Insurance Topics: Mandated Benefits* (1995).

68 See U.S. General Accounting Office, *Health Insurance Regulation: Varying State Requirements Affect Cost of Insurance* (1996).

69 See Mark A. Hall, "The Competitive Impact of Small Group Health Insurance Reform Laws," 32 *U. Mich. J. L. Ref.* 685 (2000); Thomas R. Oliver, "The Dilemmas of Incrementalism: Logical and Political Constraints in the Design of Health Insurance Reforms," 18 *J. Pol'y Analysis and Mgmt.* 652 (1999); and Thomas R. Oliver and Robert M. Fiedler, "State Government and Health Insurance Market Reform," in *Health Policy Reform in America: Innovations from the States* 47 (Howard M. Leichter ed., 2d ed. 1997).

70 See Kevin T. Stroupe, Eleanor D. Kinney, and Thomas J. Kniesner, "Does Chronic Illness Affect the Adequacy of Health Insurance Coverage?" 25 *J. Health Pol. Pol'y and L.* 309 (2000); Eleanor D. Kinney et al., "Serious Illness and Private Health Coverage: A Unique Problem Calling for Unique Solutions," 25 *J. L. Med. and Ethics* 180 (1997); Donald Light, "Life, Death, and the Insurance Companies," 330 *New Eng. J. Med.* 498 (1994); Deborah A. Stone, "The Struggle for the Soul of Health Insurance," 18 *J. Health Pol. Pol'y and L.* 287 (1993); and Wendy Zellers, Catherine McLaughlin, and Kevin Frick, "Small Business Health Insurance: Only the Healthy Need Apply," *Health Aff.*, spring 1992, at 174.

71 See U.S. General Accounting Office, *Health Insurance Portability: Reform Could Ensure Continued Coverage for Up to 25 Million Americans* (1995); and U.S. General Accounting Office, *Variation in Recent State Small Employer Health Insurance Reform* (1995).

72 See National Association of Insurance Commissioners, *The Regulation of Health Risk-Bearing Entities* (1997).

73 See *Health Care Quality and Consumer Protection: Hearings before the Senate Committee on Labor and Human Resources,* 105th Cong., 1st Sess. 66 (1997) (statement of Kathleen Sebelius, National Association of Insurance Commissioners).

74 See National Association of Insurance Commissioners, *NAIC Model Laws, Regulations, and Guidelines* (2001).

75 See John S. Conniff, "Regulating Managed Health Care Provider Sponsored Organizations," 16 *J. Ins. Reg.* 377 (1998); Edward Hirshfeld, "Provider Sponsored Organizations and Provider Service Networks—Rationale and Regulation," 22 *Am. J. L. and Med.* 263 (1996); Allison Overbay and Mark Hall, *Insurance Regulation of Providers That Bear Risk,* 22 *Am. J. L. and Med.* 361 (1996); and Charles D. Weller, "The Secret Life of the Dominant Form of Managed Care: Self-Insured ERISA Networks," 6 *Health Matrix* 305 (1996). See also E. Haavi Morreim, "Benefits Decisions in ERISA Plans: Diminishing Deference to Fiduciaries and an Emerging Problem for Provider-Sponsored Organizations," 65 *Tenn. L. Rev.* 511 (1998).

76 Employee Retirement Income Security Act of 1974, §503, Pub. L. No. 93-406, 88 Stat. 832 (codified as amended at 29 U.S.C. §§1001 et seq.).

77 Id. at §§1002(1)–(3).

78 Id. at §1104.

79 Id. at §§1101(a) and 1021–25.

80 Id. at §§1021(a) and 1022(a).

81 See Richard Rouco, "Available Remedies under ERISA Section 502(a)," 45 *Ala. L. Rev.* 631 (1994).

82 29 U.S.C. §1132(a) (1994 and Supp. V 1999).

83 Id. at §1132(a)(3).

84 Id. at §1132(a)(6).

85 481 U.S. 41 (1987).

86 29 U.S.C. §1102(1) (1994 and Supp. V 1999).

87 Id. at §1144(a).

88 Id. at §1144(b).

89 Id. at §1144(c).

90 See Metropolitan Life Ins. Co. v. Massachusetts, 471 U.S. 724 (1985).

91 See, e.g., Robert N. Covington, "Amending ERISA's Preemption Scheme," 8 *Kan. J. L. and Pub. Pol'y* 1 (1999); Karen A. Jordan, "The Shifting Preemption Paradigm: Conceptual and Interpretive Issues," 51 *Vand. L. Rev.* 1149 (1998); Peter D. Jacobson and Scott D. Pomfret, "Form, Function, and Managed Care Torts: Achieving Fairness and Equity in ERISA Jurisprudence," 35 *Hous. L. Rev.* 985 (1998); Margaret G. Farrell, "ERISA Preemption and Regulation of Managed Health Care: The Case of Managed Federalism," 23 *Am. J. L. and Med.*

251 (1997); and Catherine L. Fisk, "The Last Article about the Language of ERISA Preemption: A Case Study of the Failure of Textualism," 33 *Harv. J. on Legis.* 35 (1996).

92 481 U.S. 41 (1987).

93 See, e.g., Donald T. Bogan, "Protecting Patient Rights Despite ERISA: Will the Supreme Court Allow States to Regulate Managed Care?" 74 *Tul. L. Rev.* 951 (2000); Karen A. Jordan, "Tort Liability for Managed Care: The Weakening of ERISA's Protective Shield," 25 *J. L. Med. and Ethics* 160, 163 (1997); Barry R. Furrow, "Managed Care Organizations and Patient Injury: Rethinking Liability," 31 *Ga. L. Rev.* 419 (1997); and Jack K. Kilcullen, "Groping for the Reins: ERISA, HMO Malpractice, and Enterprise Liability," 22 *Am. J. L. and Med.* 7 (1997). See also U.S. General Accounting Office, *Employer-Based Managed Care Plans: ERISA's Effect on Remedies for Benefit Denials and Medical Malpractice* (1998).

94 See De Buono v. NYSA-ILA Medical and Clinical Services Fund, 520 U.S. 806 (1997); California Division of Labor Standards Enforcement, N.A., Inc., 519 U.S. 316 (1997); and Boggs v. Boggs, 520 U.S. 833 (1997). See also New York State Conference of Blue Cross Blue Shield Plans v. Travelers Ins., Inc., 514 U.S. 645 (1995).

95 See Alice A. Noble and Troyen A. Brennan, "The Stages of Managed Care Regulation: Developing Better Rules," 24 *J. Health Pol. Pol'y and L.* 1275 (1999); and Robert N. Covington, supra note 91.

96 See Chirba-Martin and Brennan, supra note 22; Gottlich, supra note 22; Mariner, "Problems with Employer-Provider Health Insurance," supra note 22; and Stone, "Why the States Can't Solve the Healthcare Crisis," supra note 22. See also James E. Holloway, "ERISA, Preemption, and Comprehensive Federal Health Care: A Call for 'Cooperative Federalism' to Preserve the States' Role in Formulating Health Care Policy," 16 *Campbell L. Rev.* 405 (1994); Alan I. Widiss and Larry Gostin, "What's Wrong with the ERISA 'Vacuum'? The Case against Unrestricted Freedom for Employers to Terminate Employee Health Care Plans and to Decide What Coverage Is to Be Provided When Risk Retention Plans Are Established for Health Care," 41 *Drake L. Rev.* 635 (1992); and Mary Anne Bobinski, "Unhealthy Federalism: Barriers to Increasing Health Care Access for the Uninsured," 24 *U.C. Davis L. Rev.* 255 (1990). See generally Patricia Butler and Karl Polzer, *Private-Sector Health Coverage: Variation in Consumer Protections under ERISA and State Law* (1996); and U.S. General Accounting Office, *Employer-Based Health Plans: Issues, Trends, and Challenges Posed by ERISA* (1995).

97 See National Association of Insurance Commissioners, *NAIC White Paper: ERISA: A Call for Reform: Recommendations of the National Association of Insurance Commissioners* 9 (1995).

98   See U.S. General Accounting Office, *Employer-Based Health Plans,* supra note 96, at 17–18 (1995).

99   See id. at 12–14.

100 See generally Weller, supra note 75.

101 946 F.2d 401 (5th Cir. 1991), cert. denied, 506 U.S. 981 (1992).

102 See id. at 408.

103 111 F.3d 358 (4th Cir. 1997), cert. denied, 524 U.S. 936 (1998).

104 See id. at 365.

105 Consolidated Budget Reconciliation Act of 1985, Pub. L. No. 99-272, §10001, 100 Stat. 222 (codified as amended at 29 U.S.C. §§1161 and 1162).

106 The Mental Health Parity Act of 1996 and the Newborns' and Mothers' Health Protection Act of 1996, in Pub. L. No. 104-204, 110 Stat. 2944 (codified at 29 U.S.C. §1185).

107 Health Insurance Portability and Accountability Act of 1997, Pub. L. No. 104-191, 110 Stat. 1936 (codified at scattered sections of 26, 29, and 42 U.S.C.). See U.S. General Accounting Office, *Implementation of HIPAA: Progress Slow in Enforcing Federal Standards in Nonconforming States* (2000); and U.S. General Accounting Office, *Health Insurance Standards: New Federal Law Creates Challenges for Consumers, Insurers, Regulators* (1998).

108 29 U.S.C. §§1182(a) and (b) (1994 and Supp. V 1999).

109 Social Security Amendments of 1965, Pub. L. No. 89-97, 79 Stat. 286 (codified as amended at 42 U.S.C. §1395 (Medicare)).

110 42 U.S.C. §§1395c, i-2, and o (1994 and Supp. V 1999).

111 Id. at §1395c.

112 Id. at §1395y(a)(1).

113 Id. at §§1395c–i.

114 Id. at §§1395j–w.

115 Id. at §1395t.

116 Id. at §1395i.

117 Id. at §1395w-21.

118 U.S. General Accounting Office, *Medicare Managed Care Plans,* supra note 54.

119 42 U.S.C. §§1395h and u (fiscal intermediaries and carriers) and §§1320c-1–c-12 (peer review organizations) (1994 and Supp. V 1999).

120 Id. at §1395bb. See Timothy S. Jost, "Medicare and the Joint Commission on Accreditation of Healthcare Organizations: A Healthy Relationship?" 57 *L. and Contemp. Probs.* 15 (1994).

121 42 U.S.C. §1395w-21 (1994 and Supp. V 1999).

122 Social Security Amendments of 1965, Pub. L. No. 89-97, 79 Stat. 286 (codified as amended at 42 U.S.C. §1396).

123 U.S. Census Bureau, supra note 1, at 1 (fig. 1).

124 42 U.S.C. §1396a(a) (1994 and Supp. V 1999).

125 Id. at §1396.

126 See *Medicare and Medicaid Guide* (CCH) ¶¶14211–14381 (1999); and Congressional Research Service, *Medicaid Source Book: Background Data and Analysis, 1993 Update* 187 (1993).

127 See John K. Iglehart, "Federal Policies and the Poor," 307 *New Eng. J. Med.* 836 (1982).

128 See Kinney, "Rule and Policy Making under the Medicaid Program," supra note 17.

129 42 U.S.C. §1396a(a)(10) (1994 and Supp. V 1999).

130 Id. at §1396a(a)(10)(A)(ii).

131 Pub. L. No. 104-193, 110 Stat. 2105 (codified at 42 U.S.C. §1305).

132 42 U.S.C. §602(a)(1) (Supp. V 1999). See Tonya L. Brito, "From Madonna to Proletariat: Constructing a New Ideology of Motherhood in Welfare Discourse," 44 *Vill. L. Rev.* 415 (1999); and Sara Rosenbaum and Kathleen A. Maloy, "The Law of Unintended Consequences: The 1996 Personal Responsibility and Work Opportunity Reconciliation Act and Its Impact on Medicaid for Families with Children," 60 *Ohio St. L. J.* 1443 (1999).

133 42 U.S.C. §1396(a) (Supp. V 1999).

134 Id. at §1396a(10)(C).

135 See "Medicaid State Plan Summaries," *Medicare and Medicaid Guide* (CCH) ¶ 15501 (1999).

136 42 U.S.C. §§1396a(a)(1)–(17) (1994 and Supp. V 1999).

137 Id. at §1396a(a)(10)(E)(iv) and (v).

138 Id. at §1396a(a)(1)(10).

139 Id. at §§1396a(a)(10)(B) (categorically needy), 1396a(a)(10)(B) (medically needy), and 1396b(m)(1)(A)(i) (comparability for HMO and non-HMO benefits).

140 Id. at §§1396a(a)(1)–(5).

141 See Congressional Research Service, *Medicaid Source Book*, supra note 126, at 1.

142 Omnibus Budget Reconciliation Act of 1981, Pub. L. No. 97-35, §2175, 95 Stat. 357, 809–11 (1981) (codified as amended at 42 U.S.C. §1396n(b)(1)). See Michael S. Sparer, *Medicaid and the Limits of State Health Reform* (1996); Robert E. Hurley, Deborah A. Freund, and John E. Paul, *Managed Care in Medicaid: Lessons for Policy and Program Design* (1993); and Bovbjerg and Holahan, supra note 46.

143 Balanced Budget Act of 1997, §§4702–4, Pub. L. No. 105-33, 111 Stat. 522 (to be codified at 42 U.S.C. §1396u-2); Medicaid Program, Medicaid Managed Care: Proposed Rule, 63 Fed. Reg. 52,021, 52,049–50 (Sept. 29, 1998); Sidney D. Watson, "Commercialization of Medicaid," 45 *St. Louis U. L.J.* 53 (2001).

144 42 U.S.C. §1315 (1994 and Supp. V 1999).

145 See John Holahan et al., *Health Policy for the Low-Income Population: Major*

Findings from the "Assessing the New Federalism" (1998); Lisa Axelrod, "The Trend toward Medicaid Managed Care: Is the Government Selling Out the Medicaid Poor?" 7 *B.U. Pub. Int. L. J.* 251 (1998); Thomas J. Anton, "New Federalism and Intergovernmental Fiscal Relationships: The Implications for Health Policy," 22 *J. Health Pol. Pol'y and L.* 691 (1997); Judith M. Rosenberg and David T. Zaring, "Managing Medicaid Waivers: Section 1115 and State Health Care Reform," 32 *Harv. J. on Legis.* 545 (1995); and John Holahan et al., "Insuring the Poor through Section 1115 Medicaid Waivers," *Health Aff.*, spring 1995, at 200.

146 Balanced Budget Amendments of 1997, Pub. L. No. 105-33, §4901(a), 111 Stat. 552 (codified at 42 U.S.C. §1397aa). See Brian K. Bruen and Frank Ullman, *Children's Health Insurance Programs: Where States Are, Where They Are Headed* (1998); and Sarah Rosenbaum et al., "The Children's Hour: The State Children's Health Insurance Program," *Health Aff.*, Jan.–Feb. 1998, at 75.

147 Pub. L. No. 105-33, §4901(a), 111 Stat. 552 (codified at 42 U.S.C. §1397aa).

148 42 U.S.C. §1397aa (Supp. V 1999).

149 Id. at §1397aa.

150 See Kenneth E. Thorpe and Curtis S. Florence, "Covering Uninsured Children and Their Parents: Estimated Costs and Numbers of Newly Insured," 56 *Med. Care Res. and Rev.* 197, 201 (1999).

151 Department of Health and Human Services, Indian Health Service, *Fact Sheet* (2000).

152 10 U.S.C. §§1071 et seq. (1994 and Supp. V 1999).

153 U.S. General Accounting Office, *Defense Health Care: TRICARE Resource Sharing Program Failing to Achieve Expected Savings* (1997).

154 38 U.S.C. §§1701 et seq. (1994 and Supp. V 1999). See U.S. General Accounting Office, *VA Health Care: Progress and Challenges in Providing Care to Veterans* (1999); and Gerald A. Williams, "A Primer on Veterans' Benefits for Legal Assistance Attorneys," 47 *A.F.L. Rev.* 163 (1999).

155 38 U.S.C. §§1705 and 1710 (1994 and Supp. V 1999).

156 See Shruti Rajan, "Publicly Subsidized Health Insurance: A Typology of State Approaches," *Health Aff.*, May–June 1998, at 101; and Pamela Paul-Shaheen, "The States and Health Reform: The Road Traveled and Lessons Learned from the Seven That Took the Lead," 23 *J. Health Pol. Pol'y and L.* 319, 353 (1998). See generally John Holahan and Len Nichols, "State Health Policy in the 1990s," in *Health Policy, Federalism, and the American States* 39 (Robert F. Reich and William D. White eds., 1996).

157 See Colleen M. Grogan, "Hope in Federalism? What Can the States Do and What Are They Likely to Do?" 20 *J. Health Pol. Pol'y and L.* 477 (1995); Howard M. Leichter, "State Governments and Their Capacity for Healthcare Reform," in *Health Policy, Federalism, and the American States,* supra note 156,

at 151; Trish Riley, "Can We Count on the States to Cover the Poor and Uninsured?" in *The Future U.S. Healthcare System: Who Will Care for the Poor and Uninsured?* 273 (Stuart H. Altman et al. eds., 1998); and Raymond C. Scheppach, "The State Health Agenda: Austerity, Efficiency, and Monitoring the Emerging Market," in *The Future U.S. Healthcare System,* supra, at 285.

158 U.S. Census Bureau, supra note 1, at 1 (fig. 1).

159 See, e.g., Olveen Carrasquillo et al., "Going Bare: Trends in Health Insurance Coverage, 1989 through 1996," 89 *Am. J. Pub. Health* 36 (1998); Linda J. Blumberg and David Liska, *The Uninsured in the United States: A Status Report* 6 (1996); and Karen Davis et al., "Health Insurance: The Size and Shape of the Problem," 32 *Inquiry* 196 (1995).

160 "Working Families Struggle to Get Needed Care and Pay Medical Bills," *Commonwealth Fund Q.,* winter 1997, at 1.

161 See Jensen et al., "The New Dominance of Managed Care," supra note 53; Blumberg and Liska, supra note 159; Cynthia B. Sullivan and Thomas Rice, "The Health Insurance Picture in 1990," *Health Aff.,* summer 1991, at 104; Bovbjerg et al., supra note 5; Jensen et al., "Cost-Sharing and the Changing Pattern of Employer-Sponsored Health Benefits," supra note 60; and U.S. General Accounting Office, *Employment-Based Health Insurance,* supra note 60.

162 See Ginsburg et al., supra note 60; Michael Chernew et al., "The Demand for Health Insurance Coverage by Low-Income Workers: Can Reduced Premiums Achieve Full Coverage?" 32 *HSR: Health Services Res.* 453 (1997); Phillip Cooper and Barbara Steinberg Schone, "More Offers, Fewer Takers for Employment-Based Health Insurance: 1987 and 1996," *Health Aff.,* Nov.– Dec. 1997, at 142; M. Susan Marquis and Steven H. Long, "Worker Demand for Health Insurance in the Non-Group Market," 14 *J. Health Econ.* 47 (1995); Steven H. Long and M. Susan Marquis, "The Uninsured 'Access Gap' and the Cost of Universal Coverage," *Health Aff.,* spring 1994, at 211; and Gabel et al., "Job-Based Health Insurance in 2000," supra note 52.

163 See *Employment and Health Benefits: A Connection at Risk* (Marilyn Field and Harold Shapiro eds., 1993); Mary E. O'Connell, "On the Fringe: Rethinking the Link between Wages and Benefits," 67 *Tul. L. Rev.* 1421 (1993); and Edward J. McCaffery, "The Burdens of Benefits," 44 *Vill. L. Rev.* 445 (1999).

4 Relevant Law and Theory

1 Employee Retirement Income Security Act of 1974, Pub. L. No. 93-406, 88 Stat. 832 (codified as amended at 29 U.S.C. §§1001 et seq.).

2 Richard B. Stewart, "The Reformation of American Administrative Law," 88 *Harv. L. Rev.* 1669 (1975). See also David Truman, *The Governmental Process:*

Political Interests and Public Opinion (1951); and Robert Dahl, *A Preface to Democratic Theory* (1956).

3 See Daniel A. Farber and Philip P. Frickey, *Law and Public Choice: A Critical Introduction* 17 (1991); Gary Minda, *Postmodern Legal Movements: Law and Jurisprudence at Century's End* 96–97 (1995); and Susan Rose-Ackerman, "Progressive Law and Economics—and the New Administrative Law," 98 *Yale L. J.* 341 (1988).

4 See Mancur Olsen, *The Logic of Collective Action* (1965); Anthony Downs, *An Economic Theory of Democracy* (1957); James M. Buchanan and Gordon Tullock, *The Calculus of Consent* (1962); George J. Stigler, "The Theory of Economic Regulation," 2 *Bell J. Econ. and Mgmt. Sci.* 3 (1971); and Gary S. Becker, "A Theory of Competition among Pressure Groups for Political Influence," 98 *Q. J. Econ.* 371 (1983).

5 See Jerry L. Mashaw, *Greed, Chaos, and Governance: Using Public Choice to Improve Public Law* (1997); Glen O. Robinson, *American Bureaucracy: Public Choice and Public Law* (1991); John P. Heinz et al., *The Hollow Core: Private Interests in National Policy-Making* (1993); Kay Lehman Schozman and John T. Tierney, *Organized Interests and American Democracy* (1986); "Symposium on the Theory of Public Choice," 74 *Va. L. Rev.* 167 (1988); Cass R. Sunstein, "Interest Groups in American Public Law," 38 *Stan. L. Rev.* 29 (1985); and Richard B. Stewart, "The Discontents of Legalism: Interest Group Relations in Administrative Regulation," 1985 *Wis. L. Rev.* 655 (1985).

6 See *Regulation of the Healthcare Professions* (Timothy S. Jost ed., 1997).

7 See Eleanor D. Kinney, "Administrative Law Issues in Professional Regulation," in *Regulation of the Healthcare Professions*, supra note 6, at 103.

8 See Council on Ethical and Judicial Affairs, American Medical Association, *Code of Medical Ethics* (1996). See generally William M. Sage, "Physicians as Advocates," 35 *Hous. L. Rev.* 1529 (1999); David Orentlicher, "The Role of Professional Self-Regulation," in *Regulation of the Healthcare Professions*, supra note 6, at 129; and David Orentlicher, "Health Care Reform and the Patient-Physician Relationship," 5 *Health Matrix* 141 (1995).

9 See David Young, "Accounting and Financial Management for Health Care Facilities," in *Health Care Corporate Law: Financing and Liability* (Mark A. Hall ed., 1994).

10 See "Symposium: Private Accreditation in the Regulatory State," 57 *L. and Contemp. Probs.* (1994); Douglas C. Michael, "Federal Agency Use of Audited Self-Regulation as a Regulatory Technique," 47 *Admin. L. Rev.* 171 (1995); and Timothy S. Jost, "The Joint Commission on the Accreditation of Hospitals: Private Regulation of Health Care and the Public Interest," 24 *B.C. L. Rev.* 835 (1983).

11 Model HMO Act, in National Association of Insurance Commissioners, *NAIC Model Laws, Regulations, and Guidelines* (1998).

12 See Barbara A. Shickich, "Legal Characteristics of the Health Maintenance Organization," in *Health Care Facilities Law* §16 (Anne M. Dellinger ed., 1991).

13 See Eleanor D. Kinney, "Private Accreditation as a Substitute for Direct Government Regulation in Public Health Insurance Programs: When Is It Appropriate?" 57 *L. and Contemp. Probs.* 47 (1994); and Jost, "The Joint Commission on the Accreditation of Hospitals," supra note 10.

14 See Kinney, "Private Accreditation as a Substitute for Direct Government Regulation," supra note 13; and Jost, "The Joint Commission on the Accreditation of Hospitals," supra note 10.

15 See Kinney, "Private Accreditation as a Substitute for Direct Government Regulation," supra note 13; and Sandra H. Johnson, "Quality-Control Regulation of Home Health Care," 26 *Hous. L. Rev.* 901, 935 (1989).

16 See Timothy S. Jost, "Oversight of the Quality of Medical Care: Regulation, Management, or the Market?" 37 *Ariz. L. Rev.* 825 (1995); and Timothy Stoltzfus Jost, "The Necessary and Proper Role of Regulation to Assure the Quality of Health Care," 25 *Hous. L. Rev.* 525 (1988).

17 Barry A. Furrow et al., *Health Law* §§1-4, 4-23, 4-24 (1995).

18 See William M. Sage, "Regulating through Information: Disclosure Laws and American Health Care," 99 *Colum. L. Rev.* 1701 (1999); and Neil B. Cohen and Aaron D. Twerski, "Comparing Medical Providers: A First Look at the New Era of Medical Statistics," 58 *Brook. L. Rev.* 5 (1992). See also Frances H. Miller, "Health Care Information Technology and Informed Consent: Computers and the Doctor-Patient Relationship," 31 *Ind. L. Rev.* 1019 (1998); Shoshanna Sofaer, "Informing and Protecting Consumers under Managed Competition," *Health Aff.*, Supp. 1993, at 76; and Paul B. Ginsburg and Glenn T. Hammons, "Competition and the Quality of Care: The Importance of Information," 25 *Inquiry* 108 (1988).

19 Elaine M. Hadden and Blaire A. French, *Nonprofit Organizations: Rights and Liabilities for Members, Directors, and Officers* 76 (1987).

20 See Henry B. Hansmann, "Reforming Nonprofit Corporation Law," 129 *U. Pa. L. Rev.* 497 (1981); and Henry B. Hansmann, "The Role of Nonprofit Enterprise," 89 *Yale L. J.* 835 (1980).

21 Hadden and French, supra note 19, at 22–25.

22 I.R.C. §501 (1994).

23 Hadden and French, supra note 19, at 22–29.

24 See John Columbo and Mark Hall, *The Charitable Tax Exemption* (1995).

25 Harry G. Henn and John R. Alexander, *Laws of Corporations and Other Business Enterprises* §133 (3d ed. 1993).

26 See Michele M. Garvin, "Health Maintenance Organizations," in *Health Care Corporate Law: Managed Care* (Mark Hall and William Brewbaker III eds., 1996); and Joanne B. Stern, "The Conversion of HMOs from Non-Profit to For-

Profit Status: Background, Methodology, and Problems," 26 *St. Louis U. L. J.* 711 (1982).

27 See, e.g., Mark Schlesinger, Bradford Gray, and Elizabeth Bradley, "Charity and Community: The Role of Nonprofit Ownership in a Managed Health Care System," 21 *J. Health Pol. Pol'y and L.* 697 (1996); Malik M. Hasan, "Let's End the Nonprofit Charade," 334 *New Eng. J. Med.* 1055 (1996); Phillip M. Nudelman and Linda M. Andrews, "The 'Value Added' of Not-for-Profit Health Plans," 334 *New Eng. J. Med.* 1057 (1996); and Nina J. Crimm, "Evolutionary Forces: Changes in For-Profit and Not-for-Profit Health Care Delivery Structures; a Regeneration of Tax Exemption Standards," 37 *B.C. L. Rev.* 1 (1995).

28 See, e.g., Rosemary Stevens, *In Sickness and in Wealth: American Hospitals in the Twentieth Century* (1989); Joseph Rogers Hollingsworth and Ellen Jane Hollingsworth, *Controversy about American Hospitals: Funding, Ownership, and Performance* (1987); Phyllis E. Bernard, "Privatization of Rural Public Hospitals: Implications for Access and Indigent Care," 47 *Mercer L. Rev.* 991 (1996); and M. Gregg Bloche, "Corporate Takeover of Teaching Hospitals," 65 *S. Cal. L. Rev.* 1035 (1992).

29 See Michael Peregrine, "Charitable Trust and the Evolving Nature of the Nonprofit Hospital Corporation," 30 *J. Health and Hosp. L.* 11 (1997); Lisa C. Ikemoto, "When a Hospital Becomes Catholic," 47 *Mercer L. Rev.* 1087 (1996); and Kathleen Boozang, "Deciding the Fate of Religious Hospitals in the Emerging Health Care Market," 31 *Hous. L. Rev.* 1429 (1995).

30. I.R.C. §501(c)(3) (1994).

31 See Lawrence E. Singer, "The Conversion Conundrum: The State and Federal Response to Hospitals' Changes in Charitable Status," 23 *Am. J. L. and Med.* 221 (1997).

32 See Bradford H. Gray, *The Profit Motive and Patient Care* (1991). See generally Paul Starr, *The Social Transformation of American Medicine* (1982).

33 See M. Gregg Bloche, "Health Policy below the Waterline: Medical Care and Charitable Exemption," 80 *Minn. L. Rev.* 299 (1995); John Columbo and Mark Hall, "The Future of Tax Exemption for Nonprofit Hospitals and Other Health Care Providers," 2 *Health Matrix* 1 (1992); David A. Hyman, "The Conundrum of Charitability: Reassessing Tax Exemption for Hospitals," 16 *Am. J. L. and Med.* 327 (1988); Theodore R. Marmor, Mark Schlesinger, and Richard W. Smithey, "A New Look at Nonprofits: Health Care Policy in a Competitive Age," 3 *Yale J. on Reg.* 313 (1986); and Robert Charles Clark, "Does the Nonprofit Form Fit the Hospital Industry?" 93 *Harv. L. Rev.* 1416 (1980). See also Mark A. Hall and John D. Columbo, "The Charitable Status of Nonprofit Hospitals: Toward a Donative Theory of Tax Exemption," 66 *Wash. L. Rev.* 307 (1991). See also Utah County v. Intermountain Health Care, Inc., 709 P.2d 265 (Utah 1985).

34 See Institute of Medicine, *For-Profit Enterprise in Health Care* (Bradford Gray ed., 1986); and Arnold Relman, "The New Medical-Industrial Complex," 303 *New Eng. J. Med.* 963 (1980).

35 I.R.C. §501(c)(6) (1994).

36 I.R.C. §501(c)(3) (1994). See generally Bruce R. Hopkins, *The Law of Tax Exempt Organizations* (1987).

37 I.R.C. §501(c)(3) (1994).

38 See, e.g., Jeffrey S. Lubbers, *A Guide to Federal Agency Rulemaking* 93–107 (3d ed. 1998); Arthur Earl Bonfield, "State Administrative Policy Formulation and the Choice of Lawmaking Methodology," 42 *Admin. L. Rev.* 121 (1990); Richard K. Berg, "Re-Examining Policy Procedures: The Choice between Rulemaking and Adjudication," 38 *Admin. L. Rev.* 149 (1986); Glen O. Robinson, "The Making of Administrative Policy: Another Look at Rulemaking and Adjudication and Administrative Procedure Reform," 118 *U. Pa. L. Rev.* 485 (1970); and Bernard Schwartz, "Administrative Terminology and the Administrative Procedure Act," 48 *Mich. L. Rev.* 57 (1949).

39 Pub. L. No. 404, 60 Stat. 237, Ch. 324, §§1–12, codified by Pub. L. No. 89-554 (1966), in 5 U.S.C. §§551–59, 701–6 (1994 and Supp. V 1999). See "Symposium: The Administrative Procedure Act: A Fortieth Anniversary Symposium," 72 *Va. L. Rev.* 215 (1986).

40 National Conference of Commissioners on Uniform State Laws, *Model State Administrative Procedures Act* (1981).

41 Kenneth Culp Davis, "An Approach to Problems of Evidence in the Administrative Process," 55 *Harv. L. Rev.* 364 (1942).

42 See Jerry L. Mashaw, " 'Rights' in the Federal Administrative State," 92 *Yale L. J.* 1129 (1983). See also Cass Sunstein, *After the Rights Revolution: Reconceiving the Regulatory State* (1990).

43 Stewart, "The Reformation of American Administrative Law," supra note 2.

44 Mashaw, " 'Rights' in the Federal Administrative State," supra note 42.

45 See William Van Alstyne, "Cracks in 'the New Property': Adjudicative Due Process in the Administrative State," 62 *Cornell L. Rev.* 445, 445–46 (1977); and Charles A. Reich, "The New Property," 73 *Yale L. J.* 733 (1964).

46 5 U.S.C. §554(a) (1994) (invoking APA hearing procedures (id. at §§556–57) when Congress requires an on-the-record hearing).

47 Id. at §553(a)(2).

48 *Goldberg v. Kelly,* 397 U.S. 254 (1970).

49 See Lubbers, supra note 38; Cornelius M. Kerwin, *Rulemaking: How Government Agencies Write Law and Make Policy* (1994); and Arthur E. Bonfield, *State Administrative Rulemaking* (1986).

50 See Bernard Schwartz, *Administrative Law* §51 (2d ed. 1989). See also Ernest Gellhorn and Glen O. Robinson, "Rulemaking 'Due Process': An Inconclusive Dialogue," 48 *U. Chi. L. Rev.* 201 (1981).

51 See Robert F. Williams, "In the Supreme Court's Shadow: Legitimacy of State Rejection of Supreme Court Reasoning and Result," 35 *S.C. L. Rev.* 353 (1984).

52 5 U.S.C. §553 (1994).

53 See the administrative codes of Alabama, Alaska, California, Connecticut, Florida, Idaho, Illinois, Indiana, Kansas, Maryland, Massachusetts, Minnesota, Nevada, New York, North Carolina, Ohio, Oregon, Pennsylvania, South Carolina, Virginia, and Wyoming.

54 See Lubbers, supra note 38, at 3–6; and Robert L. Rabin, "Federal Regulation in Historical Perspective," 38 *Stan. L. Rev.* 1189 (1986).

55 See Paul R. Verkuil, "The Emerging Concept of Administrative Procedure," 78 *Colum. L. Rev.* 258 (1978).

56 See, e.g., "Symposium: The Contribution of the D.C. Circuit to Administrative Law," 40 *Admin. L. Rev.* 507 (1988); and Daniel J. Gifford, "Rulemaking and Rulemaking Review: Struggling toward a New Paradigm," 32 *Admin. L. Rev.* 577 (1980).

57 See Neil R. Eisner, "Agency Delay in Informal Rulemaking," 3 *Admin. L. J.* 7 (1989).

58 Negotiated Rulemaking Act of 1990, Pub. L. No. 101-648, 104 Stat. 4969 (codified at 5 U.S.C. §§561–70). See Administrative Conference of the United States, *Negotiated Rulemaking Sourcebook* (2d ed. 1995); Henry H. Perritt Jr., "Administrative Alternative Dispute Resolution: The Development of Negotiated Rulemaking and Other Processes," 14 *Pepp. L. Rev.* 863 (1987); and Philip J. Harter, "Negotiating Regulations: A Cure for Malaise," 71 *Geo. L. J.* 1 (1982).

59 See, e.g., Robert E. Litan and William D. Nordhaus, *Reforming Federal Regulation* (1983); Stephen Breyer, *Regulation and Its Reform* (1983); Jerry L. Mashaw, "Reinventing Government and Regulatory Reform: Studies in the Neglect and Abuse of Administrative Law," 57 *U. Pitt. L. Rev.* 405 (1996); Thomas O. McGarity, "Regulatory Reform in the Reagan Era," 45 *Md. L. Rev.* 253 (1986); and Christopher C. Demuth and Douglas H. Ginsburg, "White House Review of Agency Rulemaking," 99 *Harv. L. Rev.* 1075 (1986).

60 See Mark Seidenfeld, "Demystifying Deossification: Rethinking Recent Proposals to Modify Judicial Review of Notice and Comment Rulemaking," 75 *Tex. L. Rev.* 483 (1997); Richard J. Pierce Jr., "Seven Ways to Deossify Agency Rulemaking," 47 *Admin. L. Rev.* 59 (1995); and Thomas O. McGarity, "Some Thoughts on 'Deossifying' the Rulemaking Process," 41 *Duke L. J.* 1385 (1992).

61 See William F. Leahy, "The Fate of the Legislative Veto after *Chadha*," 53 *Geo. Wash. L. Rev.* 168 (1984); E. Donald Elliott, "*INS v. Chadha:* The Administrative Constitution, the Constitution, and the Legislative Veto," 1983 *Sup. Ct. Rev.* 125; and Harold H. Bruff, "Presidential Management of Agency Rulemaking," 57 *Geo. Wash. L. Rev.* 533 (1989).

62 See Barry R. Furrow, "Governing Science: Public Risks and Private Remedies," 131 *U. Pa. L. Rev.* 1403 (1983); David L. Bazelon, "Coping with Technology

through the Legal Process," 62 *Cornell L. Rev.* 817 (1977); and Arthur Kantrowitz, "Controlling Technology Democratically," 63 *Am. Scientist* 505 (1975).

63 435 U.S. 519 (1978).

64 See, e.g., Cooley B. Howarth Jr., "Informal Agency Rulemaking and the Courts: A Theory for Procedural Review," 61 *Wash. U. L. Q.* 891 (1984); Richard B. Stewart, "*Vermont Yankee* and the Evolution of Administrative Procedure," 91 *Harv. L. Rev.* 1805 (1978); and Antonin Scalia, "*Vermont Yankee:* The APA, the D.C. Circuit, and the Supreme Court," 1978 *Sup. Ct. Rev.* 345.

65 See Stephen Williams, "Hybrid Rulemaking under the Administrative Procedure Act: A Legal and Empirical Analysis," 42 *U. Chi. L. Rev.* 401 (1975).

66 See Vermont Yankee Nuclear Power Corp. v. Natural Resources Defense Council, 435 U.S. 519 (1978); and U.S. v. Florida East Coast Ry., 410 U.S. 224 (1973). See also Loren A. Smith, "Judicialization: The Twilight of Administrative Law," 1985 *Duke L. J.* 427.

67 See Peter L. Strauss, "The Rulemaking Continuum," 41 *Duke L. J.* 1463 (1992).

68 5 U.S.C. §553(a)(2) (1994 and Supp. V 1999).

69 Administrative Conference of the United States, Recommendation No. 69-8, Elimination of Certain Exemptions from the APA Rulemaking Requirements, 38 Fed. Reg. 19,782 (1973). See Arthur Earl Bonfield, "Public Participation in Federal Rulemaking Relating to Public Property, Loans, Grants, Benefits, or Contracts," 118 *U. Pa. L. Rev.* 540 (1970).

70 See Robert A. Anthony, "'Interpretive' Rules, 'Legislative' Rules, and 'Spurious' Rules: Lifting the Smog," 8 *Admin. L. J. Am. U.* 1 (1994); Jeffrey S. Lubbers and Nancy G. Miller, "The APA Procedural Rule Exemption: Looking for a Way to Clear the Air," 6 *Admin. L. J. Am. U.* 482 (1992); Robert A. Anthony, "Interpretative Rules, Policy Statements, Guidances, Manuals, and the Like: Should Federal Agencies Use Them to Bind the Public?" 41 *Duke L. J.* 1311 (1992); and Robert A. Anthony, "Which Agency Interpretations Should Bind Citizens and the Courts?" 7 *Yale J. on Reg.* 1 (1990).

71 Freedom of Information Act, Pub. L. No. 89-487, 80 Stat. 250 (1966) (codified as amended at 5 U.S.C. §552 (1994 and Supp. V 1999)).

72 See Teresa Dale Pupillo, "Note: The Changing Weather Forecast: Government in the Sunshine in the 1990s—an Analysis of State Sunshine Laws," 71 *Wash. U. L. Q.* 1165 (1993).

73 See Michael Asimow, "Public Participation in the Adoption of Interpretative Rules and Policy Statements," 75 *Mich. L. Rev.* 520 (1977); and Michael Asimow, "Nonlegislative Rulemaking and Regulatory Reform," 1985 *Duke L. J.* 381.

74 See Charles H. Koch, *Administrative Law and Practice* §§2.23–2.24 (2d ed. 1997); and Kenneth C. Davis and Richard J. Pierce Jr., *Administrative Law Treatise* §9.5 (3d ed. 1994).

75 397 U.S. 254 (1970).

76 See Schwartz, *Administrative Law,* supra note 50, at §§5.15–5.16.

77 See, e.g., Henry Friendly, "Some Kind of Hearing," 123 *U. Pa. L. Rev.* 1267 (1975); Lawrence Tribe, "Structural Due Process," 10 *Harv. C. R.–C. L. L. Rev.* 269 (1975); Mark Tushnet, "The Newer Property: Suggestions for the Revival of Substantive Due Process," 1975 *Sup. Ct. Rev.* 261; and Van Alstyne, supra note 45. See generally Neil Duxbury, "Faith in Reason: The Process Tradition in American Jurisprudence," 15 *Cardozo L. Rev.* 601 (1993); and Robert S. Summers, "Evaluating and Improving Legal Processes--a Plea for 'Process Values,' " 60 *Cornell L. Rev.* 1 (1974).

78 424 U.S. 319 (1976).

79 See, e.g., Ingraham v. Wright, 430 U.S. 651 (1977); Board of Curators, University of Missouri v. Horiwitz, 435 U.S. 78 (1978); Parrott v. Taylor, 451 U.S. 527 (1981); and Walters v. Nat'1 Ass'n of Radiation Survivors, 473 U.S. 305 (1985).

80 See Cynthia R. Farina, "Conceiving Due Process," 3 *Yale J. L. and Feminism* 189 (1991); Joel Handler, "Discretion in Social Welfare: The Uneasy Position in the Rule of Law," 92 *Yale L. J.* 1270 (1983); Jerry L. Mashaw, "The Supreme Court's Due Process Calculus for Administrative Adjudication in *Mathews v. Eldridge:* Three Factors in Search of a Theory of Value," 44 *U. Chi. L. Rev.* 28 (1976); and Richard B. Saphire, "Specifying Due Process Values: Toward a More Responsive Approach to Procedural Protection," 127 *U. Pa. L. Rev.* 111 (1978).

81 See, e.g., Jerry L. Mashaw, *Due Process in the Administrative State* (1985); Jerry L. Mashaw, *Bureaucratic Justice* (1983); Richard H. Fallon Jr., "Some Confusions about Due Process, Judicial Review, and Constitutional Remedies," 93 *Colum. L. Rev.* 309 (1993); Judith Resnik, "Due Process: A Public Dimension," 39 *U. Fla. L. Rev.* 405 (1987); Timothy P. Terrell, "Liberty and Responsibility in the Land of 'New Property': Exploring the Limits of Procedural Due Process," 39 *U. Fla. L. Rev.* 351 (1987); Martin H. Redish and Lawrence C. Marshall, "Adjudicatory Independence and the Values of Procedural Due Process," 95 *Yale L. J.* 455 (1986); Edward L. Rubin, "Due Process and the Administrative State," 72 *Cal. L. Rev.* 1044 (1984); and Jerry L. Mashaw, "Administrative Due Process: The Quest for a Dignitary Theory," 61 *B.U. L. Rev.* 885 (1981).

82 See, e.g., Richard B. Stewart and Cass R. Sunstein, "Public Programs and Private Rights," 95 *Harv. L. Rev.* 1193 (1982); Stephen Williams, "Liberty and Property: The Problem of Government Benefits," 12 *J. Legal Stud.* 1 (1983); and Richard A. Epstein, "No New Property," 56 *Brook. L. Rev.* 747 (1990).

83 See E. Allan Lind and Tom R. Tyler, *The Social Psychology of Procedural Justice* (1988) (summarizing this research).

84 See John Thibaut and Laurens Walker, *Procedural Justice as Fairness: A Psychological Analysis* (1975).

85 See, e.g., Cynthia Farina, "On Misusing 'Revolution' and 'Reform': Procedural Due Process and the New Welfare Act," 50 *Admin. L. Rev.* 591 (1998); Re-

becca E. Zietlow, "Giving Substance to Process: Countering the Due Process Counterrevolution," 75 *Denv. U. L. Rev.* 9 (1997); and Richard J. Pierce Jr., "The Due Process Counterrevolution of the 1990s?" 96 *Colum. L. Rev.* 1973 (1996). See also "Symposium: The Legacy of *Goldberg v. Kelly:* A Twenty Year Perspective," 56 *Brook. L. Rev.* 1 (1990).

86   119 S.Ct. 977 (1999).

87   See, e.g., Grijalva v. Shalala, 152 F.3d 1115 (9th Cir. 1998), vacated by 526 U.S. 1096 (1999); and Catanzano v. Wing, 103 F.3d 223 (2d Cir. 1996).

88   35 F.3d 106 (2d Cir. 1994). See Pierce, "The Due Process Counterrevolution of the 1990s?" supra note 85.

89   133 F. Supp. 2d 549 (E.D. Mich. 2001).

90   42 U.S.C. §1983 (1994 and Supp. V 1999).

91   See, e.g., Personal Responsibility and Work Opportunity Act of 1996, Pub. L. No. 104-193, §103(a), 110 Stat. 2105 (to be codified at 42 U.S.C. §401(a)) (the new welfare program); and Balanced Budget Amendments of 1997, Pub. L. No. 105-33, §2102(b)(4), 111 Stat. 554 (to be codified at 42 U.S.C. §1397bb) (the Children's Health Insurance Program).

92   See Phillip Harter, "Points on a Continuum: Dispute Resolution Procedures and the Administrative Process," 1 *Admin. L. J. Am. U.* 141 (1987).

93   Administrative Dispute Resolution Act of 1990, Pub. L. No. 101-552, 104 Stat. 2736 (codified as amended at 5 U.S.C. §556(c)).

94   See Administrative Conference of the United States, *Sourcebook: Federal Agency Use of Alternative Means of Dispute Resolution* (1987); and Cynthia D. Dauber, "The Ties That Do Not Bind: Nonbinding Arbitration in Federal Administrative Agencies," 9 *Admin. L. J. Am. U.* 165 (1995).

95   See Wendy K. Mariner, "Standards of Care and Standard Form Contracts: Distinguishing Patient Rights and Consumer Rights in Managed Care," 15 *J. Contemp. Health L. and Pol'y* 1 (1998); and Maxwell J. Mehlman, "Fiduciary Contracting: Limitations on Bargaining between Patients and Health Care Providers," 51 *U. Pitt. L. Rev.* 365 (1990).

96   See Council on Ethical and Judicial Affairs, American Medical Association, "Ethical Issues in Managed Care," 273 *JAMA* 330 (1995).

97   See Sage, "Physicians as Advocates," supra note 8.

98   See Kenneth S. Abraham, *Distributing Risk: Insurance, Legal Theory, and Public Policy* 101–32 (1986); and Robert E. Keeton and Alan I. Widiss, *Insurance Law: A Guide to Fundamental Principles, Legal Doctrines, and Commercial Practices* §§6.2 and 6.3(a)(2) (1988). See generally Malcom Clarke, *Policies and Perceptions of Insurance* (1997); and Kenneth S. Abraham, "A Theory of Insurance Policy Interpretation," 95 *Mich. L. Rev.* 531 (1996).

99   See John S. Conniff, "Regulating Managed Health Care Provider Sponsored Organizations," 16 *J. Ins. Reg.* 377 (1998); Allison Overbay and Mark Hall, "Insurance Regulation of Providers That Bear Risk," 22 *Am. J. L. and Med.*

361 (1996); Edward Hirshfeld, "Provider Sponsored Organizations and Provider Service Networks—Rationale and Regulation," 22 *Am. J. L. and Med.* 263 (1996); and Charles D. Weller, "The Secret Life of the Dominant Form of Managed Care: Self-Insured ERISA Networks," 6 *Health Matrix* 305 (1996).

100 See generally Bertram Harnett and Irving I. Lesnick, *The Law of Life and Health Insurance* (1995).

101 Keeton and Widiss, supra note 98, at §2.6a.

102 Kaiser Family Foundation and Health Research and Educational Trust, *Employer Health Benefits: 1999 Annual Survey* (2000).

103 Jody Freeman, "The Private Role in Public Grievance," 75 *N.Y.U. L. Rev.* 543 (2000).

104 Id.

105 119 S.Ct. 977 (1999).

106 Jill A. Marsteller et al., "The Resurgence of Selective Contracting Restrictions," 22 *J. Health Pol. Pol'y and L.* 1133 (1997).

107 Id.; Karen A. Jordan, "Managed Competition and Limited Choice of Providers: Countering Negative Perceptions through a Responsibility to Select Quality Network Physicians," 27 *Ariz. St. L. J.* 875 (1995).

108 See *Conflicts of Interest in Clinical Practice and Research* (Roy G. Spece et al. eds., 1996); Marc A. Rodwin, "Conflicts in Managed Care," 332 *New Eng. J. Med.* 604 (1995); Council on Ethical and Judicial Affairs, American Medical Association, "Ethical Issues in Managed Care," supra note 96; and Ezekiel J. Emanuel and Nancy N. Dubler, "Preserving the Physician-Patient Relationship in the Era of Managed Care," 273 *JAMA* 323 (1992). For law review articles on the subject, see Orentlicher, "Health Care Reform and the Patient-Physician Relationship," supra note 8; Marc A. Rodwin, "Strains in the Fiduciary Metaphor: Divided Physician Loyalties and Obligations in a Changing Health Care System," 21 *Am. J. L. and Med.* 241 (1995); and Mary Anne Bobinski, "Autonomy and Privacy: Protecting Patients from Their Physicians," 55 *U. Pitt. L. Rev.* 291 (1994).

109 See, e.g., David I. Samuals, *Capitation: New Opportunities in Healthcare Delivery* (1996); Steven D. Pearson et al., "Ethical Guidelines for Physician Compensation Based on Capitation," 339 *New Eng. J. Med.* 689 (1998); Frances H. Miller, "Forward: The Promise and Problems of Capitation," 22 *Am. J. L. and Med.* 167 (1996); David Orentlicher, "Paying Physicians to Do Less: Financial Incentives to Limit Care," 30 *U. Rich. L. Rev.* 155 (1996); Alan Hillman, "Financial Incentives for Physicians in HMOs," 317 *New Eng. J. Med.* 1743 (1987); and Alan L. Hillman, Mark V. Pauly, and Joseph J. Kerstein, "How Do Financial Incentives Affect Physicians' Clinical Decisions and the Financial Performance of Health Maintenance Organizations?" 321 *New Eng. J. Med.* 86 (1989).

110 See Edmund Pellegrino, "Rationing Health Care: The Ethics of Gatekeeping," 2 *J. Contemp. Health L. and Pol'y* 23 (1988).

111 See Mariner, supra note 95; and Mehlman, supra note 95.

112 See Judith Resnick, "Many Doors? Closing Doors? Alternative Dispute Resolution and Adjudication," 10 *Ohio St. J. on Disp. Resol.* 211 (1995); Michelle G.
Hermann, "The Dangers of ADR: A Three-Tiered System of Justice," 3 *J.
Contemp. Legal Issues* 117 (1989–90); and Richard Delgado et al., "Fairness
and Formality: Minimizing the Risk of Prejudice in Alternative Dispute Reso-
lution," 1985 *Wis. L. Rev.* 1359. See generally Kathy L. Cerminara, "Contextualizing ADR in Managed Care: A Proposal Aimed at Easing Tensions and
Resolving Conflict," 33 *Loy. U. Chi. L.J.* (forthcoming 2002); Carrie Menkel-
Meadow, "What Will We Do When Adjudication Ends? A Brief Intellectual
History of ADR," 44 *UCLA L. Rev.* 1613 (1997); Edward Brunet, "Question-
ing the Quality of Alternative Dispute Resolution," 62 *Tul. L. Rev.* 1 (1987);
Harry T. Edwards, "Alternative Dispute Resolution: Panacea or Anathema?"
99 *Harv. L. Rev.* 688 (1986); Jethro K. Lieberman and James F. Henry, "Les-
sons from the Alternative Dispute Resolution Movement," 53 *U. Chi. L. Rev.*
424 (1986); and Richard Abel, "The Contradiction of Informal Justice," in 1
The Politics of Informal Justice 267 (Richard Abel ed., 1982). See also Marc
Galanter and John Lande, "Private Courts and Public Authority," 12 *Stud. in
L. Pol. and Soc'y* 393 (1992).

113 See, e.g., Diane Archer and Mal Schechter, "Dispute Resolution and the Med-
icare Consumer," 34 *Forum* 37 (1997); Karen J. Brodsky and Stephen A.
Somers, "Conflicts Inherent to Medicaid Managed Care Governance and the
Building Blocks for Resolution," 34 *Forum* 33 (1997); and Alan W. Houseman,
"ADR, Justice, and the Poor," 30 *Forum* 9 (1993).

114 See Jay E. Grenig, *Alternative Dispute Resolution* §1.11 (1997).

115 See Galanter and Lande, supra note 112.

116 See Paul H. Rubin, *Tort Reform by Contract* (1993).

117 See, e.g., Clark C. Havighurst, *Health Care Choices: Private Contracts as Instru-
ments of Health Reform* (1995); Clark C. Havighurst, "Prospective Self-Denial:
Can Consumers Contract Today to Accept Health Care Rationing Tomor-
row?" 140 *U. Pa. L. Rev.* 1755 (1992); and Clark C. Havighurst, "Decentraliz-
ing Decision Making: Private Contract versus Professional Norms," in *Market
Reforms in Health Care: Current Issues, New Directions, Strategic Decisions* (Jack
Meyer ed., 1983). See also Eleanor D. Kinney, Book Review (*Health Care
Choices: Private Contracts as Instruments of Health Reform,* by Clark C. Havig-
hurst), 17 *J. Legal Med.* 331 (1996).

118 Havighurst, *Health Care Choices,* supra note 117, at 12.

119 This paragraph was originally published in Kinney, Book Review, supra note
117. I am indebted to Arnold Rosoff for masterful editorial improvements in
this description of consumer reactions to the terms of health plan contracts.

120 See Robert J. Blendon et al., "Understanding the Managed Care Backlash,"

July–Aug. 1998, at 80; and Atul Gawande et al., "Does Dissatisfaction with Health Plans Stem from Having No Choice?" *Health Aff.*, Sept.–Oct. 1998, at 184.

121 See Clark C. Havighurst, "Contract Failure in the Market for Health Services," 29 *Wake Forest L. Rev.* 47 (1994).

122 119 S.Ct. 977 (1999).

123 *Restatement (Second) of Torts* §917 (1977); W. Page Keeton et al., *Prosser and Keeton on the Law of Torts* §1 (5th ed. 1984).

124 *Restatement (Second) of Torts,* supra note 123, at §285.

125 The standard of care, as well as its proof and application, is markedly different in a medical malpractice case than in the conventional negligence case. Negligence law leaves the definition of the standard of care and the determination of breach of the standard to members of the medical profession. See Eleanor D. Kinney and Marilyn M. Wilder, "Medical Standard Setting in the Current Malpractice Environment: Problems and Possibilities," 22 *U.C. Davis L. Rev.* 421 (1989).

126 See Furrow et al., supra note 17, at §§12-1 and 12-14. See also, e.g., Hurley v. Eddingfield, 59 N.E. 1058 (Ind. 1901) (physicians); and Campbell v. Mincy, 542 F.2d 573 (6th Cir. 1976); LeJeune Road Hospital, Inc. v. Watson, 171 So.2d 202 (Fla. Ct. App. 1965); and Wilmington General Hospital v. Manlove, 174 A.2d 135 (Del. 1961) (hospitals).

127 Council on Ethical and Judicial Affairs, American Medical Association, "Caring for the Poor," 269 *JAMA* 2533 (1993); American Medical Association, *Principles of Medical Ethics* §VI (1980).

128 See Furrow et al., supra note 17, at §12-1.

129 See Maria O'Brien Hylton, "Some Preliminary Thoughts on the Deregulation of Insurance to Advantage the Working Poor," 24 *Fordham Urb. L. J.* 687 (1997); Karen Rothenberg, "Who Cares? The Evolution of the Legal Duty to Provide Emergency Care," 26 *Hous. L. Rev.* 21 (1989); and Jeffrey E. Fine, "Opening the Closed Doors: The Duty of Hospitals to Treat Emergency Patients," 24 *Wash. U. J. Urb. and Contemp. L.* 123 (1983).

130 See William M. Shernoff et al., *Insurance Bad Faith Litigation* §30.02(3) (1996); Keeton and Widiss, supra note 98, at 628–30; Alan I. Widiss, "Obligating Insurers to Inform Insureds about the Existence of Rights and Duties regarding Coverage for Losses," 1 *Conn. Ins. L. J.* 67 (1995); and Marvin Milich, "The Evolution of the Tort of Bad Faith Breach of Contract: Current Trends and Future Trepidation," 94 *Com. L. J.* 418 (1989).

131 See Kenneth S. Abraham, *Insurance Law and Regulation: Cases and Materials* 429 (2d ed. 1995).

132 See, e.g., Clark C. Havighurst, "Vicarious Liability: Relocating Responsibility for the Quality of Medical Care," 26 *Am. J. L. and Med.* 7 (2000); J. Clark

Kelso, *Alternative Approaches to Liability: Models for Health Plan Liability* (Kaiser Family Foundation, 1999); William S. Brewbaker III, "Medical Malpractice and Managed Care Organizations: The Implied Warranty of Quality," 60 *L. and Contemp. Probs.* 117 (1997); Barry R. Furrow, "Managed Care Organizations and Patient Injury: Rethinking Liability," 31 *Ga. L. Rev.* 419 (1997); Diane J. Bearden and Brian J. Maedgen, "Emerging Theories of Liability in the Managed Health Care Industry," 47 *Baylor L. Rev.* 285 (1995); Sharon M. Glenn, "Tort Liability of Integrated Health Care Delivery Systems: Beyond Enterprise Liability," 29 *Wake Forest L. Rev.* 305 (1994); and William A. Chittenden III, "Malpractice Liability and Managed Health Care: History and Prognosis," 26 *Tort and Ins. L. J.* 451 (1991).

133 See generally Peter Schuck, *Suing Government: Citizen Remedies for Official Wrongs* (1983).

134 See Bivens v. Six Unknown Agents of the Federal Bureau of Narcotics, 403 U.S. 388 (1971).

135 28 U.S.C. §§1346(b) and 2671–80 (1994 and Supp. V 1999).

136 Id. at §2680(a).

137 See Peter Huber, *The Legal Revolution and Its Consequences* (1988); and Stephen J. Carroll and Nicholas Pace, *Assessing the Effects of Tort Reforms* (1987).

138 See Theodore Eisenberg and James A. Henderson, "Inside the Quiet Revolution in Products Liability," 39 *UCLA L. Rev.* 731 (1992).

139 See *Restatement (Second) of Torts*, supra note 123, at §901; and Keeton et al., supra note 123, at §§46–52.

140 See *Tort Law and the Public Interest: Competition, Innovation, and Consumer Welfare* (Peter Schuck ed., 1991); and Kenneth Abraham and Lance Liebman, "Private Insurance, Social Insurance, and Tort Reform: Toward a New Vision of Compensation for Illness and Injury," 93 *Colum. L. Rev.* 75 (1993). See generally G. Edward White, *Tort Law in America: An Intellectual History* (1980).

141 See, e.g., Deborah Jones Merritt and Kathryn Barry, "Is the Tort System in Crisis? New Empirical Evidence," 60 *Ohio St. L. J.* 315 (1999); Deborah R. Hensler, "The Real World of Tort Litigation," in *Everyday Practices and Trouble Cases* (Austin Sarat et al. eds., 1998); Marc Galanter, "Real World Torts: An Antidote to Anecdote," 55 *Md. L. Rev.* 1093 (1996); Deborah R. Hensler, "Reading the Tort Litigation Tea Leaves: What's Going on in the Civil Liability System?" 16 *Just. Sys. J.* 139 (1993); Michael J. Saks, "Do We Really Know Anything about the Behavior of the Tort Litigation System—and Why Not?" 140 *U. Pa. L. Rev.* 1147 (1992); Marc Galanter, "The Day after the Litigation Explosion," 46 *Md. L. Rev.* 3 (1986); Mark Galanter, "Reading the Landscape of Disputes: What We Know and Don't Know (and Think We Know) about Our Allegedly Contentious and Litigious Society," 31 *UCLA L. Rev.* 4 (1983); and Deborah R. Hensler, *Summary of Research Results on the Tort System* (1986).

142   See Eleanor D. Kinney, "Medical Malpractice Reform in the 1990s: Past Dis-
      appointments, Future Success?" 1 *J. Health Pol. Pol'y and L.* 99 (1995); and
      Randall R. Bovbjerg, "Legislation on Medical Malpractice: Further Develop-
      ments and a Preliminary Report Card," 2 *U.C. Davis L. Rev.* 499 (1989).

143   See Patricia Danzon, *Medical Malpractice: Theory, Evidence, and Public Policy*
      (1985); Bovbjerg, supra note 142.

144   See Kinney, "Medical Malpractice Reform in the 1990s," supra note 142.

145   See, e.g., Jeffrey O'Connell and James F. Neale, "HMO's Cost Containment and
      Early Offers: New Malpractice Threats and a Proposed Reform," 14 *J. Con-
      temp. Health L. and Pol'y* 287, 295 (1998); William M. Sage, "Enterprise Lia-
      bility and the Emerging Managed Health Care System," 60 *L. and Contemp.
      Probs.* 159 (1997); Randall R. Bovbjerg and Frank A. Sloan, "No-Fault for
      Medical Injury: Theory and Evidence," 67 *U. Cin. L. Rev.* 53 (1998); and
      Barbara A. Brill, "An Experiment in Patient Injury Compensation: Is Utah the
      Place?" 1996 *Utah L. Rev.* 987 (1996).

146   See, e.g., P. H. Rubin, supra note 116; Havighurst, *Health Care Choices*, supra
      note 117; and Richard Epstein, "Medical Malpractice: The Case for Con-
      tract," 1976 *Am. Bar Found. Res. J.* 87. But see Kinney, Book Review, supra
      note 117.

147   See Robert A. Berenson, "Dispute Resolution of Malpractice in Managed
      Care," 34 *Forum* 49 (1997); Thomas B. Metzloff, "The Unrealized Potential of
      Malpractice Arbitration," 31 *Wake Forest L. Rev.* 203 (1996); Thomas B. Metz-
      loff, "Resolving Malpractice Disputes: Imaging the Jury's Shadow," 54 *L. and
      Contemp. Probs.* 43 (1991); Thomas B. Metzloff, "Researching Litigation: The
      Medical Malpractice Example," 51 *L. and Contemp. Probs.* 199 (1988); and
      Neil D. Schor, "Health Care Providers and Alternative Dispute Resolution:
      Needed Medicine to Combat Medical Malpractice Claims," 4 *Ohio St. J. on
      Disp. Resol.* 65 (1988).

148   See P. H. Rubin, supra note 116; "Symposium: Medical Malpractice: Can the
      Private Sector Provide Relief?" 49 *L. and Contemp. Probs.* 1 (1986); and Ep-
      stein, "Medical Malpractice," supra note 146.

149   See, e.g., Robert A. Baruch Bush and Joseph P. Folger, *The Promise of Media-
      tion: Responding to Conflict through Empowerment and Recognition* (1994); Wil-
      liam L. Ury, Jean M. Brett, and Stephen B. Goldberg, *Getting Disputes Re-
      solved: Designing Systems to Cut the Costs of Conflict* (1988); Robert A. Baruch
      Bush, "The Dilemmas of Mediation Practice: A Study of Ethical Dilemmas
      and Policy Implications," 1994 *J. Disp. Resol.* 1; and Edward A. Dauer et al.,
      "Strategies and Tools for Cost-Effective Dispute Management," 11 *Alterna-
      tives to High Cost Litig.* 154 (1993).

150   Grenig, supra note 114, at §§1.2 and 1.12.

151   See Jerold S. Auerbach, *Justice without Law* (1983).

1 The material in this chapter has been presented in Eleanor D. Kinney, "Tapping and Resolving Consumer Concerns about Health Care," 26 *Am. J. L. and Med.* 335 (2000).

2 See Avedis Donabedian, "Evaluating the Quality of Medical Care," 44 *Milbank Mem. Fund Q.* 166 (1966); Avedis Donabedian, *The Definition of Quality and Approaches to Its Assessment* 4–6 (1980); and Avedis Donabedian, *The Criteria and Standards of Quality* (1982).

3 Avedis Donabedian, *The Definition of Quality,* supra note 2, at 4.

4 Id.

5 Id. at 4–6.

6 Id. at 5.

7 Id.

8 See Avedis Donabedian, "Quality, Cost, and Clinical Decisions," 468 *Annals of Internal Med.* 196 (1983).

9 See Leslie Pickering Francis, "Consumer Expectations and Access to Health Care," 140 *U. Pa. L. Rev.* 1881 (1992).

10 See, e.g., E. Haavi Morreim, "Medicine Meets Resource Limits: Restructuring the Legal Standard of Care," 59 *U. Pitt. L. Rev.* 1 (1997); Maxwell J. Mehlman, "The Patient-Physician Relationship in an Era of Scarce Resources: Is There a Duty to Treat?" 25 *Conn. L. Rev.* 349 (1993); John A. Siliciano, "Wealth, Equity, and the Unitary Medical Malpractice Standard," 77 *Va. L. Rev.* 439 (1991); E. Haavi Morreim, "Cost Containment and the Standard of Medical Care," 75 *Cal. L. Rev.* 1719 (1987); and Randall R. Bovbjerg, "The Medical Malpractice Standard of Care: HMOs and Customary Practice," 1975 *Duke L. J.* 1375.

11 See Robert H. Miller and Harold S. Luft, "Does Managed Care Lead to Better or Worse Quality Care?" *Health Aff.,* Sept.–Oct. 1997, at 17; and Robert H. Miller and Harold S. Luft, "Managed Care Plan Performance since 1980: A Literature Analysis," 271 *JAMA* 1512 (1994).

12 See James R. Posner, "Trends in Medical Malpractice Insurance, 1970–1985," 49 *L. and Contemp. Probs.* 37 (1986).

13 See U.S. Congress, Office of Technology Assessment, *Defensive Medicine and Medical Malpractice* (1994); Steven Zucherman et al., "Information on Malpractice: A Review of the Empirical Research on Major Policy Issues," 49 *L. and Contemp. Probs.* 85 (1986); Patricia M. Danzon, "The Frequency and Severity of Medical Malpractice Claims: New Evidence," 49 *L. and Contemp. Probs.* 57 (1986); and Patricia M. Danzon, *Medical Malpractice: Theory, Evidence, and Public Policy* (1985).

14 See LaRae Huycke and Mark M. Huycke, "Characteristics of Potential Plaintiffs in Malpractice Litigation," 120 *Annals of Internal Med.* 792 (1994); Roy

Penchansky and Carol Macnee, "Initiation of Medical Malpractice Suits," 32 *Med. Care* 813 (1994); Gerald B. Hickson et al., "Factors That Prompted Families to File Medical Malpractice Claims Following Perinatal Injuries," 267 *JAMA* 1359 (1992); Marilyn L. May and Daniel B. Stengel, "Who Sues Their Doctors? How Patients Handle Medical Grievances," 24 *L. and Soc'y Rev.* 105 (1990); Molly McNulty, "Are Poor Patients More Likely to Sue for Malpractice?" 262 *JAMA* 1391 (1989); David Ross Garr and Frank J. Marsh, "Medical Malpractice and the Primary Care Physician: Lowering the Risks," 79 *S. Med. J.* 1289 (1986); and Frank A. Sloan et al., *Suing for Medical Malpractice* (1993). See generally Urban Institute, *Medical Malpractice: Problems and Reforms* (1995).

15 See Troyen A. Brennen et al., "Incidence of Adverse Events and Negligence in Hospitalized Patients—Results of the Harvard Medical Practice Study I," 324 *New Eng. J. Med.* 370 (1991); Troyen A. Brennen et al., "Relation between Malpractice Claims and Adverse Events Due to Negligence," 325 *New Eng. J. Med.* 245 (1991); and Paul Weiler et al., *A Measure of Malpractice* (1993). See also David M. Studdard et al., "Can the United States Afford a 'No-Fault' System of Compensation for Medical Injury?" 60 *L. and Contemp. Probs.* 1 (1997).

16 See Lucian L. Leape, "Error in Medicine," 272 *JAMA* 1851 (1994).

17 See Frank A. Sloan et al., "The Road from Medical Injury to Claims Resolution: How No-Fault and Tort Differ," 60 *L. and Contemp. Probs.* 35 (1997).

18 See Gerald B. Hickson et al., "Development of an Early Identification and Response Model of Malpractice Prevention," 60 *L. and Contemp. Probs.* 7, 19 (1997).

19 Institute of Medicine, *To Err Is Human: Building a Safer Health System* (1999).

20 Id. at 1.

21 See Hickson et al., "Development of an Early Identification and Response Model," supra note 18; Wendy Levinson et al., "Physician-Patient Communication: The Relationship with Malpractice Claims among Primary Care Physicians and Surgeons," 277 *JAMA* 553 (1997); Wendy Levinson, "Physician Patient Communication: A Key to Malpractice Prevention," 262 *JAMA* 1619 (1994); and Howard B. Beckman et al., "The Doctor-Patient Relationship and Malpractice," 154 *Archives of Internal Med.* 1365 (1994).

22 See Hickson et al., "Development of an Early Identification and Response Model," supra note 18, at 19.

23 See Hickson et al., "Factors That Prompted Families to File Medical Malpractice Claims," supra note 14.

24 See Sandra H. Johnson, "End-of-Life Decision Making: What We Don't Know, We Make Up; What We Do Know, We Ignore," 31 *Ind. L. Rev.* 13 (1998). See also Robert Gatter, "Unnecessary Adversaries at the End of Life: Mediating End-of-Life Treatment Disputes to Prevent Erosion of Physician-Patient Relationships," 79 *B.U. L. Rev.* 1091 (1999).

25 See SUPPORT Investigators, "A Controlled Trial to Impede Care for Seriously Ill

Hospitalized Patients: The Study to Understand Prognosis and Preferences for Outcomes and Risks of Treatment (SUPPORT)," 274 *JAMA* 1591 (1995).

26 Id. See also Johnson, supra note 24, at 41–47; and T. P. Gallanis, "Write and Wrong: Rethinking the Way We Communicate Health-Care Decisions," 31 *Conn. L. Rev.* 1015 (1999).

27 Donabedian, *The Definition of Quality,* supra note 2, at 4.

28 Id.

29 *Restatement (Second) of Torts* (1965), at §§313, 436-36A (negligent infliction of emotional distress), and 46 (intentional infliction of emotional distress).

30 See Eleanor D. Kinney, "Resolving Consumer Grievances in a Managed Care Environment," 6 *Health Matrix* 147, 157–61 (1996).

31 See, e.g., Sara Rosenbaum et al., "Who Should Determine When Health Care Is Medically Necessary?" 340 *New Eng. J. Med.* 229 (1999); J. Gregory Lahr, "What Is the Method to Their 'Madness'? Experimental Treatment Exclusions in Health Insurance Policies," 13 *J. Contemp. Health L. and Pol'y* 613 (1997); and Mark A. Hall and Gerald F. Anderson, "Health Insurers' Assessment of Medical Necessity," 140 *U. Pa. L. Rev.* 1637 (1992).

32 See William P. Peters and Mark C. Rogers, "Variation in Approval by Insurance Companies of Coverage for Autologous Bone Marrow Transplantation for Breast Cancer," 330 *New Eng. J. Med.* 473 (1994); and Lawrence C. Kleinman et al., "Adherence to Prescribed Explicit Criteria during Utilization Review: An Analysis of Communications between Attending and Reviewing Physicians," 278 *JAMA* 497 (1997). See generally William M. Sage, "Physicians as Advocates," 35 *Hous. L. Rev.* 1529, 1545 and n. 61 (1999).

33 U.S. General Accounting Office, *HMO Complaints and Appeals, Most Key Procedures in Place, but Others Valued by Consumers Largely Absent* 3 (1998).

34 Id.

35 Id.

36 Karen Pollitz et al., *External Review of Health Plan Decisions: An Overview of Key Program Features in the States and Medicare* 17 (1998).

37 Id. at 18.

38 American Bar Association, Commission on Legal Problems of the Elderly, *Understanding Health Plan Dispute Resolution Practices* (2000).

39 Id. at 2.

40 See William M. Sage, "Judicial Opinions Involving Health Insurance Coverage: Trompe l'Oeil or Window on the World?" 31 *Ind. L. Rev.* 49 (1998); Mark A. Hall et al., "Judicial Protection of Managed Care Consumers: An Empirical Study of Insurance Coverage Disputes," 26 *Seton Hall L. Rev.* 1055 (1996); and Hall and Anderson, supra note 31.

41 See Maxwell J. Mehlman, "Getting a Handle on Coverage Decisions: If Not Case Law, Then What?" 31 *Ind. L. Rev.* 75 (1998).

42 See Barry R. Furrow et al., *Health Law* §12-1 (1st ed. 1995).

43 See Joel S. Weissman and Arnold M. Epstein, *Falling through the Safety Net: Insurance Status and Access to Health Care* 55–112 (1994).

44 See, e.g., Nina Bernstein, "State Faults Hospital in Death of Baby Who Was Denied Care," *N.Y. Times,* Oct. 26, 1998, at A21; Karen Brandon, "Some Poor Face Cash Demand during Labor; Those Who Can't Pay Often Denied Epidural," *Chi. Trib.,* Oct. 1, 1998, at 1; and Sharon Bernstein, "4 Hospitals Required Cash for Epidurals," *L.A. Times,* Aug. 28, 1998, at A1.

45 See National Health Law Program, "Health Access: An Issue Whose Time Has Come," 26 *Clearinghouse Rev.* 1211 (1993); and Jane Perkins et al., "Health Care Rights of the Poor: An Introduction," 23 *Clearinghouse Rev.* 825 (1989). See also National Health Law Program, "Reflections on 25 Years of Health Law Advocacy," 26 *Clearinghouse Rev.* 110 (1992).

46 See Hickson et al., "Development of an Early Identification and Response Model," supra note 18, at 19.

47 See Katherine R. Levit et al., "National Health Expenditures, 1996," *Health Care Fin. Rev.,* fall 1997, at 161, 174.

48 See Gail A. Jensen et al., "The New Dominance of Managed Care: Insurance Trends in the 1990s," *Health Aff.,* Jan.–Feb. 1997, at 125.

49 See Levit et al., supra note 47, at 177.

50 See, e.g., Carol Gentry, "*New England Journal:* Hospital Lets Poor Patients Pay Their Bills in Kind," *Wall St. J.,* Jan. 28, 1998, at N1; and John G. Carlton, "Tenant Denied Loan for Surgery; Woman in Pain Was Turned Down Twice," *St. Louis Post-Dispatch,* Oct. 26, 1997, at 1A. See also Brandon, supra note 44; N. Bernstein, supra note 44; and S. Bernstein, supra note 44.

51 See, e.g., Eleanor D. Kinney et al., "Serious Illness and Private Health Coverage: A Unique Problem Calling for Unique Solutions," 25 *J. L. Med. and Ethics* 190 (1997).

52 See Robert Wood Johnson Foundation, *Chronic Care in America: A Twenty-first Century Challenge* 10–12 (1996).

53 See Robert J. Blendon et al., "Paying Medical Bills in the United States: Why Health Insurance Isn't Enough," 271 *JAMA* 949 (1994).

54 See Hickson et al., "Development of an Early Identification and Response Model," supra note 18, at 19.

55 See Earl Hollingsworth et al., "Note: The Ohio Small Claims Court: An Empirical Study," 42 *U. Cin. L. Rev.* 469 (1973); and Elizabeth Purdum, "Examining the Claims of a Small Claims Court: A Florida Case Study," 65 *Judicature* 25 (1981).

56 See Hollingsworth et al., supra note 55, at 513 (table 10).

57 See, e.g., Neil Vidmar, "The Small Claims Court: A Reconceptualization of Disputes and an Empirical Investigation," 18 *L. and Soc. Rev.* 515 (1984); Barbara Yngvesson and Patricia Hennessey, "Small Claims, Complex Disputes: A Review of the Small Claims Literature," 9 *L. and Soc. Rev.* 219 (1975); Archi-

bald S. Alexander, "Small Claims Courts in Montana: A Statistical Study," 44 *Mont. L. Rev.* 227 (1983); and William G. Haemmel, "The North Carolina Small Claims Court—an Empirical Study," 9 *Wake Forest L. Rev.* 503 (1973).

58 Marc L. Berk and Alan C. Monheit, "The Concentration of Health Expenditures: An Update," *Health Aff.,* Mar.–Apr. 1992, at 145.

59 See Kinney et al., supra note 51; Donald Light, "Life, Death, and the Insurance Companies," 330 *New Eng. J. Med.* 498 (1994); and Deborah A. Stone, "The Struggle for the Soul of Health Insurance," 18 *J. Health Pol. Pol'y and L.* 287 (1993).

60 William L. F. Felstiner et al., "The Emergence and Transformation of Disputes: Naming, Blaming, Claiming . . . ," 14 *L. and Soc. Rev.* 631 (1980–81).

61 Id. at 633–35.

62 Id. at 636.

63 See, e.g., Herbert M. Kritzer et al., "Aftermath of Injury: Cultural Factors in Compensation Seeking in Canada and the United States," 25 *L. and Soc'y Rev.* 499 (1991); and Richard L. Abel, "The Real Tort Crisis—Too Few Claims," 48 *Ohio St. L. J.* 443, 448–52 (1987).

64 See Albert O. Hirschman, *Voice and Loyalty: Responses to Decline in Firms, Organizations, and States* (1970); and Albert O. Hirschman, "Exit, Voice, and Loyalty: Further Reflections and a Survey of Recent Contributions," 13 *Soc. Sci. Info.* 7 (1980) (reprinted in 58 *Milbank Mem. Fund Q.* 7 (1980)). See also Marc A. Rodwin, *Promoting Accountable Managed Health Care: The Potential Role for Consumer Voice* (2000).

65 See Rodwin, supra note 64; Marc A. Rodwin, "The Neglected Remedy: Strengthening Consumer Voice in Managed Care," *Am. Prospect,* Sept.–Oct. 1997, at 45; Marc A. Rodwin, "Consumer Protection and Managed Care: The Need for Organized Consumers," *Health Aff.,* May–June 1996, at 110; and Marc A. Rodwin, "Consumer Protection and Managed Care: Issues, Reform Proposals, and Trade-Offs," 32 *Hous. L. Rev.* 1319 (1996).

66 See Barry A. Furrow et al., *Health Law* §4-24-4-26 (2d ed. 2000).

67 See Eleanor D. Kinney, "Private Accreditation as a Substitute for Direct Government Regulation in Public Health Insurance Programs: When Is It Appropriate?" 57 *L. and Contemp. Probs.* 47, 50–55 (1994); and Timothy S. Jost, "The Joint Commission on Accreditation of Hospitals: Private Regulation of Healthcare and the Public Interest," 24 *B.C. L. Rev.* 835, 841-49 (1983).

68 See Furrow et al., *Health Law* (2d ed.), supra note 66.

69 See Kinney, "Private Accreditation," supra note 67, at 55–64. See also Timothy S. Jost, "Medicare and the Joint Commission on Accreditation of Healthcare Organizations: A Healthy Relationship?" 57 *L. and Contemp. Probs.* 15, 18 (1994).

70 See Timothy S. Jost, "Oversight of the Competence of Healthcare Professionals," in *Regulation of the Healthcare Professions* 17 (Timothy S. Jost ed., 1997);

and William M. Sage and Linda H. Aiken, "Regulating Interdisciplinary Practice," in *Regulation of the Healthcare Professions*, supra, at 11.

71   42 U.S.C. §§1320(c)1–12 (1994 and Supp. V 1999). See Furrow et al., *Health Law* (2d ed.), supra note 66, at §§3–26.

72   Larry S. Gage and William H. E. von Oehsen, *Managed Care Manual: Medicaid, Medicare, and State Health Reform* 5–49 (1997–98 ed. 1998).

73   Federal Health Maintenance Organization Act of 1973, Pub. L. No. 93-222, 87 Stat. 914 (1973) (codified as amended at 42 U.S.C. §§300e et seq.). See generally Barbara Allan Shickich, "Legal Characteristics of the Health Maintenance Organization," in *Healthcare Facilities Law: Critical Issues for Hospitals, HMOs, and Extended Care Facilities* 1051, 1098–1107 (Anne M. Dellinger ed., 1991).

74   See John K. Iglehart, "The National Committee for Quality Assurance," 335 *New Eng. J. Med.* 995 (1996); and Arnold Epstein, "Performance Reports on Quality—Prototypes, Problems, and Prospects," 333 *New Eng. J. Med.* 57 (1995). See generally Barry R. Furrow, "Regulating the Managed Care Revolution: Private Accreditation and a New System Ethos," 43 *Vill. L. Rev.* 361 (1998).

75   See Troyen A. Brennan and Donald M. Berwick, *New Rules: Regulation, Markets, and the Quality of American Health Care* 152 (1996); and Mara M. Melum and Marie K. Sinioris, *Total Quality Management: The Health Care Pioneers* (1992).

76   See Jay L. Lebow, "Consumer Assessments of the Quality of Medical Care," 12 *Med. Care* 328 (1974); and John E. Ware and Mary K. Snyder, "Dimensions of Patient Attitudes regarding Doctors and Medical Care Services," 13 *Med. Care* 669 (1975).

77   See, e.g., Paul D. Cleary and Barbara J. McNeil, "Patient Satisfaction as an Indicator of Quality Care," 25 *Inquiry* 25 (1988); and Allyson Ross Davies and John E. Ware, "Involving Consumers in Quality Assessment," *Health Aff.,* spring 1988, at 33.

78   See, e.g., Joanne E. Turnbull and William E. Hembree, "Consumer Information, Patient Satisfaction Surveys, and Public Reports," 11 *Am. J. Med. Qual.* S42 (1996); Anthony Scott and Richard D. Smith, "Keeping the Customer Satisfied: Issues in the Interpretation and Use of Patient Satisfaction Surveys," 6 *J. Qual. Health Care* 353 (1994); Barry D. Weiss and Janet H. Senf, "Patient Satisfaction Survey Instrument for Use in Health Maintenance Organizations," 28 *Med. Care* 434 (1990); and Harold S. Luft, "HMOs and the Quality of Care," 25 *Inquiry* 147 (1988).

79   National Committee for Quality Assurance, *Health Plan Employer Data and Information Set 3.0* (HEDIS 3.0) (1998).

80   See generally John V. Jacobi, "Patients at a Loss: Protecting Health Care Consumers through Data Driven Quality Assurance," 45 *U. Kan. L. Rev.* 705 (1997).

81 See Linda Skaggs, "Note: Hospital Risk Management Programs in the Age of Health Care Reform," 4 *Kan. J. L. and Pub. Pol'y* 89 (1995); Steven L. Salman, "Risk Management Processes and Functions," in *Handbook of Health Care Risk Management* 149 (Glenn T. Troyer and Steven L. Salman eds., 1986); and Layton Severson and Malcolm S. Parsons, "Claims Management," in *Handbook of Health Care Risk Management,* supra, at 235. See generally James E. Orlikoff and Audrey M. Vanagunas, *Malpractice Prevention and Liability Control for Hospitals* (1988); and Ruth Kilduff, *Clinical Risk Management: A Practical Approach* (1985).

82 See Severson and Parsons, supra note 81, at 252.

83 See Erica Wood and Naomi Karp, " 'Fitting the Forum to the Fuss' in Acute and Long-Term Care Facilities," 29 *Clearinghouse Rev.* 621 (1995).

84 See Severson and Parson, supra note 81, at 236; and Garr and Marsh, supra note 14.

85 See Thomas B. Metzloff, "Resolving Malpractice Disputes: Imaging the Jury's Shadow," 54 *L. and Contemp. Probs.* 43 (1991); and Thomas B. Metzloff, "Researching Litigation: The Medical Malpractice Example," 51 *L. and Contemp. Probs.* 199 (1988).

86 See Owen M. Fiss, "Against Settlement," 93 *Yale L. J.* 1073 (1984); and Stephen McG. Bundy, "The Policy in Favor of Settlement in an Adversary System," 44 *Hastings L. J.* 1 (1992).

87 See Hickson et al., "Development of an Early Identification and Response Model," supra note 18; Edward A. Dauer and Leonard J. Marcus, "Adapting Mediation to Link Resolution of Medical Malpractice Disputes with Health Care Quality Improvement," 60 *L. and Contemp. Probs.* 185 (1997); Orley H. Lindgren et al., "Medical Malpractice Risk Management Early Warning Systems," 54 *L. and Contemp. Probs.* 23 (1991); and Laura L. Morlock and Faye E. Malitz, "Do Hospital Risk Management Programs Make a Difference? Relationships between Risk Management Program Activities and Hospital Malpractice Claims Experience," 54 *L. and Contemp. Probs.* 1 (1991).

88 See Hickson et al., "Development of an Early Identification and Response Model," supra note 18.

89 See Dauer and Marcus, supra note 87.

90 See id. at 203–5.

91 See Henry S. Farber and Michelle J. White, "A Comparison of Formal and Informal Dispute Resolution in Medical Malpractice," 23 *J. Legal Stud.* 777 (1994).

92 See, e.g., Judith Wilson Ross et al., *Health Care Ethics Committees: The Next Generation* 2–3 (1993); and "Symposium: Hospital Ethics Committees and the Law: Introduction," 50 *Md. L. Rev.* 742 (1991).

93 See Robin Fretwell Wilson, "Hospital Ethics Committees as the Forum of Last Resort: An Idea Whose Time Has Not Come," 76 *N.C. L. Rev.* 353 (1998);

Jonathan D. Moreno, "Institutional Ethics Committees: Proceed with Caution," 50 *Md. L. Rev.* 895 (1991); Susan M. Wolf, "Ethics Committees and Due Process: Nesting Rights in a Community of Caring," 50 *Md. L. Rev.* 798 (1991); David C. Blake, "The Hospital Ethics Committee: Health Care's Moral Conscience or White Elephant?" 22 *Hastings Center Rep.* 5 (1992); and George J. Annas, "Ethics Committees: From Ethical Comfort to Ethical Cover," 21 *Hastings Center Rep.* 18 (1991).

94 See Diane E. Hoffman, "Evaluating Ethics Committees: A View from Outside," 71 *Milbank Mem. Fund Q.* 677 (1993).

95 See Nancy N. Dubler and Leonard J. Marcus, *Mediating Biomedical Disputes* (1994); Diane Hoffman and Naomi Karp, "Mediating Bioethics Disputes," *Disp. Resol. Mag.*, spring 1996, at 10; Diane E. Hoffman, "Mediating Life and Death Decisions," 36 *Ariz. L. Rev.* 821 (1994); and Lynne Sims-Taylor, "Reasoned Compassion in a More Humane Forum: A Proposal to Use ADR to Resolve Medical Treatment Decisions," 9 *Ohio St. J. on Disp. Resol.* 333 (1994).

6 The Universe of Medical Standards and Other Policies
Regarding Health Care

1 Some material in this chapter appears in Eleanor D. Kinney, "The Brave New World of Medical Standards of Care," *J. L. Med. and Ethics* 323 (2001).

2 See, e.g., David Orentlicher, "Practice Guidelines: A Limited Role in Resolving Rationing Decisions," 46 *J. Am. Geriatrics Soc'y* 369 (1998); Robert H. Brook, "Practice Guidelines: To Be or Not to Be," 348 *Lancet* 1005 (1996); Kathleen N. Lohr, "Guidelines for Clinical Practice: What They Are and Why They Count," 23 *J. L. Med. and Ethics* 49 (1995); Robert L. Kane, "Creating Practice Guidelines: The Dangers of Over-Reliance on Expert Judgment," 23 *J. L. Med. and Ethics* 62 (1995); Sandra J. Tanenbaum, "Knowing and Acting in Medical Practice: The Epistemological Politics of Outcomes Research," 19 *J. Health Pol. Pol'y and L.* 27 (1994); and Robert H. Brook, "Practice Guidelines and Practicing Medicine: Are They Compatible?" 262 *JAMA* 3017 (1990).

3 See James S. Roberts, Jack G. Coale, and Robert R. Redman, "A History of the Joint Commission on Accreditation of Hospitals," 258 *JAMA* 936 (1987); and Timothy S. Jost, "The Joint Commission on Accreditation of Hospitals: Private Regulation of Health Care and the Public Interest," 24 *B.C. L. Rev.* 835, 849–52 (1983).

4 See generally Eleanor D. Kinney, "Private Accreditation as a Substitute for Direct Government Regulation in Public Health Insurance Programs: When Is It Appropriate?" 57 *L. and Contemp. Probs.* 47 (1994).

5 Federal Health Maintenance Organization Act of 1973, Pub. L. No. 93-222, 87 Stat. 914 (1973) (codified as amended at 42 U.S.C. §300e (1994)). See generally

Barbara Allan Shickich, "Legal Characteristics of the Health Maintenance Organization," in *Healthcare Facilities Law: Critical Issues for Hospitals, HMOs, and Extended Care Facilities* 1051, 1098–1107 (Anne M. Dellinger ed., 1991).

6   See Arnold P. Epstein, "Performance Report on Quality—Prototypes, Problems, and Prospects," 333 *New Eng. J. Med.* 57, 58 (1995); John K. Iglehart, "The National Committee for Quality Assurance," 335 *New Eng. J. Med.* 995, 996 (1996); and Barry R. Furrow, "Regulating the Managed Care Revolution: Private Accreditation and a New System Ethos," 43 *Vill. L. Rev.* 361 (1998).

7   Paul Starr, *The Social Transformation of American Medicine* 338–63 (1982); Troyen A. Brennan and Donald M. Berwick, *New Rules: Regulation, Markets, and the Quality of American Health Care* 105–7 (1996). See also John Ehrenreich and Barbara Ehrenreich, *The Health Empire: Power, Politics, and Profits* (1970); Donald Fredrickson, "Health and the Search for Knowledge," in *Doing Better and Feeling Worse: Health in the United States* 159 (John Knowles ed., 1977); and Robert Ebert, "Medical Education in the United States," in *Doing Better and Feeling Worse*, supra, at 171.

8   See Angela Roddey Holder, *Medical Malpractice Law* 53–57 (1975).

9   Avedis Donabedian, "Evaluating the Quality of Medical Care," 44 *Milbank Mem. Fund Q.* 166 (1966).

10 See Avedis Donabedian, *The Definition of Quality and Approaches to Its Assessment* 79–84 (1980); and Avedis Donabedian, *The Criteria and Standards of Quality* (1982).

11 See David Blumenthal, "Part 1: Quality of Care—What Is It?" 335 *New Eng. J. Med.* 891 (1996); and Robert H. Brook, Elizabeth A. Mcglynn, and Patricia D. Cleary, "Part 2: Measuring Quality of Care," 335 *New Eng. J. Med.* 966 (1996).

12 See Brennan and Berwick, supra note 7, at 108–9. See generally E. Evelyn Flook and Paul J. Sanazaro, *Health Services Research and R&D in Perspective* (1973); and *Health Services Research: Key to Health Policy* (Eli Ginsberg ed., 1991).

13 See Tanenbaum, supra note 2; and Daniel M. Fox, "Health Policy and the Politics of Research in the United States," 15 *J. Health Pol. Pol'y and L.* 481 (1990). See generally Brennan and Berwick, supra note 7, at 109-22.

14 See, e.g., Jack E. Wennberg and Alan M. Gittelsohn, "Small Area Variations in Health Care Delivery: A Population-Based Health Information System Can Guide Planning and Regulatory Decision Making," 182 *Sci.* 1102 (1973); and Jack E. Wennberg, Jean L. Freeman, and William J. Culp, "Are Hospital Services Rationed in New Haven or Over-Utilized in Boston?" 1 *Lancet* 1185 (1987).

15 See, e.g., David Eddy, "Variations in Physician Practice: The Role of Uncertainty," *Health Aff.*, summer 1984, at 74; Robert Brook and Katherine Lohr, "Efficacy, Effectiveness, Variations, and Quality: Boundary Crossing Research," 23 *Med. Care* 710 (1985); and David Eddy and John Billings, "The Quality of Medical Evidence: Implications for Quality of Care," *Health Aff.*, spring 1988, at 19. See also Timothy S. Jost, "Oversight of the Quality of Medical Care: Regula-

tion, Management, or the Market?" 37 *Ariz. L. Rev.* 825 (1995); Maxwell J. Mehlman, "Assuring the Quality of Medical Care: The Impact of Outcome Measurement and Practice Standards," 18 *L. Med. and Health Care* 328 (1990); and Barry R. Furrow, "The Changing Role of the Law in Promoting Quality in Health Care: From Sanctioning Outlaws to Managing Outcomes," 26 *Hous. L. Rev.* 147 (1989).

16 See Arnold S. Rehlman, "The Third Revolution in Medical Care," 319 *New Eng. J. Med.* 1220 (1988); Paul Ellwood, "Shattuck Lecture: Outcomes Management: A Technology of Patient Experience," 318 *New Eng. J. Med.* 1549 (1988); and Steven Schroeder, "Outcome Assessment 70 Years Later: Are We Ready?" 316 *New Eng. J. Med.* 160 (1986).

17 U.S. General Accounting Office, *Report Cards: A Useful Concept but Significant Issues Need to Be Addressed* (1994). See also Mark R. Chassin, "Assessing Strategies for Quality Improvement," *Health Aff.,* May–June 1997, at 151; and Paul B. Ginsburg and Glenn T. Hammons, "Competition and the Quality of Care: The Importance of Information," 25 *Inquiry* 108 (1988).

18 See Mark R. Chassin, "Standards of Care in Medicine," 25 *Inquiry* 437 (1988); and Eleanor D. Kinney and Marilyn M. Wilder, "Medical Standard Setting in the Current Malpractice Environment: Problems and Possibilities," 22 *U.C. Davis L. Rev.* 421, 422–38 (1989).

19 See Council of Medical Specialties, *Standards of Quality in Patient Care: The Importance and Risks of Standard Setting* (1987). See also J. Sanford Schwartz, "The Role of Professional Medical Societies in Reducing Practice Variations," *Health Aff.,* summer 1984, at 90.

20 Institute of Medicine, *Crossing the Quality Chasm: A New Health System for the Twenty-first Century* (2001).

21 See Judith M. Feder, *Medicare: The Politics of Federal Hospital Insurance* 34 (1977); and Herman Miles Somers and Anne Ramsay Somers, *Medicare and the Hospitals: Issues and Prospects* 111–19, 259–61 (1967).

22 See *Regulation of the Health Care Professions* (Timothy S. Jost ed., 1997) (professionals); and Kinney, supra note 4 (institutions).

23 See David Tennenbaum, "Blue Cross and Blue Shield Association's Perspective on the Common Diagnostic Testing Guidelines," 4 *J. Gen. Internal Med.* 553 (1989).

24 See, e.g., Colleen M. Grogan et al., "How Will We Use Clinical Guidelines? The Experience of Medicare Carriers," 19 *J. Health Pol. Pol'y and L.* 7 (1994); and David Eddy, "Benefit Language: Criteria That Will Improve Quality while Reducing Costs," 275 *JAMA* 650 (1996). See also Eleanor D. Kinney, "National Coverage Policy in the Medicare Program: Problems and Proposals for Change," 32 *St. Louis U. L. J.* 869 (1988).

25 See William Roper et al., "Effectiveness in Health Care: An Initiative to Evaluate and Improve Medical Practice," 319 *New Eng. J. Med.* 1197 (1988).

26 Physician Payment Review Commission, *Report to Congress* 230 (1988). See Eddy, "Benefit Language," supra note 24.

27 See Roper et al., supra note 25; and William L. Roper and Glenn M. Hackbarth, "HCFA's Agenda for Promoting High-Quality Care," *Health Aff.*, spring 1988, at 91.

28 Omnibus Budget Reconciliation Act of 1989, Pub. L. No. 101-239, §6103, 103 Stat. 2189 (codified at 42 U.S.C. §299, adding Title IX to the Public Health Service Act, and 42 U.S.C. §1142 to the Social Security Act).

29 See H.R. Rep. No. 247, 101st Cong., 1st Sess. 3, reprinted in 1989 U.S.C.C.A.N. 2101, 2104. See also Agency for Health Care Policy and Research, *Clinical Practice Guidelines* (1995).

30 See Congressional Research Service, *Report for Congress: Outcomes Research, Clinical Practice Guidelines, and the Agency for Health Care Policy and Research* (1994). See also William R. Trail and Brad A. Allen, "Government Created Medical Practice Guidelines," 10 *J. L. and Health* 231 (1996).

31 See Eleanor D. Kinney, "Behind the Veil Where the Action Is: Private Policy Making and American Health Care," 51 *Admin. L. Rev.* 145, 166-69 (1999).

32 Stephen C. Schoenbaum and David N. Sundwall, *Using Clinical Practice Guidelines to Evaluate Quality of Care* (United States Agency for Health Care Policy and Research, Office of the Forum for Quality and Effectiveness in Health Care, 1995). See also Cliff R. Gaus, "Future Directions for the Agency for Health Care Policy and Research," 11 *Am. J. Med. Quality* s26 (1996).

33 Healthcare Research and Quality Act of 1999, Pub. L. No. 106-129, §(b)(2), 113 Stat. 1653 (codified at 42 U.S.C. §§299 et seq.).

34 See Timothy S. Jost, "The Necessary and Proper Role of Regulation to Assure the Quality of Health Care," 25 *Hous. L. Rev.* 525, 530–31 (1988).

35 See Anthony L. Komaroff, "Quality Assurance in 1984," 23 *Med. Care* 723, 724–26 (1985); and Brennan and Berwick, supra note 7, at 41.

36 See Brennan and Berwick, supra note 7, at 124–33; and Mara M. Melum and Marie K. Sinioris, *Total Quality Management: The Health Care Pioneers* (1992). Some classics in the field of TQM/CQI are W. Edward Deming, *Out of Crisis* (1982); Joseph M. Juran, *Managerial Breakthrough: A New Concept of the Manager's Job* (1964); and Walter A. Shewhart, *Economic Control of Quality of Manufactured Product* (1931). See generally Harrison M. Wadsworth et al., *Modern Methods for Quality Control and Improvement* (1989).

37 See, e.g., Donald M. Berwick et al., *Curing Health Care: New Strategies for Quality Improvement* (1990); Donald M. Berwick, "Controlling Variation in Health Care: A Consultation from Walter Shewhart," 29 *Med. Care* 1212 (1991); Glenn Laffel and David Blumenthal, "The Case for Using Industrial Quality Management Science in Health Care Organizations," 262 *JAMA* 2869 (1989); and Donald M. Berwick, "Continuous Improvement as an Ideal in Health Care," 320 *New Eng. J. Med.* 53 (1989).

38 Deming, supra note 36, at 177–78.

39 See Berwick et al., supra note 37; *Putting Research to Work in Quality Improvement and Quality Assurance* (Mary L. Grady et al. eds., 1993); and Brennan and Berwick, supra note 7, at 30.

40 See Ellen Marszalek-Gaucher and Richard J. Coffey, *Transforming Healthcare Organizations: How to Achieve and Sustain Organizational Excellence* (1990); and Brennan and Berwick, supra note 7.

41 See Joint Commission on Accreditation of Healthcare Organizations, *An Introduction to Quality Improvement in Health Care* (1991); and Dennis S. O'Leary, "Agenda for Change Fosters CQI Concepts," 2 *J. Comm'n Persp.* 3 (1992).

42 H.R. 3600, Health Security Act, 104th Cong., 1st Sess. (1993). See Timothy S. Jost, "Health System Reform: Forward or Backward?" 271 *JAMA* 1580 (1994).

43 See Physician Payment Review Commission, *Annual Report to Congress* 109–20 (1995); and U.S. General Accounting Office, supra note 17.

44 See Institute of Medicine, *Medicare: A Strategy for Quality Assurance* (Kathleen N. Lohr ed., 1990); Congressional Office of Technology Assessment, *The Quality of Medical Care: Information for Consumers* (1988); and Robert Brook and Katherine Lohr, "Monitoring Quality of Care in the Medicare Program," 258 *JAMA* 3138 (1987).

45 See, e.g., Robert H. Miller and Harold S. Luft, "Does Managed Care Lead to Better or Worse Quality of Care?" *Health Aff.*, Sept.–Oct. 1997, at 7; and Harold S. Luft, "HMOs and the Quality of Care," 25 *Inquiry* 147 (1988).

46 See Brennan and Berwick, supra note 7, at 159–62; and Iglehart, supra note 6.

47 See Epstein, supra note 6, at 57.

48 See Betty Leyerle, *The Private Regulation of American Health Care* 43–47 (1994).

49 See David Ellis, *Technology and the Future of Medical Care: Preparing the Next Thirty Years* (2000).

50 See, e.g., Maxwell J. Mehlman, "Getting a Handle on Coverage Decisions: If Not Case Law, Then What?" 31 *Ind. L. Rev.* 75 (1998); Christine W. Parker, "Practice Guidelines and Private Insurers," 23 *J. L. Med. and Ethics* 57 (1995); Grogen et al., supra note 24; Mark A. Hall and Gerald F. Anderson, "Health Insurers' Assessment of Medical Necessity," 140 *U. Pa. L. Rev.* 1637 (1992); Kinney, "National Coverage Policy in the Medicare Program," supra note 24; and Sally Hart Wilson, "Benefit Cutbacks in the Medicare Program through Administrative Agency Fiat without Protections: Litigation Approaches on Behalf of Beneficiaries," 16 *Gonz. L. Rev.* 533, 550–51 (1981).

51 See Institute of Medicine, *The Computer-Based Patient Record: An Essential Technology for Health Care* (rev. ed. 1987).

52 See Clement J. McDonald et al., "The Regenstrief Medical Record System: A Quarter Century Experience," 54 *Int'l J. Med. Informatics* 225 (1999).

53 See Institute of Medicine, *The Computer-Based Patient Record*, supra note 51, at 120–21; and R. D. Andrews and C. Beauchamp, "A Clinical Database Manage-

ment System for Improved Integration of the Veterans Affairs Hospital Information System," 13 *J. Med. Sys.* 309 (1989).

54 See Ellis, supra note 49.

55 See Andrews and Beauchamp, supra note 53.

56 See, e.g., J. Marc Overhage et al., "Computer Reminders to Implement Preventative Care Guidelines for Hospitalized Patients," 156 *Archives of Internal Med.* 1551 (1996); E. Andrew Balas et al., "The Clinical Value of Computerized Information Services: A Review of 98 Randomized Clinical Trials," 5 *Archives of Fam. Med.* 271 (1996); William M. Tierney et al., "Computerizing Guidelines to Improve Care and Patient Outcomes: The Example of Heart Failure," 2 *J. Am. Med. Informatics Ass'n* 316 (1995); Robert B. Elson and Donald P. Connelly, "Computerized Patient Records in Primary Care: Their Role in Mediating Guideline-Driven Physician Behavior Change," 4 *Archives of Fam. Med.* 698 (1995); D. M. Rind et al., "Effect of Computer-Based Alerts on the Treatment and Outcomes of Hospitalized Patients," 154 *Archives of Internal Med.* 1511 (1994); Clement J. McDonald et al., "Reminders to Physicians from an Introspective Computer Medical Record," 100 *Annals of Internal Med.* 130 (1984); and Clement J. McDonald, "Computer Reminders, the Quality of Care, and the Nonperfectability of Man," 295 *New Eng. J. Med.* 1351 (1976).

57 See Ellis, supra note 49.

58 See Charles M. Clark Jr. et al., "A Systematic Approach to Risk Stratification and Intervention within a Managed Care Environment Improves Diabetes Outcomes and Patient Satisfaction," 24 *Diabetes Care* 1079 (2001).

59 See "Organizations of Medical Quality," 270 *JAMA* 174 (1993).

60 See John T. Kelly and James E. Swartwout, "Development of Practice Parameters by Physician Organizations," 16 *Qual. Rev. Bull.* 54 (1990).

61 See Council of Medical Specialties, supra note 19; and Schwartz, supra note 19.

62 National Committee for Quality Assurance, *Health Plan Employer Data and Information Set* (2001). See also National Committee for Quality Assurance, *The State of Managed Care Quality* (1999).

63 See, e.g., Mehlman, "Getting a Handle on Coverage Decisions," supra note 50; Parker, supra note 50; Grogan et al., supra note 24; and Hall and Anderson, supra note 50.

64 See John H. Fergeson, "The NIH Consensus Development Program," 21 *Joint Comm'n J. Qual. Improvement* 332 (1995).

65 See Congressional Research Service, supra note 30; and Trail and Allen, supra note 30.

66 See Roper et al., supra note 25; and Roper and Hackbarth, supra note 27.

67 See Donabedian, "Evaluating the Quality of Medical Care," supra note 9.

68 Donabedian, *The Definition of Quality,* supra note 10, at 5.

69 See, e.g., ECRI, *2001 Healthcare Standards Directory* (2001); Faulkner and Gray, Inc., *Faulkner and Gray's 1998 Practice Guidelines CD-ROM* (1998); Laura

Newman, *The 1999 Medical Outcomes and Guidelines Sourcebook: A Progress Report and Resource Guide on Medical Outcomes Research and Practice Guidelines: Developments, Data, and Documentation* (1998); Margaret C. Toepp et al., *Directory of Clinical Practice Guidelines: Titles, Sources, and Updates* (1998); and Joseph M. Rees and Sherry J. Saunders, *Standards of Medical Care: The Comparative Guide to Medical Practice Guidelines and Outcomes Research* (1997).

70 See Institute of Medicine, *Clinical Practice Guidelines: Directions for a New Program* 8 (1990).

71 See Kenneth S. Abraham, *Distributing Risk* 2 (1986).

72 See Steven Leichter, "The Silent Standards in Diabetes Care: Millman and Robertson," 19 *Clinical Diabetes* 140 (2000).

73 See Gail Jensen et al., "The New Dominance of Managed Care: Insurance Trends in the 1990s," *Health Aff.*, Jan.–Feb. 1997, at 125; Cynthia B. Sullivan and Thomas Rice, "The Health Insurance Picture in 1990," *Health Aff.*, summer 1991, at 104; and Gail Jensen et al., "Cost-Sharing and the Changing Pattern of Employer-Sponsored Health Benefits," 65 *Milbank Mem. Fund Q.* 4 (1987).

74 See, e.g., Paul Joskow, *Controlling Hospital Costs: The Role of Government Regulation* (1981); and *The Role of Health Insurance in the Health Services Sector* (Richard Rosett ed., 1976).

7 Processes for Making Policies Regarding Health Care

1 Many ideas and analyses in this chapter have been published previously in Eleanor D. Kinney, "Behind the Veil Where the Action Is: Private Policy-Making and American Health Care," 51 *Admin. L. Rev.* 145 (1999).

2 See, e.g., Harold J. Krent, "Fragmenting the Unitary Executive: Congressional Delegations of Administrative Authority outside the Federal Government," 85 *Nw. U. L. Rev.* 62 (1990); Kurt L. Hanslowe, "Regulation by Visible Public and Invisible Private Government," 40 *Tex. L. Rev.* 88 (1961); Louis L. Jaffe, "Law Making by Private Groups," 51 *Harv. L. Rev.* 201 (1937); and "Note: Delegation of Governmental Power to Private Groups," 32 *Colum. L. Rev.* 80 (1932).

3 See Jody Freeman, "Collaborative Governance in the Administrative State," 45 *UCLA L. Rev.* 1 (1997); Douglas C. Michael, "Federal Agency Use of Audited Self-Regulation as a Regulatory Technique," 47 *Admin. L. Rev.* 171 (1995); and Harold I. Abramson, "A Fifth Branch of Government: The Private Regulators and Their Constitutionality," 16 *Hastings Const. L. Q.* 165 (1989).

4 See, e.g., Mark R. Chassin, "Standards of Care in Medicine," 25 *Inquiry* 437 (1988); David M. Eddy and John Billings, "The Quality of Medical Evidence: Implications for Quality of Care," *Health Aff.*, spring 1988, at 19; Robert H. Brook and Kathleen N. Lohr, "Efficacy, Effectiveness, Variations, and Quality:

Boundary Crossing Research," 23 *Med. Care* 710 (1985); and John H. Wasson et al., "Clinical Prediction Rules: Applications and Methodological Standards," 313 *New Eng. J. Med.* 793 (1985).

5 See Chassin, supra note 4.

6 See, e.g., David M. Eddy, "Practice Policies: Where Do They Come From?" 263 *JAMA* 1265 (1990); and David M. Eddy, "Variations in Physician Practice: The Role of Uncertainty," *Health Aff.*, summer 1984, at 74. See also David M. Eddy, "Designing Practice Policy: Standards, Guidelines, and Options," 263 *JAMA* 3077 (1990); and David M. Eddy, "Practice Policies—Guidelines for Methods," 263 *JAMA* 1839 (1990).

7 See American Medical Association, *Board of Trustees Report JJ: Practice Parameters* (1990).

8 See Institute of Medicine, *Clinical Practice Guidelines: Directions for a New Program* 8 (1990).

9 The quotations in this paragraph are taken from id. at 12.

10 See Joint Commission on the Accreditation of Healthcare Organizations, *Proposed Standards Related to the Use of Clinical Practice Guidelines* http://www.jcaho.org/pubedmul/publicat/std_rel.htm (visited Sept. 9, 1998).

11 See Stanley B. Jones, "Medicare Influence on Private Insurance: Good or Ill?" *Health Care Fin. Rev.*, winter 1996, at 153.

12 See Eleanor D. Kinney, "Rule and Policy-Making under the Medicaid Program: A Challenge to Federalism," 51 *Ohio St. L. J.* 855 (1990).

13 42 U.S.C. §1397aa (Supp. V 1999).

14 See Kinney, "Rule and Policy-Making under the Medicaid Program," supra note 12.

15 Health Care Financing Administration, *Carriers Manual* (1998); Health Care Financing Administration, *Coverage Issues Manual* (1998), in *Medicare and Medicaid Guide* (CCH) ¶27201 (1998). See generally Timothy S. Jost, "Governing Medicare," 51 *Admin. L. Rev.* 39 (1998); and Eleanor D. Kinney, "National Coverage Policy under the Medicare Program: Problems and Proposals for Change," 32 *St. Louis U. L. J.* 869, 879–83 (1988).

16 See, e.g., Timothy P. Blanchard, " 'Medical Necessity' Denials as a Medicare Part B Cost-Containment Strategy: Two Wrongs Don't Make It Right or Rational," 34 *St. Louis U. L. J.* 939 (1990); Kinney, "National Coverage Policy under the Medicare Program," supra note 15; and Sally Hart Wilson, "Benefit Cutbacks in the Medicare Program through Administrative Agency Fiat without Protections: Litigation Approaches on Behalf of Beneficiaries," 16 *Gonz. L. Rev.* 533 (1981).

17 Medicare, Medicaid, and SCHIP Benefits Improvement and Protection Act, Pub. L. No. 106-554, Appendix F, §§521, 522, 114 Stat. 2763, 276A-463 (2000) (to be codified at 42 U.S.C. §§1395y(a)(1)(A) and 1935ff).

18 Id.

19 Id.

20 Id. at §522.

21 See Eleanor D. Kinney, "Setting Limits: A Realistic Assignment for the Medicare Program?" 33 *St. Louis U. L. J.* 631 (1989).

22 42 U.S.C. §360c (1994 and Supp. V 1999).

23 See Administrative Conference of the United States, Recommendation 87-8, National Coverage Determinations under the Medicare Program, 52 Fed. Reg. 49,144 (1987); American Bar Association, *Recommendations on Medicare Procedures by the ABA House of Delegates* (Aug. 1988); U.S. General Accounting Office, *Medicare Part B: Regional Variation in Denial Rates for Medical Necessity* (1994); and U.S. General Accounting Office, *Medicare—Technology Assessment and Medical Coverage Decisions* (1994).

24 [1987-1 Transfer Binder] *Medicare and Medicaid Guide* (CCH) ¶36033 (E.D. Cal. Feb. 20, 1987) (settlement agreement and release of claims).

25 Procedures for Medical Services Coverage Decisions, Request for Comments, 52 Fed. Reg. 15,560 (Apr. 29, 1987).

26 Criteria and Procedures for Making Medical Service Coverage Decisions That Relate to Health Care Technology, 54 Fed. Reg. 4302 (proposed Jan. 30, 1989).

27 Establishment of the Medicare Coverage Advisory Committee and Request for Nominations for Members, 63 Fed. Reg. 68,780 (Dec. 14, 1998).

28 See *Medicare Appeals Processes: Hearings before the Subcommittee on Health of the House Committee on Ways and Means,* 105th Cong., 2d Sess. (Apr. 23, 1998); *The Medicare Coverage Process and Beneficiary Processes: Hearings before the Subcommittee on Health House Committee on Ways and Means,* 106th Cong., 1st Sess. (Apr. 22, 1999).

29 Procedures for Making National Coverage Decisions, 64 Fed. Reg. 22,619 (Apr. 27, 1999).

30 42 U.S.C. §§1395ff(b)(3)(B) and (b)(4) (1994 and Supp. V 1999).

31 H.R. Rep. No. 1012, 99th Cong., 2d Sess. 350–51 (1986).

32 See Kinney, "National Coverage Policy under the Medicare Program," supra note 15.

33 42 U.S.C. §1395ff(b) (1994 and Supp. V 1999).

34 See, e.g., Warder v. Shalala, 149 F.3d 73 (1st Cir. 1998); and St. Francis Health Care Center v. Shalala, 205 F.3d 937 (6th Cir. 2000).

35 See Edward B. Hirshfeld, "Should Third Party Payers of Health Care Services Disclose Cost Control Mechanisms to Potential Beneficiaries?" 14 *Seton Hall Legis. J.* 115 (1990); and Judith Feinberg, "Note: Utilization Review as the Practice of Medicine: Scaling the Wall of ERISA," 9 *B.U. Pub. Int. L. J.* 89 (1999).

36 See Jon Gabel, "Ten Ways HMOs Have Changed during the 1990s," *Health Aff.,* May–June 1997, at 134.

37 See Jody Freeman, "Private Parties, Public Functions, and the New Administrative Law," in *Recrafting the Rule of Law* 331, 369 (David Dyzenhaus ed., 1999).

38 Charles Tiefer and William A. Shook, *Government Contract Law*, at chs. 1, 8 (1999).

39 See Sara Rosenbaum et al., *Negotiating the New Health System: A Nationwide Study of Medicaid Managed Care Contracts* (2d ed. 1999).

40 119 S.Ct. 977 (1999).

41 See Kenneth S. Abraham, *Insurance Law and Regulation: Cases and Materials* (3d ed. 1999).

42 See Kathleen Heald Ettlinger et al., *State Insurance Regulation* (1995).

43 42 U.S.C. §§1395w-27(e), (g), and (i) and 1395w-28(e)(4) (Supp. V 1999).

44 Id. at §1935w-23(c).

45 Id. at §1395b-6(b)(2).

46 See John T. McDonough, "Tracking the Demise of State Hospital Rate Setting," *Health Aff.*, Jan.–Feb. 1997, at 13.

47 Massachusetts Medical Society v. Dukakis, 815 F.2d 790, cert. denied, 108 S.Ct. 229 (1987). See Sylvia Law and Barry Ensminger, "Negotiating Physicians' Fees: Individual Patients or Society?" 61 *N.Y.U. L. Rev.* 1 (1986).

48 See *Strategic Choices for a Changing Health Care System* (Stuart H. Altman and Uwe E. Reinhardt eds., 1996); Gail A. Jensen et al., "The New Dominance of Managed Care: Insurance Trends in the 1990s," Jan.–Feb. 1997, at 125; and Kenneth E. Thorpe, "The Health System in Transition: Care, Cost, and Coverage," 22 *J. Health Pol. Pol'y and L.* 339 (1997). See also Johnathan Weiner and Gregory de Lissovy, "Razing a Tower of Babel: A Taxonomy for Managed Care and Health Insurance Plans," 18 *J. Health Pol. Pol'y and L.* 75 (1993).

49 See Edward Hirshfeld, "Provider Sponsored Organizations and Provider Service Networks—Rationale and Regulation," 22 *Am. J. L. and Med.* 263 (1996).

50 See David Orentlicher, "Health Care Reform and the Patient-Physician Relationship," 5 *Health Matrix* 141 (1995); Marc A. Rodwin, "Strains in the Fiduciary Metaphor: Divided Physician Loyalties and Obligations in a Changing Health Care System," 21 *Am. J. L. and Med.* 241 (1995); and Mary Anne Bobinski, "Autonomy and Privacy: Protecting Patients from Their Physicians," 55 *U. Pitt. L. Rev.* 291 (1994).

51 42 U.S.C. §1395g (1994 and Supp. V 1999).

52 Id. at §1395(f).

53 Id. at §1395ff(b)(4).

54 476 U.S. 667 (1986).

55 529 U.S. 1. (2000).

56 42 U.S.C. §§1395oo(g)(2) and 1395w-4(i)(1) (1994 and Supp. V 1999).

57 Id. at §§1395ww (regulating hospital payment rates), 1395w-4 (regulating physician payment rates). See Medicare Advisory Commission, *Report to Congress: Medicare Payment Policy* (1998). See generally Eleanor D. Kinney, "Making Hard Choices under the Medicare Prospective Payment System: One Admin-

istrative Model for Allocating Medical Resources under a Government Health Insurance Program," 19 *Ind. L. Rev.* 1151 (1986).

58 42 U.S.C. §1395b-6 (Supp. III 1997).

59 See American Diabetes Association, *Diabetes Info,* http://www.diabetes.org/dia betesinfo.html. (visited Oct. 26, 1998).

60 Diabetes Control and Complications Trial Research Group, "The Effects of Intensive Treatment of Diabetes on the Development and Progression of Long-Term Complications in Insulin-Dependent Diabetes Mellitus," 329 *New Eng. J. Med.* 977 (1993).

61 See generally Charles M. Clark Jr. and D. Anthony Lee, "Prevention and Treatment of the Complications of Diabetes Mellitus," 332 *New Eng. J. Med.* 1210 (1995); and David M. Nathan, "Long-Term Complications of Diabetes Mellitus," 328 *New Engl. J. Med.* 1676 (1993).

62 See *National Diabetes Education Program: A Joint Program Sponsored by the National Institutes of Health and the Centers for Disease Control and Prevention,* http://www.niddk.nih.gov/health/diabetes/ndep/ndep.htm (visited Oct. 19, 1998).

63 See Charles M. Clark Jr. and Eleanor D. Kinney, "Standards for the Care of Diabetes: Origins, Uses, and Implications for Third Party Payment," 15 *Diabetes Care* 1 (Supp. 1992).

64 See, e.g., American Diabetes Association, *Physician's Guide to Non–Insulin Dependent (Type II) Diabetes: Diagnosis and Treatment* (2d ed. 1989); and American Diabetes Association, *Physician's Guide to Insulin Dependent (Type I) Diabetes: Diagnosis and Treatment* (1989). The ADA also worked with the NIH in the development of guidelines. See Department of Health and Human Services, National Institutes of Health, National Diabetes Advisory Board, *The Prevention and Treatment of Five Complications of Diabetes: A Guide for Primary Care Practitioners* (1983). See also Department of Health and Human Services, National Institutes of Health, Office of Medical Applications of Research, *Diet and Exercise in Non-Insulin-Dependent Diabetes Mellitus* (1986) (report of an NIH consensus conference).

65 See American Diabetes Association, *Professional Section Councils,* http://www.diabetes.org/councils.htm (visited Oct. 20, 1998).

66 See, e.g., American Diabetes Association, "Screening for Diabetic Retinopathy," 16 *Diabetes Care* 16 (1993); and American Diabetes Association, National Kidney Foundation, "Consensus Development Conference on the Diagnosis and Management of Nephropathy in Patients with Diabetes Mellitus," 17 *Diabetes Care* 1357 (1994). See also American Diabetes Association, "Standards of Medical Care for Patients with Diabetes Mellitus," 12 *Diabetes Care* 365 (1989).

67 See Sheldon Greenfield et al., "Outcomes of Patients with Hypertension and Non-Insulin-Dependent Diabetes Mellitus Treated by Different Systems and

Specialties: Results from the Medical Outcomes Study," 274 *JAMA* 1436 (1995).

68 See Steven Leichter, "The Silent Standards in Diabetes Care: Millman and Robertson," 19 *Clinical Diabetes* 140 (2000).

69 See, e.g., Terisa Fama et al., "Do HMOs Care for the Chronically Ill?" *Health Aff.,* Jan.–Feb. 1995, at 234; and Dana Safran, Alvin Tarlov, and William Rogers, "Primary Care Performance in Fee-for-Service and Prepaid Health Care Systems: Results from the Medical Outcomes Study," 271 *JAMA* 1579 (1994).

70 See Charles M. Clark Jr. et al., "A Systematic Approach to Risk Stratification and Intervention within a Managed Care Environment Improves Diabetes Outcomes and Patient Satisfaction," 24 *Diabetes Care* 1079 (2001).

71 Balanced Budget Act of 1997, §§4921–23, 111 Stat. 574 (1997).

72 See Diabetes Dateline, supra note 71.

8 Regimes for Tapping and Resolving Consumer Concerns about Health Care

1 Much of the material in this chapter was previously published in Eleanor D. Kinney, "Tapping and Resolving Consumer Concerns about Health Care," 26 *Am. J. L. and Med.* 335 (2000).

2 "Health Carrier Grievance Procedure Model Act," in *NAIC Model Laws, Regulations, and Guidelines* (1996).

3 Id. at 3.G.

4 Medicaid Managed Care, 66 Fed. Reg. 6228, 6335 (2001) (to be codified at 42 C.F.R. pt. 438).

5 Id.

6 National Committee for Quality Assurance, "Draft MCO Accreditation 2000" (1999) (unpublished).

7 American Bar Association, Commission on Legal Problems of the Elderly, *Understanding Health Plan Dispute Resolution* (2000).

8 See American Bar Association, Commission on Legal Problems of the Elderly, "When the HMO Says No: Internal Health Plan Practices," in *Resolving Consumer Disputes* 24–44 (1999); Erica Wood and Naomi Karp, " 'Fitting the Forum to the Fuss' in Acute and Long-Term Care Facilities," 29 *Clearinghouse Rev.* 621 (1995); and CPR Institute for Dispute Resolution, *Managed Conflict in Health Care Organizations: A Handbook* (1995). See generally Cathy A. Costatino and Christina Sickles Merchant, *Designing Conflict Management Systems: A Guide to Creating Productive and Healthy Organizations* (1996).

9 American Bar Association, *Understanding Health Plan Dispute Resolution,* supra note 7, at 1.

10 Jay E. Grenig, *Alternative Dispute Resolution* §§16.20–16.22, 16.30–16.34 (1997); Brad Honoroff, "Lessons from Mediating Health Care Disputes," *Forum*, Dec. 1997, at 45.

11 Medicare+Choice Program, 65 Fed. Reg. 40,170 (June 29, 2000 (to be codified at pts. 417 and 422)).

12 See American Bar Association, "When the HMO Says No," supra note 8.

13 See, e.g., Ellen J. Waxman and Howard Gadlin, "A Breed Apart: An Ombudsman Serves as a Buffer between and among Individuals and Large Institutions," *Disp. Resol. Mag.*, summer 1998, at 21; and Shirley A. Wiegand, "A Just and Lasting Peace: Supplanting Mediation with the Ombuds Model," 12 *Ohio St. J. on Disp. Resol.* 95 (1996). See also *International Handbook of the Ombudsman: Evolution and Present Function* (Gerald E. Caiden ed., 1983).

14 Waxman and Gadlin, supra note 13, at 21.

15 See Administrative Conference of the United States, *The Ombudsman: A Primer for Federal Agencies* (1991). See also Paul R. Verkuil, "The Ombudsman and the Limits of the Adversary System," 75 *Colum. L. Rev.* 845 (1975); and Walter Gellhorn, *The Ombudsman Concept in the United States: Our Kind of Ombudsman* (1970).

16 42 U.S.C. §3027(a)(12) (1994 and Supp. V 1999). See Institute of Medicine, *An Evaluation of the Long-Term Care Ombudsman Programs of the Older Americans Act* (Jo Harris-Wehling, Jill C. Feasley, and Carroll L. Estes eds., 1995); and Elizabeth B. Herrington, "Strengthening the Older Americans Act's Long-Term Care Protection Provisions: A Call for Further Improvement of Important State Ombudsman Programs," 5 *Elder L. J.* 321 (1997). See also Anthony Szczygiel, "Long Term Care Coverage: The Role of Advocacy," 44 *U. Kan. L. Rev.* 721 (1996).

17 See generally Center for Health Care Rights, *Managed Care Ombudsman Programs: New Approaches to Assist Consumers and Improve the Health Care System* (1996).

18 See Wiegand, supra note 13, at 103.

19 See, e.g., Roderick B. Mathew, "The Role of ADR in Managed Health Care Disputes," *Disp. Resol. J.*, Aug. 1999, at 10; Alan Bloom et al., "Alternative Dispute Resolution in Health Care," 16 *Whittier L. Rev.* 61 (1995); James W. Reeves, "ADR Relieves Pain in Health Care Disputes," *Disp. Resol. J.*, Sept. 1994, at 14; and Stephen Meili and Tamara Packard, "Alternative Dispute Resolution in a New Health Care System: Will It Work for Everyone?" 10 *Ohio St. J. on Disp. Resol.* 23 (1994). See also Leonard J. Marcus et al., *Renegotiating Health Care: Resolving Conflict to Build Collaboration* 317–63 (1995).

20 See Robert A. Berenson, "Dispute Resolution of Malpractice in Managed Care," *Nat'l. Inst. Disp. Resol. Forum*, Dec. 1997, at 49, 51; and Thomas B. Metzloff, "Alternative Dispute Resolution Strategies in Medical Malpractice," 9 *Alaska L. Rev.* 429 (1992).

21 See Stephen B. Goldberg and Frank E. A. Sander, *Dispute Resolution: Negotiation, Mediation, and Other Processes* (2d ed. 1992).

22 See Reeves, supra note 20.

23 See, e.g., Thomas B. Metzloff, "The Unrealized Potential of Malpractice Arbitration," 31 *Wake Forest L. Rev.* 203 (1996); and Neil D. Schor, "Note: Health Care Providers and Alternative Dispute Resolution: Needed Medicine to Combat Medical Malpractice Claims," 4 *Ohio St. J. on Disp. Resol.* 65 (1988).

24 See Patricia I. Carter, "Binding Arbitration in Malpractice Disputes: The Right Prescription for HMO Patients?" 18 *Hamline J. Pub. L. and Pol'y* 423 (1997); Amy Elliot, "Arbitration and Managed Care: Will Consumers Suffer If the Two Are Combined?" 10 *Ohio St. J. on Disp. Resp.* 417, 434 (1995); and Jacqueline R. Baum, "Note: Medical Malpractice Arbitration: A Patient's Perspective," 61 *Wash. U. L. Q.* 123 (1983).

25 See, e.g., Buraczynski v. Eyring, 919 S.W.2d 314 (Tenn. 1996); Sosa v. Paulos, 924 P.2d 357 (Utah 1996); Engalla v. Permanente Medical Group, Inc., 43 Cal. Rptr. 2d 621 (1995), review granted, 905 P.2d 416 (Cal. 1995); Cannon v. Lane, 867 P.2d 1235 (Okla. 1993); Broemmer v. Abortion Services of Phoenix, Ltd., 840 P.2d 1013 (Ariz. 1992) (en banc); and Moore v. Fragatos, 321 N.W.2d 781 (Mich. App. 1982). But see Coon v. Nicola, 21 Cal. Reptr. 2d 846 (Cal. App. 5 Dist. 1993) (ruling that a retroactive arbitration agreement was not a contract of adhesion).

26 See, e.g., St. Paul Fire and Marine Ins. Co. v. Nat'l Chiropractic Mut. Ins. Co., 496 N.W.2d 411 (Minn. Ct. App. 1993); Herbert v. Kaiser Found. Hosp., 215 Cal. Rptr. 477 (Cal. Ct. App. 1985); Wilson v. Kaiser Found. Hosp., 190 Cal. Rptr. 649 (Cal. Ct. App. 1983); Hawkins v. Kaiser Hosp., 152 Cal. Rptr. 491 (Cal. Ct. App. 1979); and Madden v. Kaiser Found. Hosp., 131 Cal. Rptr. 882 (Cal. 1976). See generally Mark R. Kroeker, "Finding the Parameters: The Scope of Arbitration Agreements in Medical Service Contracts in California," 1994 *J. Disp. Resol.* 159.

27 See Henry S. Farber and Michelle J. White, "A Comparison of Formal and Informal Dispute Resolution in Medical Malpractice," 23 *J. Legal Stud.* 777 (1994).

28 See Elizabeth Rolph, Erik Miller, and John E. Rolph, "Arbitration Agreements in Health Care: Myths and Reality," 60 *L. and Contemp. Probs.* 153 (1997).

29 See id.

30 See U.S. General Accounting Office, *Medical Malpractice: Alternatives to Litigation* 8 (1992).

31 See, e.g., William F. Fox Jr., *Understanding Administrative Law* 151–68 (3d ed. 1997); Kenneth Culp Davis and Richard J. Pierce Jr., *Administrative Law Treatise* §§9.1–9.8 (3d ed. 1994); Peter H. Shuck, *Foundations of Administrative Law* 111–22 (1994); Charles H. Koch, *Administrative Law and Practice* §§2.23–2.24 (2d ed. 1997); and Bernard Schwartz, *Administrative Law* §5.1 (3d ed. 1991).

32 See Pollitz et al., supra note 19. See also Geraldine Dallek and Karen Pollitz, *External Review of Health Plan Decisions: An Update* (2000); and Kesselheim, supra note 19.

33 National Association of Insurance Commissioners, *Issues Involving External Grievance Review Procedures* (2000); Karen Pollitz et al., *External Review of Health Plan Decisions: An Overview of Key Program Features in the States and Medicare* (1998). See also Aaron Seth Kesselheim, "Comment: What's the Appeal? Trying to Control Managed Care Medical Necessity Decisionmaking through a System of External Appeals," 149 *U. Pa. L. Rev.* 873 (2001).

34 Utilization Review Model Act, in National Association of Insurance Commissioners, *NAIC Model Laws, Regulations, and Guidelines* (2001), at I-73-1.

35 Health Carrier Grievance Procedure Model Act, in National Association of Insurance Commissioners, supra note 34, at I-72-1.

36 National Association of Insurance Commissioners, supra note 34, at I-73-13–I-73-16.

37 See Pollitz et al., supra note 19.

38 See Barbara Allan Shickich, "Legal Characteristics of the Health Maintenance Organization," in *Healthcare Facilities Law: Critical Issues for Hospitals, HMOs, and Extended Care Facilities* §16.9 (Anne M. Dellinger ed., 1991). See also Michael E. Ginsberg, "Recent Legislation: HMO Grievance Processes," 37 *Harv. J. on Legis.* 237 (2000).

39 Susan J. Stayn, "Securing Access to Care in Health Maintenance Organizations: Toward a Uniform Model of Grievance and Appeal Procedures," 94 *Colum. L. Rev.* 1674, 1703 and nn. 204–5 (1994). See also U.S. General Accounting Office, *HMO Complaints and Appeals, Most Key Procedures in Place, but Others Valued by Consumers Largely Absent* 3 (1998).

40 See Model HMO Act, in National Association of Insurance Commissioners, supra note 34, at III-430-1. See generally Shickich, supra note 38, at §16.4; and Ginsberg, supra note 38.

41 Model HMO Act, supra note 40, at III-430-1.

42 Id. at III-432-1.

43 Id.

44 See Stayn, supra note 39, at 1702–3 and n. 203.

45 See Federal Health Maintenance Organization Act of 1973, 87 Stat. 914 (1973) (codified as amended at 42 U.S.C. §§300e et seq.). See generally Shickich, supra note 38, at §16.11.

46 See 42 U.S.C. §300e(c)(5) (1994 and Supp. V 1999). See also Stayn, supra note 39, at 1702–3.

47 See Kinney, "Tapping and Resolving Consumer Concerns about Health Care," supra note 1, at 359–60.

48 See U.S. General Accounting Office, *HMO Complaints and Appeals*, supra note 39, at 3.

49 See U.S. General Accounting Office, *Indemnity Health Plans: Key Features of Consumer Complaint and Appeal Systems* 4 (1998).

50 Utilization Review Model Act, supra note 34, at I-73-1.

51 Health Carrier Grievance Procedure Model Act, supra note 35, at I-72-1.

52 See Kathleen Heald Ettlinger et al., *State Insurance Regulation* 89–127 (1995).

53 See *Health Care Quality and Consumer Protection: Hearings before the Senate Committee on Labor and Human Resources,* 105th Cong., 1st Sess. (1997) (statement of Kathleen Sebelius, National Association of Insurance Commissioners).

54 Model Unfair Claims Settlement Practices Act, in National Association of Insurance Commissioners, supra note 34, at V-900-1.

55 See Ettlinger et al., supra note 52, at 3–4, 43–45, 102–3. See also *Health Care Quality and Consumer Protection,* supra note 53, at 66 (statement of Kathleen Sebelius, National Association of Insurance Commissioners).

56 See U.S. General Accounting Office, *Indemnity Health Plans,* supra note 49.

57 See Ettlinger et al., supra note 52, at 89–127.

58 See id.

59 See U.S. General Accounting Office, *Indemnity Health Plans,* supra note 49; and U.S. General Accounting Office, *HMO Complaints and Appeals,* supra note 39.

60 See 29 U.S.C. §1133 (1994 and Supp. V 1999). See also Kathy L. Cerminara, "Protecting Participants in and Beneficiaries of ERISA-Governed Managed Health Care Plans," 29 *U. Memphis L. Rev.* 317 (1999); *Health Care Quality: Grievance Procedures: Hearings before the Senate Committee on Labor and Human Resources,* 105th Cong., 1st Sess. 7 (1998) (testimony of Olena Berg, assistant secretary of the Pension and Welfare Benefits Administration, Department of Labor).

61 See 29 U.S.C. §1133 (1994 and Supp. V 1999). See also Tracy E. Miller, "Center Stage on the Patient Protection Agenda: Grievance and Appeal Rights," 26 *J. L. Med. and Ethics* 89, 95 (1998); and *Health Care Quality: Grievance Procedures,* supra note 60, at 7 (testimony of Olega Berg, assistant secretary of the Pension and Welfare Benefits Administration, Department of Labor).

62 29 C.F.R. §§2560.503-1(e), (g) (1999).

63 Id. at §2560.503-1(g).

64 Id. at §2560.503-1(j).

65 See *Health Care Quality: Grievance Procedures,* supra note 60, at 7 (testimony of Olena Berg, assistant secretary of the Pension and Welfare Benefits Administration, Department of Labor); and U.S. General Accounting Office, *Employer-Based Health Plans: Issues, Trends, and Challenges Posed by ERISA* (1995). See also E. Haavi Morreim, "Benefits Decisions in ERISA Plans: Diminishing Deference to Fiduciaries and an Emerging Problem for Provider-Sponsored Organizations," 65 *Tenn. L. Rev.* 511, 524–53 (1998).

66 Request for Information, Claims Procedures for Employee Benefit Plans, 62

Fed. Reg. 47,262 (1997) (proposed Sept. 8, 1997) (to be codified at 29 C.F.R. pt. 2560).

67 Claims Procedures, 65 Fed. Reg. 70246 (2000) (to be codified at 29 C.F.R. pt. 2560).

68 Id. at 70250–52.

69 Id. at 70252–55.

70 Memorandum on Federal Agency Compliance with the Patient Bill of Rights, 1 Pub. Papers 260 (Feb. 20, 1998).

71 Id.

72 5 U.S.C. §§8902–13 (1994 and Supp. V 1999); 5 C.F.R. §§890.103, 890.105– 890.107 (1999).

73 Office of Personnel Management, Federal Employee Health Benefit Program, Standard Contract, §1.9. See American Association of Health Plans, "HMO Quality and Access Standards: Federal Standards, State Guidelines, and Private Accreditation Requirements" (1997) (unpublished).

74 See 32 C.F.R. §199.10 (1999).

75 See 29 U.S.C. §1003(b) (1994 and Supp. V 1999).

76 *Medicare Appeals Processes: Hearings before the Subcommittee on Health of the House Committee on Ways and Means,* 105th Cong., 2d Sess. 9 (Apr. 23, 1998) (statement of Michael Hash, deputy administrator, Health Care Financing Administration).

77 Medicare, Medicaid, and SCHIP Benefits Improvement and Protection Act of 2000, Pub. L. No. 106-554, Appendix F, 114 Stat. 2763, 2763A-463 (2000) (to be codified at 42 U.S.C. §1395ff).

78 42 U.S.C. §§1395ff, 1395u (1996). See Phyllis E. Bernard, "Social Security and Medicare Adjudication at HHS: Two Approaches to Administrative Justice in an Ever Expanding Bureaucracy," 3 *Health Matrix* 339 (1993); and Eleanor D. Kinney, "The Medicare Appeals System for Coverage and Payment Disputes: Achieving Fairness in a Time of Constraint," 1 *Admin. L. J.* 1 (1986). See also Timothy P. Blanchard, "Medical Necessity Denials as a Medicare Part B Cost-Containment Strategy: Two Wrongs Don't Make It Right or Rational," 34 *St. Louis U. L. J.* 939 (1990).

79 42 U.S.C. §1320 (1996).

80 Id. at §1395ff.

81 Id. at §1395u.

82 Medicare, Medicaid, and SCHIP Benefits Improvement and Protection Act of 2000, Pub. L. No. 106-554, Appendix F, 114 Stat. 2763, 2763A-463 (2000) (to be codified at 42 1395ff). See *Guide to Medicare Coverage Decision-Making and Appeals* (Eleanor D. Kinney ed., 2002).

83 Balanced Budget Act of 1997 §4001 (to be codified at 42 U.S.C. §1395w-21(e)– (g)). See Geraldine Dallek, *Consumer Protections in Medicare+Choice* (Kaiser Family Foundation 1998); National Association of Insurance Commissioners,

Medicare Managed Care: A Regulatory Overview (1997); Jennefer E. Gladieux, "Medicare+Choice Appeal Procedures: Reconciling Due Process Rights and Cost Containment," 25 *Am. J. L. and Med.* 61 (1994).

84   Balanced Budget Act of 1997 §4002 (to be codified at 42 U.S.C. §1395w-21).

85   Id. at §4001 (to be codified at 42 U.S.C. §1852(g)(4)).

86   42 U.S.C. §1395mm(c)(5) (1994 and Supp. V 1999); 42 C.F.R. §§417.600–417.638 (1999). See Department of Health and Human Services, Office of the Inspector General, *Medicare HMO Appeal and Grievance Processes--Overview* (1996). See also Stayn, supra note 39, at 1691; Alfred J. Chiplin and Patricia B. Nemore, "Due Process Considerations for Medicare and Medicaid Beneficiaries in Managed Care Systems," 29 *Clearinghouse Rev.* 629 (1995); Eleanor D. Kinney, "Medicare Managed Care from the Beneficiary's Perspective," 26 *Seton Hall L. Rev.* 1163, 1179 (1996); Medicare Rights Center, *Medicare Appeals and Grievances: Strategies for System Simplification and Informed Consumer Decision-Making* (1996); Carol S. Jimenez, "Medicare HMOs: A Consumer Perspective," 26 *Seton Hall L. Rev.* 1195 (1996); Sally Hart Wilson, "An Introduction to Medicare Managed Care: Appeal Rights and Other Remedies," 8 *Elder L. Rep.* 1 (1997); and Geraldine Dallek and Ron Pollack, "Medicare Managed Care: Securing Beneficiary Protections," in *Policy Options for Reforming the Medicare Program* (Stuart H. Altman et al. eds., 1997). See also Jennifer L. Wright, "Unconstitutional or Impossible: The Irreconcilable Gap between Managed Care and Due Process in Medicaid and Medicare," 17 *J. Contemp. Health L. and Pol'y* 135 (2000); and Medicare Rights Center, *Systemic Problems with Medicare HMOs: Case Studies from the Medicare Rights Center HMO Hotline* (1998).

87   [1989 Transfer Binder] *Medicare and Medicaid Guide* (CCH) ¶37809 (C.D. Cal. Mar. 14, 1989).

88   See Stayn, supra note 39, at 1694 and n. 135.

89   See Center for Health Dispute Resolution, http://www.healthappeal.com/ (visited Sept. 2, 2000).

90   152 F.3d 1115 (9th Cir. 1998), aff'g, 946 F. Supp. 747 (D. Ariz. 1996); Christopher G. Gegwich, "Note: Medicare Managed Care: A New Constitutional Right to Due Process for Denials of Care under *Grijalva v. Shalala*," 8 *Hofstra L. Rev.* 185 (1999).

91   119 S.Ct. 977 (1999).

92   Id. See Pub. L. No. 105-33, §§4001–2, 111 Stat. 275–330 (codified at 42 U.S.C. §§1395(e)–(g)); and Establishment of the Medicare+Choice Program, 63 Fed. Reg. 34,968, 35,021 (1998) (to be codified at scattered sections of 42 C.F.R. pt. 422).

93   119 S.Ct. 977 (1999).

94   See Improvements to the Medicare+Choice Appeal and Grievance Procedures, 66 Fed. Reg. 7593 (proposed Jan. 24, 2001).

95 Medicare, Medicaid, and SCHIP Benefits Improvement and Protection Act of 2000, Pub. L. No. 106-554, Appendix F, 114 Stat. 2763, 2763A-463 (2000) (to be codified at 42 U.S.C. §1395ff).

96 See Balanced Budget Act of 1997 §4001 (to be codified at 42 U.S.C. §139); and Establishment of the Medicare+Choice Program, 63 Fed. Reg. 34968, 35021 (1998) (to be codified at scattered sections of 42 C.F.R. pt. 422).

97 716 F.2d 23 (D.C. Cir. 1983).

98 42 C.F.R. §434.32 (1999). See Health Care Financing Administration, "A Health Care Quality Improvement System for Medicaid Managed Care—a Guide for States" (Mar.–Nov. 1993), reprinted in *Medicare and Medicaid Guide* (CCH) ¶41669 (July 6, 1993).

99 See, Deborah M. Chasan-Sloan, "Managed Care, the Poor, and the Constitution: Are Due Process Rights Ailing under Medicaid Managed Care?" 8 *Geo. J. on Poverty L. and Pol'y* 283 (2001); Wright, supra note 86; Jane Perkins, "Resolving Complaints in Medicaid Managed Care: The 'Brutal Need' for Consumer Protections," *Nat'l. Inst. Disp. Resol. Forum*, Dec. 1997, at 25, 25–28; and Jane Perkins et al., *Making the Consumer's Voice Heard in Medicaid Managed Care: Increasing Participation, Protection, and Satisfaction* (1996). See also Louise G. Trubek, "The Social HMO for Low-Income Families: Consumer Protection and Community Participation," 26 *Seton Hall L. Rev.* 1143 (1996).

100 Balanced Budget Act of 1997 §§4702–4 (to be codified at 42 U.S.C. §1396u-2); Sidney D. Watson, "Commercialization of Medicaid," 45 *St. Louis U. L.J.* 53 (2001).

101 Medicaid Managed Care, 66 Fed. Reg. 6228 (2001) (to be codified at 42 C.F.R. pts. 400, 430–31, 434–35, 438, 440, 447).

102 See 42 U.S.C. §1396a(a)(3) (1994 and Supp. V 1999); and 42 C.F.R. §§431.200–431.250 (1999).

103 Medicaid Managed Care, 66 Fed. Reg. 6228 (2001) (to be codified at 42 C.F.R. pts. 400, 430–31, 434–35, 438, 440, 447).

104 42 C.F.R. §431.205 (1999).

105 38 U.S.C. §7101 (1994 and Supp. V 1999).

106 Id. at §7104. See U.S. Department of Veterans Affairs, Board of Veterans Appeals, *Understanding the Appeals Process*, http://www.va.gov/vbs/bva/pamphlet.htm (visited Aug. 29, 2000); and James T. O'Reilly, "Burying Caesar: Replacement of the Veterans Appeals Process Is Needed to Provide Fairness to Claimants," 53 *Admin. L. Rev.* 223 (2001).

107 38 U.S.C. §§511(a) and 7104(a) (1994 and Supp. V 1999); 38 C.F.R. §20.101(b) (1999).

108 38 U.S.C. §§7105(a), 7107(d)(e), and 7109 (1994 and Supp. V 1999). See U.S. Department of Veterans Affairs, supra note 106.

109 38 U.S.C. §7109 (1994).

110 See generally Rand E. Rosenblatt, "The Courts, Health Care Reform, and the

Reconstruction of American Social Legislation," 18 *J. Health Pol. Pol'y and L.* 439 (1993).

111 See 29 U.S.C. §1132(a) (1994 and Supp. V 1999). See also Richard Rouco, "Available Remedies under ERISA Section 502(a)," 45 *Ala. L. Rev.* 631 (1994).

112 See 29 U.S.C. §1133 (1994 and Supp. V 1999).

113 See Barry A. Furrow et al., *Health Law* §8-6 (2d ed. 2000).

114 Claims Procedures, 65 Fed. Reg. 70246 (2000) (to be codified at 29 C.F.R. pt. 2560).

115 See 29 U.S.C. §1132(a)(3) (1994 and Supp. V 1999).

116 See Pilot Life Ins. Co. v. Dedeaux, 481 U.S. 41, 52 (1987).

117 Jones v. Kodak Medical Assistance Plan, 169 F.3d 1287 (10th Cir. 1999).

118 See 29 U.S.C. §1144(a). See generally Karen A. Jordan, "The Shifting Preemption Paradigm: Conceptual and Interpretive Issues," 51 *Vand. L. Rev.* 1149 (1998); Larry J. Pittman, "ERISA's Preemption Clause and the Health Care Industry: An Abdication of Judicial Law–Created Authority," 46 *Fla. L. Rev.* 355 (1994); Mary Ann Bobinski, "Unhealthy Federalism: Barriers to Increasing Health Care Access for the Uninsured," 24 *U.C. Davis L. Rev.* 255 (1990); and Margaret G. Farrell, "ERISA Preemption and Regulation of Managed Health Care: The Case for Managed Federalism," 23 *Am. J. L. and Med.* 251 (1997).

119 See 29 U.S.C. §1144(b) and (c) (1994 and Supp. V 1999). See also Metropolitan Life Ins. Co. v. Massachusetts, 471 U.S. 724 (1985).

120 See Metropolitan Life Ins. Co. v. Massachusetts, 471 U.S. 724 (1985).

121 See, e.g., Patricia McConnell et al., "Self-Insured Health Plans," *Health Care Fin. Rev.*, winter 1986, at 1, 2; and Gail A. Jensen and Jon R. Gabel, "The Erosion of Purchased Health Insurance," 25 *Inquiry* 328 (1988).

122 See Jon R. Gabel and Gail A. Jensen, "The Cost of Mandated Benefits," 26 *Inquiry* 419 (1989).

123 5 U.S.C. §8902(a) (1994 and Supp. V 1999).

124 10 U.S.C. §1079 (1994).

125 See Schwartz, supra note 33, at §8.2.

126 See Davis and Pierce, supra note 33, at §§11.1–11.5; and Schwartz, supra note 33, at §§8.9–8.11.

127 5 U.S.C. §§701–6 (1994).

128 See Schwartz, supra note 33, at §§9.11–9.15.

129 5 U.S.C. §706(b) (1994 and Supp. V 1999).

130 See Arthur Earl Bonfield and Michael Asimow, *State and Federal Administrative Law* §§9.1–9.4 (1989).

131 42 U.S.C. §1395ff (1994 and Supp. V 1999).

132 28 U.S.C. §1331 (1994).

133 42 U.S.C. §402(h) (1994). See Kinney, "The Medicare Appeals System," supra note 78, at 91–95.

134 476 U.S. 667 (1986).

135 Id. at 675.

136 Omnibus Budget Reconciliation Act of 1986, Pub. L. No. 99-509, §9341(a), 100 Stat. 2037 (codified as amended in 42 U.S.C. §1395ff).

137 529 U.S. 1. (2000).

138 Id. at 13.

139 42 U.S.C. §1395ff(b) (1994 and Supp. V 1999). See Eleanor D. Kinney, "National Coverage Policy under the Medicare Program: Problems and Proposals for Change," 32 *St. Louis U. L. J.* 869 (1988).

140 5 U.S.C. §§551–59 (1994).

141 42 U.S.C. §1395ff(b) (1994 and Supp. V 1999).

142 See, e.g., Heckler v. Ringer, 466 U.S. 602 (1984); National Kidney Patients Ass'n v. Sullivan, 958 F.2d 1127 (D.C. Cir. 1993), cert. denied, 113 S.Ct. 966 (1993); Abby v. Sullivan, 978 F.2d 37 (2d Cir. 1992); and Roen v. Sullivan, 764 F. Supp. 555 (D. Minn. 1991).

143 See, e.g., Hughes v. Shalala, No. C-97-20222, 1997 WL 905157 (N.D. Cal. 1997); and Kelly v. Bowen, 1987 WL 120016 (W.D. Wash. 1987).

144 28 U.S.C. §1331 (1994).

145 42 U.S.C. §405(h) (1994).

146 Civil Rights Act of 1871 §1, 42 U.S.C. §1983 (1994).

147 448 U.S. 1 (1980).

148 496 U.S. 498 (1990).

149 See Erwin Chemerinsky, *Federal Jurisdiction* §§7.4–7.7 (1994). See also Sallyanne Payton, "Medical Rationing and the Allocation of Adjudicatory Responsibility under Comprehensive Health Reform in the 103d Congress: An Administrative Lawyer's Postmortem," 47 *Admin. L. Rev.* 381 (1995).

150 38 U.S.C. §§7251, 7261 (1994).

151 38 U.S.C. §7292 (1994).

152 See Eleanor D. Kinney, "Medical Malpractice Reform in the 1990s: Past Disappointments, Future Success?" 20 *J. Health Pol. Pol'y and L.* 99 (1995); and Randall R. Bovbjerg, "Legislation on Medical Malpractice: Further Developments and a Preliminary Report Card," 22 *U.C. Davis L. Rev.* 499 (1989).

153 See, e.g., Peter Huber, *The Legal Revolution and Its Consequences* (1988); and Stephen J. Carroll and Nicholas Pace, *Assessing the Effects of Tort Reforms* (1987).

154 See, e.g., Deborah R. Hensler, *Summary of Research Results on the Tort System* (Institute for Civil Justice 1986); Deborah R. Hensler, "The Real World of Tort Litigation," in *Everyday Practices and Trouble Cases* (Austin Sarat et al. eds., 1998); Marc Galanter, "Real World Torts: An Antidote to Anecdote," 55 *Md. L. Rev.* 1093 (1996); Deborah R. Hensler, "Reading the Tort Litigation Tea Leaves: What's Going on in the Civil Liability System?" 16 *Just. Sys. J.* 139 (1993); Michael J. Saks, "Do We Really Know Anything about the Behavior of

the Tort Litigation System—and Why Not?" 140 *U. Pa. L. Rev.* 1147 (1992); Marc Galanter, "The Day after the Litigation Explosion," 46 *Md. L. Rev.* 3 (1986); and Mark Galanter, "Reading the Landscape of Disputes: What We Know and Don't Know (and Think We Know) about Our Allegedly Contentious and Litigious Society," 31 *UCLA L. Rev.* 4 (1983).

155 Federally Supported Health Centers Assistance Act of 1995, Pub. L. No. 104-73, 109 Stat. 777 (1995) (codified as amended at 42 U.S.C. §233).

156 28 U.S.C. §§2671–80 (1994).

157 Richard W. Bourne, "A Day Late, a Dollar Short: Opening a Governmental Snare Which Tricks Poor Victims Out of Medical Malpractice Claims," 62 *U. Pitt. L. Rev.* 87 (2000).

158 See Kinney, "Medical Malpractice Reform," supra note 152; and Bovbjerg, supra note 152.

159 See, e.g., Office of Technology Assessment, *Defensive Medicine and Medical Malpractice* 133–39 (1994); Dennis J. Rasor, "Mandatory Medical Malpractice Screening Panels: A Need to Reevaluate," 9 *Ohio St. J. on Disp. Resol.* 115 (1993); Jona Goldschmidt, "Where Have All the Panels Gone? A History of the Arizona Medical Liability Review Panel," 23 *Ariz. St. L. J.* 1013 (1991); and Stephen Shmanske and Tina Stevens, "The Performance of Medical Malpractice Review Panels," 11 *J. Health Pol. Pol'y and L.* 525 (1986).

160 See Eleanor D. Kinney and William P. Gronfein, "Indiana's Malpractice System: No-Fault by Accident?" 54 *L. and Contemp. Probs.* 169 (1991); and William P. Gronfein and Eleanor D. Kinney, "Controlling Large Malpractice Claims: The Unexpected Impact of Damage Caps," 16 *J. Health Pol. Pol'y and L.* 441, 442 (1991).

161 See Randall R. Bovbjerg et al., "Administrative Performance of 'No-Fault' Compensation for Medical Injury," 60 *L. and Contemp. Probs.* 71 (1997).

162 See William L. F. Felstiner, Richard L. Abel, and Austin Sarat, "The Emergence and Transformation of Disputes: Naming, Blaming, Claiming . . . ," 14 *L. and Soc. Rev.* 631 (1980–81).

163 See generally Paul Weiler et al., *A Measure of Malpractice* (1993).

164 See Frank A. Sloan et al., *Suing for Medical Malpractice* 214–17 (1993).

165 See William M. Shernoff et al., *Insurance Bad Faith Litigation* §30.02[3] (1996); Robert E. Keeton and Alan I. Widiss, *Insurance Law: A Guide to Fundamental Principles, Legal Doctrines, and Commercial Practices* 628–30 (1988); Alan I. Widiss, "Obligating Insurers to Inform Insureds about the Existence of Rights and Duties regarding Coverage for Losses," 1 *Conn. Ins. L. J.* 67 (1995); and Marvin Milich, "The Evolution of the Tort of Bad Faith Breach of Contract: Current Trends and Future Trepidation," 94 *Com. L. J.* 418 (1989).

166 See Kenneth S. Abraham, *Insurance Law and Regulation: Cases and Materials* 381–83 (3d ed. 2000).

167 See Maria O'Brien Hylton, "Some Preliminary Thoughts on the Deregulation

of Insurance to Advantage the Working Poor," 24 *Fordham Urb. L. J.* 627 (1997); Karen Rothenberg, "Who Cares? The Evolution of the Legal Duty to Provide Emergency Care," 26 *Hous. L. Rev.* 21 (1989); and Jeffrey E. Fine, "Opening the Closed Doors: The Duty of Hospitals to Treat Emergency Patients," 24 *Wash. U. J. Urb. and Contemp. L.* 123 (1983).

168 See, e.g., Mercy Medical Center v. Winnebago Cty., 206 N.W.2d 198 (Wis. 1973); Santurf v. Sipes, 447 S.W.2d 558 (Mo. 1969); and Williams v. Hospital Authority of Hall County, 168 S.E.2d 336 (Ga. App. 1969).

169 *Restatement (Second) of Torts* §323 (1965).

170 See, e.g., New Biloxi Hospital, Inc. v. Frazier, 146 So.2d 882 (Miss. 1962); Methodist Hospital v. Ball, 362 S.W.2d 475 (Tenn. Ct. App. 1961); and O'Neill v. Montefiore Hospital, 202 N.Y.S.2d 436 (1960).

171 Furrow et al., supra note 113, at §§12–14.

172 29 U.S.C. §1144 (1994 and Supp. V 1999).

173 481 U.S. 41 (1987).

174 Id. at 52.

175 See Karen A. Jordan, "Tort Liability for Managed Care: The Weakening of ERISA's Protective Shield," 25 *J. L. Med. and Ethics* 160 (1997); and Jack K. Kilcullen, "Groping for the Reins: ERISA, HMO Malpractice, and Enterprise Liability," 22 *Am. J. L. and Med.* 7 (1997). See also U.S. General Accounting Office, *ERISA's Effect on Remedies for Benefit Denials and Medical Malpractice* (1998).

176 See Jill A. Marsteller and Randall R. Bovbjerg, *Federalism and Patient Protection: Changing Roles for State and Federal Government* (1999).

177 See Corporate Health Ins., Inc. v. Texas Dep't of Ins., 12 F. Supp. 2d 597 (S.D. Tex. 1998), aff'd in part, 215 F.3d 526 (5th Cir. 2000), petition for cert. filed, 69 USLW 3317 (Oct. 24, 2000).

178 Compare Hanson v. Blue Cross Blue Shield of Iowa, 953 F. Supp. 270 (N.D. Iowa 1996); Caudill v. Blue Cross and Blue Shield of North Carolina, 999 F.2d 74 (4th Cir. 1993); and Burkey v. Government Employees Hospital Association, 983 F.2d 656 (5th Cir. 1993) (finding preemption); with Goepel v. National Postal Mail Handlers Union, 36 F.3d 306 (3d Cir. 1994); and Howard v. Group Hospital Service, 739 F.2d 1508 (10th Cir. 1984) (rejecting preemption). See also Kincade v. Group Health Services of Oklahoma, 945 P.2d 485 (Okla. 1997); Negron v. Patel, 6 F. Supp. 2d 366 (E.D. Pa. 1998); and Timothy S. Jost, "Governing Medicare," 51 *Admin. L. Rev.* 39, 56 (1999).

179 See, e.g., Ardary v. Aetna Health Plans of Cal., 98 F.3d 496 (9th Cir. 1996); and Wartenberg v. Aetna U.S. Healthcare, 2 F. Supp. 2d 273 (E.D. N.Y. 1998). See also Jost, supra note 178, at 56.

180 See Hospital Survey and Construction Act, Pub. L. No. 79-725, §622(f) 60 Stat. 1040 (1946) (codified as amended at 42 U.S.C. §291 (1995)). See also Kenneth R. Wing, "The Community Service Obligation of Hill-Burton Health Facilities," 23 *B.C. L. Rev.* 577 (1982).

181 See 42 U.S.C. §291(c) (1994).

182 391 F. Supp. 603 (E.D. La. 1970). See Rand E. Rosenblatt, "Health Care Reform and Administrative Law: A Structural Approach," 88 *Yale L. J.* 243 (1978).

183 See also Corum v. Beth Israel Medical Center, 359 F. Supp. 909 (S.D.N.Y. 1973); Newsom v. Vanderbilt University, 653 F.2d 1100 (6th Cir. 1981); and Am. Hosp. Ass'n v. Schweiker, 721 F.2d 170 (7th Cir. 1983), cert. denied sub nom., Am. Hosp. Ass'n v. Heckler, 466 U.S. 958 (1984).

184 Pub. L. No. 93-641, §4, 88 Stat. 2259 (1974) (codified as amended at 42 U.S.C. §300s-1(b)).

185 42 U.S.C. §1395dd (1994 and Supp. V 1999). See Michael J. Frank, "Tailoring EMATLA to Better Protect the Indigent: The Supreme Court Precludes One Method of Salvaging a Statute Gone Awry," 3 *Depaul J. Health Care L.* 195 (2000). See also Lawrence E. Singer, "Look What They've Done to My Law, Ma: COBRA's Implosion," 33 *Hous. L. Rev.* 113 (1996); Barry R. Furrow, "An Overview and Analysis of the Impact of the Emergency Medical Treatment and Active Labor Act," 16 *J. Legal Med.* 325 (1995); and Judith Dobertin, "Eliminating Patient Dumping: A Proposal for Model Legislation," 28 *Val. U. L. Rev.* 291 (1993).

186 42 U.S.C. §1395d(d)(1) (1994 and Supp. V 1999).

187 Id. at §1395d(d)(2)(A).

188 See, e.g., Burditt v. U.S. Dep't of Health and Human Services, 934 F.2d 1362 (5th Cir. 1991); and Melissa K. Stull, "Annotation: Construction and Application of Emergency Medical Treatment and Active Labor Act," 104 *A. L. R. Fed.* 166 (1991).

189 See, e.g., Fisher v. N.Y. Health Hosp. Corp., 989 F. Supp. 444 (E.D.N.Y. 1998); Cooper v. Gulf Breeze Hosp., Inc., 839 F. Supp. 1538 (N.D. Fla. 1993); Estate of Enck v. Beggs, 1995 WL 519148 (D. Kan. 1995); and Lopez-Soto v. Hawayek, 998 F. Supp. 41 (D.P.R. 1997). See also Demetrios G. Metropoulos, "Note: Son of COBRA: The Evolution of a Federal Malpractice Law," 45 *Stan. L. Rev.* 263 (1992).

190 See Institute of Medicine, *Health in the Context of Civil Rights* 1 (1981); and Kenneth R. Wing, "Title VI and Health Facilities: Forms without Substance," 30 *Hastings L. J.* 137 (1978).

191 See Pub. L. No. 101-335, 104 Stat. 327 (1990) (codified as amended 42 U.S.C. §§12101 et seq.). See also Mary Crossley, "Becoming Visible: The ADA's Impact on Health Care for Persons with Disabilities," 52 *Ala. L. Rev.* 51 (2000); David Orentlicher, "Destructuring Disability: Rationing of Health Care and Unfair Discrimination against the Sick," 31 *Harv. C. R.–C. L. L. Rev.* 49 (1996); and Philip G. Peters Jr., "Health Care Rationing and Disability Rights," 70 *Ind. L. J.* 491 (1995).

192   Pub. L. No. 93-112, §504, 87 Stat. 355 (1990) (codified as amended 29 U.S.C. §794).

193   See, e.g., Abbott v. Bragdon, 107 F.3d 934 (1st Cir. 1997); Woolfolk v. Duncan, 872 F. Supp. 1381 (E.D. Pa. 1995); and Glanz v. Vernick, 756 F. Supp. 632 (D. Mass. 1991).

194   United States v. University Hospital, 729 F.2d 144 (2d Cir. 1984). See Philip G. Peters Jr., "When Physicians Balk at Futile Care: Implications of the Disability Rights Laws," 91 *Nw. U. L. Rev.* 798 (1997); and E. Haavi Morreim, "Futilitarianism, Exoticare, and Coerced Altruism: The ADA Meets Its Limits," 25 *Seton Hall L. Rev.* 883 (1995).

195   See Laura J. Schacht, "The Health Care Crisis: Improving Access for Employees Covered by Self-Insured Plans under ERISA and the Americans with Disabilities Act," 45 *Wash. U. J. Urb. and Contemp. L.* 303 (1994); and H. Miriam Farber, "Subterfuge: Do Coverage Limitations and Exclusions in Employer-Provided Health Care Plans Violate the Americans with Disabilities Act?" 69 *N.Y.U. L. Rev.* 850 (1994).

196   179 F.3d 557 (7th Cir. 1999).

197   15 U.S.C. §§1011–14 (1994).

198   See Hylton, supra note 167 (listing state statutes).

199   See Furrow et al., supra note 113, at §§12–13.

200   See id.

201   Robert F. Williams, "Equality and State Constitutional Law," in *Developments in State Constitutional Law* 71 (Bradley D. McGraw et al. eds., 1985).

9   Principles of Sound Procedural Protections

1   Many ideas in this chapter have been published previously in Eleanor D. Kinney, "Behind the Veil Where the Action Is: Private Policy Making and American Health Care," 51 *Admin. L. Rev.* 145 (1999); and Eleanor D. Kinney, "Tapping and Resolving Consumer Concerns about Health Care," 26 *Am. J. L. and Med.* 335 (2000).

2   See Eleanor D. Kinney, "National Coverage Policy under the Medicare Program: Problems and Proposals for Change," 32 *St. Louis U. L. J.* 869 (1988). See also Administrative Conference of the United States, Recommendation 87-8, National Coverage Determinations under the Medicare Program, 52 Fed. Reg. 49,144 (1987).

3   See, e.g., Steven Leichter, "The Silent Standards of Care in Diabetes Care: Millman and Robertson," 17 *Clinical Diabetes* 140 (2000).

4   See Marc A. Rodwin, *Promoting Accountable Managed Health Care: The Potential Role for Consumer Voice* (2000); Marc A. Rodwin, "The Neglected Rem-

edy: Strengthening Consumer Voice in Managed Care," *Am. Prospect,* Sept.–Oct. 1997, at 45; Marc A. Rodwin, "Consumer Protection and Managed Care: The Need for Organized Consumers," *Health Aff.,* May–June 1996, at 110; and Marc A. Rodwin, "Consumer Protection and Managed Care," 22 *Hous. L. Rev.* 1319 (1996).

5 American Arbitration Association et al., *Health Care Due Process Protocol: A Due Process Protocol for Mediation and Arbitration of Health Care Disputes* (1998).

6 See, e.g., Personal Responsibility and Work Opportunity Act of 1996, Pub. L. No. 104-193, §103(a), 110 Stat. 2105 (codified at 42 U.S.C. §401(a)) (the federal/state welfare program); and Balanced Budget Amendments of 1997, Pub. L. No. 105-33, §2102(b)(4), 111 Stat. 554 (codified at 42 U.S.C. §1397(bb)) (the State Children's Health Insurance Program).

7 Colson on Behalf of Colson v. Sillman, 35 F.3d 106 (2d Cir. 1994). See Richard J. Pierce Jr., "The Due Process Counterrevolution of the 1990s?" 96 *Colum. L. Rev.* 1 (1996).

8 See E. Allan Lind and Tom R. Tyler, *The Social Psychology of Procedural Justice* (1988) (summarizing this research).

9 456 U.S. 188 (1982).

10 See Blair H. Sheppard, "Justice Is No Simple Matter: Case for Elaborating Our Model of Procedural Fairness," 49 *J. Personality and Soc. Psychol.* 953 (1985).

11 See id.

12 See id.

13 See Laurens Walker et al., "The Relationship between Procedural and Distributive Justice," 65 *Va. L. Rev.* 1401 (1979); John Thibaut and Laurens Walker, "A Theory of Procedure," 66 *Cal. L. Rev.* 541 (1978); John Thibaut et al., "Procedural Justice as Fairness," 26 *Stan. L. Rev.* 1271 (1974); and John Thibaut and Laurens Walker, *Procedural Justice as Fairness: A Psychological Analysis* (1975).

14 See Tom R. Tyler, "What Is Procedural Justice? Criteria Used by Citizens to Assess the Fairness of Legal Procedures," 22 *L. and Soc. Inquiry* 103 (1988).

15 Balanced Budget Act of 1997 §§4702–4 (codified at §1396u-2).

16 Medicaid Managed Care, 63 Fed. Reg. 52,021 (proposed Sept. 29, 1998).

17 Id. at 52,056.

18 See Carl T. Prechler, "Physicians, Surgeons, and Healers," 61 *Am. Jur.* 2d §347 (1981).

19 See President's Advisory Commission on Consumer Protection and Quality in the Health Care Industry, *Quality First: Better Health Care for All Americans* (1998); and President's Advisory Commission on Consumer Protection and Quality in the Health Care Industry, *Consumer Bill of Rights and Responsibilities: Interim Report to the President of the United States* (1997).

20 See U.S. Congress, Congressional Research Service, *CRS Issue Brief: Managed Health Care: Major Issues in the 105th Congress* (1998); and U.S. Congress, Congressional Research Service, *CRS Issue Brief for Congress: Patient Protection*

and Managed Care: Legislation in the 106th Congress (1999).

21 Norman G. Poythress et al., "Procedural Justice Judgments of Alternative Procedures for Resolving Medical Malpractice Claims," 23 *J. Applied. Soc. Psychol.* 1639 (1993).

22 119 S.Ct. 977 (1999).

23 Grijalva v. Shalala, 152 F.3d 1115 (9th Cir. 1998), vacated by 526 U.S. 1096 (1999).

24 Pub. L. No. 105-33, §§4001–2, 111 Stat. 275-330 (codified at 42 U.S.C. §§1395(e)–(g)); Establishment of the Medicare+Choice Program, 63 Fed. Reg. 34,968, 35,021 (1998) (to be codified at scattered sections of 42 C.F.R. pt. 422).

25 "$60 Million Spent to Fight HMO Reform," *Chi. Trib.,* Nov. 28, 1998, at 15.

26 See Eleanor D. Kinney, "Medical Malpractice Reform in the 1990s: Past Disappointments, Future Success?" 1 *J. Health Pol. Pol'y and L.* 99 (1995); and Randall R. Bovbjerg, "Legislation on Medical Malpractice: Further Developments and a Preliminary Report Card," 2 *U.C. Davis L. Rev.* 499 (1989).

10 A Vision of Reform

1   Shirley Eiko Sanematsu, "Comment: Taking a Broader View of Treatment Disputes beyond Managed Care: Are Recent Legislative Efforts the Cure?" 48 *UCLA L. Rev.* 1245 (2001); Karen A. Jordan, "Coverage Decisions in ERISA Plans: Assessing the Federal Legislative Solution," 65 *Mo. L. Rev.* 405 (2000); Jana Strain and Eleanor D. Kinney, "The Road Paved with Good Intentions: Problems and Potential for Employer-Sponsored Health Insurance under ERISA," 31 *Loy. U. Chi. L. Rev.* 27 (1999).

2   42 U.S.C. §1983 (1994 and Supp. V 1999).

3   See Jill A. Marsteller and Randall R. Bovbjerg, *Federalism and Patient Protection: Changing Roles for State and Federal Government* (1999).

4   See Memorandum on Federal Agency Compliance with the Patient Bill of Rights, 1 Pub. Papers 260 (Feb. 20, 1998).

5   See id.

6   See Michael Asimow, "The Administrative Judiciary: ALJs in Historical Perspective," 19 *J. Nat'l. Ass'n Admin. L. J.* 23 (1999).

7   See Carol J. DeFrances and Marika F. X. Litras, *Civil Justice Survey of State Courts: Civil Trial Cases and Verdicts in Large Counties, 1996* (U.S. Department of Justice, Bureau of Justice Statistics 1999).

8   See Deborah R. Hensler, "Science in the Court: Is There a Role for Alternative Dispute Resolution?" 54 *L. and Contemp. Probs.* 171 (1991); and Larry Ray and Anne L. Clare, "The Multi-Door Courthouse Idea: Building the Courthouse of the Future . . . Today," 1 *Ohio St. J. on Disp. Resol.* 7 (1985).

9   See Richard L. Revesz, "Specialized Courts and the Administrative Lawmaking

System," 138 *U. Pa. L. Rev.* 1111 (1990); and Ellen R. Jordan, "Specialized Courts: A Choice?" 76 *Nw. U. L. Rev.* 745 (1981).

10　See Jody Freeman, "The Private Role in Public Governance," 75 *N.Y.U. L. Rev.* 543 (2000).

11　42 U.S.C. §305g (1994).

12　See Karen Pollitz et al., *External Review of Health Plan Decisions: An Overview of Key Program Entities in the States and Medicare* (1998); Geraldine Dallek and Karen Pollitz, *External Review of Health Plan Decisions: An Update* (2000); and National Association of Insurance Commissioners, *Issues Involving External Grievance Review Procedures* (2000). See also Aaron Seth Kesselheim, "Comment: What's the Appeal? Trying to Control Managed Care Medical Necessity Decisionmaking through a System of External Appeals," 149 *U. Pa. L. Rev.* 873 (2001).

13　See, e.g., Ind. Code Ann. §34-18-10-1 (1999); La. Rev. St. Ann. §40:1299.47 (2000); and Neb. Rev. Stat. §44-2840 (2000). See also Eleanor D. Kinney, "Indiana's Malpractice System: No-Fault by Accident," 54 *L. and Contemp. Probs.* 169 (1990); and Randall R. Bovbjerg, "Legislation on Medical Malpractice: Further Developments and a Preliminary Report Card," 22 *U.C. Davis L. Rev.* 499 (1989).

14　See Pollitz et al., supra note 12.

15　See Norman G. Poythress et al., "Procedural Justice Judgments of Alternative Procedures for Resolving Medical Malpractice Claims," 23 *J. Applied Soc. Psychol.* 1639 (1993).

16　See Marc Galanter and John Lande, "Private Courts and Public Authority," 12 *Stud. in L. Pol. and Soc'y* 397 (1992).

17　See Wex Malone, Marcus Plant, and Joseph Little, *Workers' Compensation and Employment Rights* (1979).

18　See Jerry L. Mashaw and David L. Harfst, *The Struggle for Auto Safety* (1990); Robert Keeton and Jeffrey O'Connell, *After Cars Crash: The Need for Legal and Insurance Reform* (1967); and Walter J. Blum and Harry Kalven Jr., *Public Law Perspectives on a Private Law Problem* (1965).

19　See Eleanor D. Kinney, "Malpractice Reform in the 1990s: Past Disappointments, Future Success?" 20 *J. Health Pol. Pol'y and L.* 99 (1995); and Bovbjerg, supra note 13. See also U.S. Congress, Office of Technology Assessment, *Impact of Legal Reforms on Malpractice Costs* (1993).

20　See Peter Schuck, "Legal Complexity: Some Causes, Consequences, and Cures," 42 *Duke L. J.* 1 (1992). See also James A. Henderson Jr. and Theodore Eisenberg, "The Quiet Revolution in Products Liability: An Empirical Study of Legal Change," 37 *UCLA L. Rev.* 479 (1990); Larry Steven Milner, "Comment: The Constitutionality of Medical Malpractice Legislative Reform: A National Survey," 18 *Loy. U. Chi. L. J.* 1053 (1987); and Richard Turkington, "Constitutional Limitations on Tort Reform: Have State Courts Placed Insurmountable

Obstacles in the Path of Legislative Responses to the Perceived Liability Insurance Crisis?" 32 *Vill. L. Rev.* 1299 (1987).

21 Humphrey's Executor v. United States, 295 U.S. 602 (1935). See Robert E. Cushman, *The Independent Regulatory Commissions* (1972).

22 See Buckley v. Valeo, 424 U.S. 1 (1976) (an independent commission with a unique board to regulate the financing of federal elections); Morrison v. Olson, 487 U.S. 654 (1988) (unique appointment and supervision provisions for independent counsels investigating high federal officials); and Mistretta v. United States, 488 U.S. 361 (1989) (judicial commission to standardize criminal sentences). But see also Bowsher v. Syner, 478 U.S. 714 (1986) (limiting the authority of a congressional agency to manage the federal budget).

23 See Crowell v. Benson, 285 U.S. 22 (1932); Atlas Roofing Company, Inc. v. Occupational Safety and Health Review Commission, 424 U.S. 964 (1976); Middlesex County Sewerage Authority v. National Sea Clammers Association, 453 U.S. 1 (1981); Northern Pipe Line Const. Co. v. Marathon Pipe Line Co., 458 U.S. 50 (1982); Thomas v. Union Carbide Agr. Products Co., 473 U.S. 568 (1985); and Commodities Futures Trading Comm'n v. Schor, 478 U.S. 833 (1986).

24 26 U.S.C. §7441 (1994).

25 See Eleanor D. Kinney, "Private Accreditation as a Substitute for Direct Government Regulation in Public Health Insurance Programs: When Is It Appropriate?" 57 *L. and Contemp. Probs.* 47 (1994).

Index

Access to health care: concerns about, 74–77; policies to enhance, 103–107; health insurance to enhance, 23–30, 35–39. *See also* Consumer concerns about health care; Uninsured

Accountability: compromised access to the tort system and, 171–173; of health plans and providers, 163, 166, 170–173; receding constitutional protections and, 171. *See also* Principles for better ways to tap and resolve consumer disputes; Procedural reforms

Accreditation, 36, 44–45, 81–82, 86–86, 96, 118–119, 126; of health care institutions, 44–45; of HMOs, 86; private accrediting bodies, 81–82, 95–96, 98–99, 101–102, 109–114, 125, 153–154, 176. *See also* Joint Commission on the Accreditation of Healthcare Organizations (JCAHO); National Committee for Quality Assurance (NCQA); Private organizations: accrediting bodies

Adjudication, 2–3, 42, 161–174 passim, 180–189; challenging health care policies in, 156–157; fairness of adjudicative procedures, 158. *See also* Administrative law; Alternative dispute resolution (ADR); Contractual review; Grievance-and-appeal procedures; Justice; Patient protection debate; Principles for better ways to tap and resolve consumer disputes; Procedural reforms; Tapping and resolving consumer concerns

Administrative Conference of the United States, 50, 116

Administrative law, 41, 47–50, 183; adjudication, 51–53; jurisprudence, 48; model, 113, 115, 117; rulemaking, 48–51; scholarship, 49–50. *See also* Administrative Procedure Act (APA)

Administrative law judges (ALJ): federal, 136, 148; state, 183

Administrative Procedure Act (APA), 47–50, 123, 141–142; section 553 of, 48–49, 117. *See also* Administrative law; Judicial review; Rulemaking

Administrative review, 8, 131–139, 163; Medicaid, 139; Medicare, 138; veterans medical system, 139. *See also* Grievance-and-appeal procedures; Judicial review; Tapping and resolving consumer concerns

Agency for Health Care Policy and Research (AHCPR), 89, 112; Forum for Quality and Effectiveness in Health Care, 89. *See also* Health service research; Policymaking: on content and quality of health care; Quality of health care

Agency for Healthcare Quality and Research (AHQR), 90, 99. *See also* Policymaking: on content and quality of health care; Quality of health care

Aid to Families with Dependent Children (AFDC), 37. *See also* Medicaid

Alternative dispute resolution (ADR), 13, 21, 53, 59–60, 65, 129–131, 134, 159, 162–163, 165, 167, 172, 183–184, 187; empirical evidence regard-

Alternative dispute resolution (*cont.*)
ing, 130; provider ethics committees
and, 84. *See also* Contractual review;
Grievance-and-appeal procedures;
Procedural reforms; Tapping and
resolving consumer concerns
Amenities. *See* Consumer concerns
about health care: about quality;
Quality of health care
American Arbitration Association
(AAA), 13, 21, 163. *See also* Alternative dispute resolution (ADR);
Contractual review; Procedural
protections
American Association of Retired Persons (AARP), 12, 156. *See also* Consumers of health care: empowerment
of; Procedural protections
American Bar Association (ABA), 13,
21, 116, 128–129, 163; Commission
on Legal Problems of the Elderly, 75.
See also Alternative dispute resolution (ADR); Appeal: defined; complaint: defined; Contractual review;
Grievance: defined; Procedural
protections
American College of Physicians (ACP),
85, 89, 124–125. *See also* Health care
policies; Policymaking
American College of Surgeons, 85. *See
also* Accreditation
American Council of Medical Specialty Societies, 88. *See also* Standards of care
American Diabetes Association (ADA).
See Diabetes: American Diabetes
Association (ADA)
American Hospital Association, 13. *See
also* Patient protection debate
*American Manufacturers Mutual Insur-
ance Company v. Sullivan,* 52, 57, 61,
120, 138, 171. *See also* Accountability: of health plans and providers;
Administrative law: adjudication;

Grievance-and-appeal procedures;
Procedural due process of law
American Medical Association (AMA),
13, 21, 43, 85, 94, 111, 163; Practice
Parameters Forum, 94; Practice
Parameters Partnership, 94. *See also*
Procedural protections
*American Medical Security, Inc. v. Bart-
lett,* 34. *See also* Employee Retire-
ment Income Security Act (ERISA)
Americans with Disabilities Act (ADA).
See Judicial review: statutory causes
of action (federal causes)
Appeal: defined 127–128
Appeal procedures. *See* Grievance-
and-appeal procedures
Arbitration. *See* Alternative dispute
resolution (ADR); American Arbitra-
tion Association (AAA); Contractual
review
Aristotle, 4

Bad faith breach, 76, 145–147. *See also*
Consumer concerns about health
care: about access; Employee Retirement Income Security Act (ERISA):
preemption of state law; Procedural
reforms; Tapping and resolving consumer concerns; Tort law: bad faith
breach
Balanced Budget Act of 1997, 38, 125,
136, 138–139, 169–171. *See also*
Diabetes; Medicaid; Medicare
Bioethical concerns. *See* Consumer concerns about health care: about quality
Bipartisan Patient Protection Act of
2001, 16. *See also* Patient protection
debate: congressional legislative
proposals
Blue Cross and Blue Shield Association, 28, 38, 46, 89, 115
*Bowen v. Michigan Academy of Family
Physicians,* 123. *See also* Judicial
review: Medicare (payment policy)

Bush, George W., 16. *See also* Patient protection debate

Business of insurance, 33. *See also* Health insurance: regulation of; Regulation: of private health insurance

Capital expenditure review, 27. *See also* Health care cost inflation

Center for Health Care Dispute Resolution, 75, 137, 184. *See also* Grievance-and-appeal procedures: for Medicare; Patient protection debate; Principles for better ways to tap and resolve consumer disputes; Procedural reforms

Center for Health Care Rights, 12. *See also* Consumers of health care: empowerment of; Patient protection debate

Center for Medicare Advocacy, 12. *See also* Consumers of health care: empowerment of; Patient protection debate

Centers for Disease Control, 98, 124. *See also* Diabetes; Health care policies; Policymaking; Standards of care

Centers for Medicare and Medicaid Services (CMS), 77, 89–99, 102–105 (table 3), 115, 117, 123, 125, 127, 142, 155, 169, 184. *See also* Appeal: defined; Complaint: defined; Department of Health and Human Services (DHHS); Grievance: defined; Health Care Financing Administration (HCFA); Medicaid; Medicare

Children's Defense Fund, 12, 156. *See also* Consumers of health care: empowerment of; Patient protection debate

Children's Health Insurance Program. *See* Health insurance: public; State Children's Health Insurance Program (SCHIP)

Civilian Health and Medical Program of the Uniformed Services (CHAMPUS), 35, 39, 57, 141, 145, 172; TRICARE, 19, 135. *See also* Department of Defense (DOD); Health insurance: public

Civil Rights Act of 1871. *See* Section 1983, 42 U.S.C.

Clinton, William Jefferson: executive order of, 134–135, 139, 165; health reform initiative of, 2, 29. *See also* Presidential Commission on Consumer Protection and Quality in the Health Care Industry

Coalition for Consumer Protection and Quality in Health Care Reform, 12. *See also* Consumers of health care: empowerment of; Patient protection debate

Cohen, Wilber (secretary of Health, Education and Welfare), 26

Colson v. Silliman, 52, 166. *See also* Accountability: of health plans and providers; Administrative law

Commercial health insurance companies, 32–33. *See also* Health insurance: private

Competition. *See* Health care reform: managed competition

Complaint: defined, 127–128; procedures, 132–134. *See also* Procedural reforms

Consolidated Licensure for Entities Assuming Risk Initiative, 32, 131. *See also* Health insurance: regulation of; National Association of Insurance Commissioners (NAIC); Regulation: of private health insurance

Consolidated Omnibus Budget Reconciliation Act of 1985, 35. *See also* Employee Retirement Income Security Act (ERISA); Regulation: of private health insurance

Daniels, Norman, 4. *See also* Justice

Dauer, Edward A., and Leonard J. Marcus, 83. *See also* Risk management programs; Tapping and resolving consumer concerns

Deming, W. Edward, 90. *See also* Quality of health care: Total Quality Management (TQM) and Continuous Quality Improvement (CQI)

Department Appeals Board (DAB), 116, 138. *See also* Administrative review: Medicare; Department of Health and Human Services (DHHS); Medicare: coverage policies

Department of Defense (DOD), 39, 57, 135. *See also* Civilian Health and Medical Program of the Uniformed Services (CHAMPUS)

Department of Health and Human Services (DHHS), 97–98, 116, 138, 148. *See also* Departmental Appeals Board (DAB); Medicaid; Medicare; Policymaking: quality of health care

Department of Labor (DOL), 134, 140. *See also* Employee Retirement Income Security Act (ERISA)

Department of Veterans Affairs (DVA), 35, 39, 98, 139; VA health system, 39, 92. *See also* Health insurance: public

Diabetes, 109, 123–126; and accreditation, 125–126; American Diabetes Association (ADA), 95, 124–125; *Diabetes Care*, 124; Diabetes Control and Complications Trial, 124–125; Diabetes Quality Improvement Project, 125; Foundation for Accountability, 125; National Diabetes Education Program, 124; and policymaking, 125–126; standards of care for, 123–126

Dispute resolution institutions, 182–189:

—*functions of*, 185–187: enhancing independent external review, 186; facilitating diversity in dispute resolution mechanisms, 187; meeting needs of the uninsured, 185–186

—*models of*, 182–185; private dispute resolution entity, 184–185; state administrative agency, 183; state court system, 183–184

—*legal constraints on design of*, 187–189: Article III courts, 188; independent commissions and, 188; statutory compensation schemes and, 188; U.S. Tax Court, 188. *See also* Procedural reforms

Disputes: emergence and transformation of, 78–79; socio-economic and psychological factors in, 79. *See also* Tapping and resolving consumer concerns

Distributive justice. *See* Justice

Donabedian, Avedis: definition of quality, 67, 86, 100; domains of quality, 67, 70–74; "Evaluating the Quality of Medical Care," 86; taxonomy of quality criteria, 86. *See also* Quality of health care

Emergency Medical Treatment and Active Labor Act (EMTALA). *See* Judicial review: statutory causes of action (federal)

Empirical data. *See* Consumer concerns about health care; Medical malpractice; Procedural reforms

Employee Retirement Income Security Act (ERISA), 15–17, 25–28, 42, 45, 59, 63, 121, 132–134, 164; mandated benefits under, 35; preemption of state law, 33–35, 65–66, 141, 145, 172, 176, 179; section 502, 33, 140; section 503, 33, 133–134, 140. *See also* Complaint: procedures;

138–139, 164, 169; for Medicare, 136–138, 164; plan or provider ownership of, 162; for state employee health plans, 135. *See also* Adjudication; Administrative review; Model HMO Act; Patient protection debate; Principles for better ways to tap and resolve consumer concerns; Procedural reforms; Tapping and resolving consumer concerns

Grijalva v. Shalala, 137–138, 171. *See also* Accountability; Grievance-and-appeal procedures: for Medicare; Procedural due process of law

Havighurst, Clark C., 59–60. *See also* Contract law

Health-care cost inflation, 27–30; movement toward managed care, 28–30; regulatory attack on costs, 27–28

Health Care Due Process Protocol, 13, 163. *See also* American Arbitration Association (AAA); American Bar Association (ABA); American Medical Association (AMA); Procedural reforms: proposals for

Health Care Financing Administration (HCFA), 77, 99, 115–117, 122–123, 138, 155, 169. *See also* Centers for Medicare and Medicaid Services (CMS); Department of Health and Human Services (DHHS)

Health-care policies:

—*on access*, 103–104 (table 3), 105–107: formal statements of coverage, 103 (table 3), 105–107; medical review criteria, 100–102, 103–104 (table 3), 105, 107, 118, 126, 154, 158, 177; provider policies on care for the uninsured, 104 (table 3), 107

—*on costs*, 104–105 (table 3), 107–108: payment methods for public pro-

grams, 104 (table 3), 122–123; payment policy in health plan contracts, 104–105 (table 3), 107–108, 154; pricing policies of health-care providers, 105 (table 3), 108; pricing policies of health insurance and prepaid health plans, 105 (table 3), 108, 154

—*promulgation processes*, 102–105 (table 3)

—*publication of*, 15–16, 45, 157–158

—*on quality*, 100–102 (table 3), 155, 180: medical practice guidelines, 87, 89–90, 93–94, 98–99, 100–101, 102 (table 3), 107, 111–112, 114, 118–119, 124–125, 153–155, 169; medical review criteria, 100–102, 103–104 (table 3); performance measures, 100; standards of quality, 100–102 (table 3)

—*role in adjudication of consumer concerns*, 80–81

—*taxonomy of*, 101

See also Policymaking; Principles of sound policymaking procedures; Procedural reforms

Health Care Professional Credentialing Verification Model Act, 32. *See also* National Association of Insurance Commissioners (NAIC)

Health-care reform: competition, 27–28; contract as vehicle for, 59–61; managed competition, 29; President Clinton's health reform initiative, 2, 11, 29; state health reform, 31, 34–35. *See also* Justice

Health-care services. *See* Consumer concerns about health care; Quality of health-care

Health Carrier Grievance Procedure Model Act, 127, 131–133. *See also* Complaint: defined; Grievance: defined; National Association of Insurance Commissioners (NAIC)

Health insurance: cost sharing, 78; coverage, 23–25, 30, 40, 56–57, 60, 74; employer-sponsored, 25–27, 30, 45, 57, 77; expansion of, 25–27; federal, 50, 63; historical development of, 23–30; mandated benefits, 32, 35; market conduct review, 133; national, 27; private, 25–27, 30, 31–35, 40, 45, 86, 99; public, 35–40, 41, 51–54, 58–59, 61, 63, 77, 80, 86, 107, 109, 113–114, 151, 159, 170, 173, 184; regulation of, 23, 31–35, 132–133; state programs for, 39

Health Insurance Portability and Accountability Act of 1996, 35. *See also* Regulation: of private health insurance

Health maintenance organization (HMOs): mandated internal review procedures, 132; state regulation of, 129–131; tort liability of, 34, 145, 172–173. *See also* Employee Retirement Income Security Act (ERISA); Grievance: procedures; Grievance-and-appeal procedures; Judicial review; Managed care; Managed care organizations (MCOs); Model HMO Act; Patient protection debate; Procedural reforms; Tapping and resolving consumer concerns

Health Plan Employer Data and Information Set (HEDIS), 82, 91, 96, 111, 173. *See also* National Committee of Quality Assurance (NCQA); Quality of health care; Standards of care

Health plans, 35–39, 56–66; ERISA-regulated, 34–35, 130, 133–135; 140–141, 172, 176; government-sponsored, 172; preferred provider, 29; private, 31–35; public, 35–39; self-insured, 27, 34, 140; third party administrators for, 30. *See also* Consumer concerns about health care; Health insurance; Patient protection

debate; Principles of better ways to tap and resolve consumer concerns; Principles of sound policymaking procedures; Procedural protections; Tapping and resolving consumer concerns

Health services research, 87–88, 111–113, 125. *See also* Models of policymaking; Quality of health care

Hickson, Gerald B., 83. *See also* Medical malpractice; Risk management programs

Hill-Burton Community Service Assurance. *See* Judicial review: statutory causes of action (federal causes)

Hospitals: obligations of, 46–47, 62, 97; private for-profit, 46; private, not-for-profit, 46, 96–97, 148; public, 46, 148; rate regulation, 27, 153

Indiana Health Service, 39. *See also* Health insurance: public

Indiana University School of Medicine, 91

Institute of Medicine (IOM), 72, 88, 100, 107, 111–112. *See also* Health care policies: taxonomy of; Medical malpractice; Quality of health care; Standards of care

Internal Revenue Code, 30; section 501, 45–47. *See also* Corporate and tax law

Internal review, 127, 129–139, 163. *See also* Alternative dispute resolution (ADR); Contractual review

Jameson v. Bowen, 116. *See also* Policymaking

John Doe and Richard Smith v. Mutual Omaha Insurance Company, 149. *See also* Judicial review: statutory causes of action (federal causes): Americans with Disabilities Act (ADA)

National health insurance. *See* Health insurance

National Health Law Program, 12, 156. *See also* Consumers of health care: empowerment of; Patient protection debate

National Health Planning and Resources Development Act of 1974, 148. *See also* Capital expenditure review; Judicial review: statutory causes of action (federal causes): Hill-Burton community service assurance

National Institutes of Health (NIH), 24, 86, 98–99, 124. *See also* Policymaking; Quality of health care; Standards of care

National Senior Citizens Law Center, 12, 156. *See also* Consumers of health care: empowerment of; Patient protection debate

Native Americans, 14, 35, 39. *See also* Indian Health Service

Negligence. *See* Medical malpractice; Tort law: negligence

Office of Personal Management, 135, 141. *See also* Federal Employee Health Benefit Plan (FEHBP)

Older Americans Act, 129, 185. *See also* Ombudsman programs

Ombudsman programs, 129, 160–161, 183, 185. *See also* Complaint: procedures; Extralegal institutions for dispute resolution; Procedural reforms; Tapping and resolving consumer concerns

Patient: defined, 9–10

Patient Bill of Rights, 14, 165, 182. *See also* Patient protection debate; Procedural reforms

Patient protection debate, 1–2, 11–22, 27, 42, 99, 46, 66, 121, 158, 165–

166, 170; Clinton administration initiative, 14–15; congressional legislative proposals, 15–16, 21, 58, 91, 130, 170; judicial response to, 17–19; private reform proposals, 12–13; state government reform initiatives, 13–14; uninsured and, 22. *See also* Principles for better ways to tap and resolve consumer concerns; Procedural reforms

Patient satisfaction survey, 82, 161–172

Peer review organizations, 36, 136. *See also* Grievance-and-appeal procedures: Medicare

Pegram v. Herdrich, 17. *See also* Employee Retirement Income Security Act (ERISA); Patient protection debate: judicial response to

Personal Responsibility and Work Opportunity Reconciliation Act of 1996, 37. *See also* Medicaid

Physician-patient relationship, 9

Physician Payment Review Commission, 89. *See also* Policymaking: for cost policy of providers

Pilot Life Insurance v. Dedeaux, 33, 145. *See also* Employee Retirement Income Security Act (ERISA): preemption of state law; Grievance-and-appeal procedures: ERISA-regulated plans; Tort law: federal preemption of state tort causes of action

Policies. *See* Health-care policies; Standards of care

Policymakers, 100; federal agencies as, 98–99; health plan sponsors as, 98; private accrediting bodies as, 95–96; private medical organizations as, 93–95; providers as, 96–97

Policymaking, 48, 109–126, 150–158, 178–179:
—*on access to health care,* 113–120

Private organizations, 94, 110, 152; accrediting bodies, 109–113; role in policymaking and dispute resolution, 176. *See also* Corporations; Hospitals; Medical professional organizations; Medical specialty societies; Voluntary health organizations

Procedural due process of law, 48, 51–53, 58, 120, 131, 135, 167, 171, 177; scholarship on, 51–52; threats to, 52–53, 171

Procedural justice, 4–6, 9, 175. *See also* Justice; Principles for better ways to tap and resolve consumer concerns; Principles for sound policymaking procedures; Procedural due process of law; Procedural reforms

Procedural protections. *See* Procedural reforms

Procedural reforms, 150–190 passim:
—*access to tort remedies,* 165, 171–173
—*adjudicative proceedings*: development of medical facts in, 67; "discovery" in, 160–161, 169; independence and authority of decisionmakers in, 167–168; interaction of process elements in, 169; opportunity for procedural challenges of policy in, 178–179; right to judicial review in, 168–169; right to reconsideration in, 168–169; simplification and coordination of procedures of, 163–165
—*allocation of regulatory responsibility,* 175–177: clarification of federal responsibilities, 176–177; expanded role for states, 177–178
—*expertise of state courts for,* 183–184
—*legal counsel and,* 161
—*for policymaking,* 178–180: government leadership in the policymaking process, 179–180; maintenance of tort liability, 179
—*proposals for,* 11–13, 15, 25, 41–42, 81

—*relations with quality assurance and risk management,* 161–162
—*settlement in,* 161
—*tort liability and,* 171–172, 176
    See also Justice: procedural justice; Principles for better ways to tap and resolve consumer concerns; Principles for sound policymaking procedures

Provider ethics committees, 69 (table 2), 81, 84. *See also* Consumer concerns about health care: about quality; Tapping and resolving consumer concerns

Provider-sponsored networks, 32. *See also* National Association of Insurance Commissioners (NAIC); Regulation: of private health insurance

Public: distinguished from private in Western law, 41

Publication of health care policy. *See* Health-care policies: publication of; Regulation: publication as

Public Citizen Health Research Group, 12. *See also* Patient protection debate

Quality of health care: assessment of, 32, 90, 91, 161; assurance and improvement programs, 81–82; assurance of, 101, 160; elements of, 67; improvement of, 81–83, 91; interpersonal domain, 67; payer interest in, 88–90; revolution in, 85–91; technical domain, 67; Total Quality Management (TQM) and Continuous Quality Improvement (CQI), 90–91. *See also* Health-care policies: quality; Policymaking; Principles for sound policymaking procedures; Procedural reforms; Standards of care

Racketeer-Influenced and Corrupt Practice Act, 19

RAND Institute for Civil Justice, 130

Rawls, John: *A Theory of Justice. See* Justice

Regenstrief Institute for Health Care, 91; Medical Records System, 91

Regulation: of hospitals and health-care facilities, 44; of physicians and health-care professionals, 43, 81–82; private (*see* Self-regulation); of private health insurance, 31–35, 45, 132–133; publication as, 45, 180. *See also* Accreditation; Health insurance; Licensure; Regulatory law; Self-regulation

Regulatory law, 41–43. *See also* Accreditation; Licensure; Regulation; Self-regulation

Rehabilitation Act of 1973. *See* Judicial review: statutory causes of action (federal causes)

Risk management programs, 82–83, 160, 162; integration with quality assurance, 83. *See also* Medical malpractice; Principles for better ways to tap and resolve consumer concerns; Procedural reforms; Tapping and resolving consumer concerns

Robert Wood Johnson Foundation, 73, 174

Rule: interpretative, 50; legislative, 48–49; nonlegislative, 50–51. *See also* Administrative law; Policymaking; Rulemaking

Rulemaking: legislative, 48–50; nonlegislative rulemaking and policymaking, 50–51; notice-and-comment, 48–50, 113, 117, 123, 155. *See also* Administrative law; Administrative Procedure Act (APA)

Schweicker v. McClure, 167. *See also* Administrative law: adjudication; Procedural due process of law

Section 1983, 42 U.S.C., 63, 143, 177.

See also Judicial review: Medicaid; Procedural reforms

Self-regulation, 188; health care institutions, 44–45; physicians, 43. *See also* Accreditation

Shalala v. Illinois Council on Long Term Care, 123, 142. *See also* Judicial review: Medicare (payment policy)

Shewhart, Walter, 90. *See also* Quality of health care: Total Quality Management (TQM) and Continuous Quality Improvement (CQI)

Small claims court, 77–78. *See also* Consumer concerns about health care: about costs

Social Security Act, 36–37, 39, 142–143; 1965 amendments, 26; 1972 amendments, 25, 27; 1983 amendments, 28; section 205, 142–143; section 1115, 38. *See also* Judicial review: Medicaid; Medicaid; Medicare

Standard setting. *See* Policymaking

Standards of care, 85–108, 109–111, 113, 118–119, 124–126, 150–157, 170, 174, 176, 179–180; computerization of, 91–93. *See also* Accreditation; Health-care policies; Principles of sound policymaking procedures; Quality of health care

State Children's Health Insurance Program (SCHIP), 26, 35, 38–39, 53, 63, 115, 119, 166, 177. *See also* Health insurance: public

State health-care reform. *See* Health-care reform

Statutory causes of action. *See* Judicial review: statutory causes of action

Supplemental Security Income (SSI), 37. *See also* Medicaid

Tapping and resolving consumer concerns, 127–149 passim:

Eleanor D. Kinney, JD, MPH, is the Samuel R. Rosen Professor of Law and Co-director of the Center for Law and Health at Indiana University School of Law, Indianapolis. She is also Adjunct Professor of Public Health and Adjunct Professor of Public and Environmental Affairs at Indiana University. In 1999–2000, as a Fulbright Fellow, she was a visiting professor at the Institute of Latin American Integration, Faculty of Juridical and Social Sciences, National University of La Plata, in La Plata, Argentina.

Professor Kinney was formerly Assistant General Counsel of the American Hospital Association (1982–84) and a program analyst in the Office of the Secretary of the U.S. Department of Health and Human Services (1979–82). She received her law degree from Duke University School of Law (1973) and her Masters of Public Health from the University of North Carolina School of Public Health (1979).

Professor Kinney is an expert on health-care financing and regulation, medical malpractice, and long-term care. Much of her research has been funded by foundations and government agencies, including the Robert Wood Johnson Foundation and the Administrative Conference of the United States. She has had several gubernatorial appointments in Indiana, including service on the Executive Board of the Indiana State Department of Health.

Library of Congress Cataloging-in-Publication Data

Kinney, Eleanor D.
  Protecting American health care consumers / Eleanor DeArman Kinney.
    p. cm.
  ISBN 0-8223-2876-3 (cloth : alk. paper)
  1. Medical policy—United States. 2. Patients—Civil rights—United States. 3. Health care reform—United States. 4. Consumer protection—United States.
  [DNLM: 1. Health Policy—United States. 2. Consumer Advocacy—United States. 3. Health care Reform—United States. 4. Insurance, Health—United States. WA 540 AA1 K55p 2002] I. Title.
  RA394 .K56 2002
  362.1′0973—dc21   2001008586